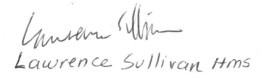

D0779455

Abernathy's
SURGICAL
SECRETS

Third Edition

ALDEN H. HARKEN, M.D.
Professor and Chairman
Department of Surgery
University of Colorado Health Sciences Center
Denver, Colorado

ERNEST E. MOORE, M.D.
Professor and Vice-Chairman
Department of Surgery
University of Colorado Health Sciences Center
Chief of Surgery
Denver General Hospital
Denver, Colorado

HANLEY & BELFUS, INC./ Philadelphia
MOSBY/ St. Louis • Baltimore • Boston • Carlsbad • Chicago • London
Madrid • Naples • New York • Philadelphia • Sydney • Tokyo • Toronto

Publisher: HANLEY & BELFUS, INC.
                      210 S. 13th Street
                      Philadelphia, PA 19107
                      (215) 546-7293
                      FAX (215) 790-9330

North American and worldwide sales and distribution:

                      MOSBY
                      11830 Westline Industrial Drive
                      St. Louis, MO 63146

In Canada: Times Mirror Professional Publishing, Ltd.
                      130 Flaska Drive
                      Markham, Ontario L6G 1B8
                      Canada

SURGICAL SECRETS   Third Edition   ISBN 1-56053-170-3

Library of Congress catalog card number   96-75883

Last digit is the print number: 9 8 7 6 5 4 3 2

In Memoriam

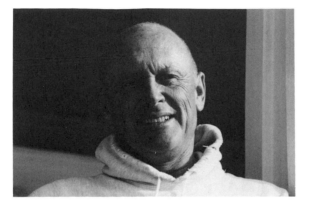

CHARLES M. ABERNATHY, M.D.

1941–1994

CONTENTS

Contents

CONTRIBUTORS

Benjamin O. Anderson, MD
Assistant Professor of Surgical Oncology, University of Washington Medical Center, Seattle, Washington

James F. Bascom, M.D.
Assistant Professor of Surgery, University of Colorado Health Sciences Center, Denver, Colorado

B. Timothy Baxter, M.D.
Associate Professor of Surgery, University of Nebraska Medical Center, Omaha, Nebraska

Denis David Bensard, M.D.
Assistant Professor of Surgery, University of Colorado Health Sciences Center, Denver, Colorado

Walter L. Biffl, M.D.
Resident in Surgery, University of Colorado Health Sciences Center, Denver, Colorado

Kerry Brega, M.D.
Assistant Professor of Neurosurgery, University of Colorado Health Sciences Center; Chief of Neurosurgery, Denver General Hospital, Denver, Colorado

Elizabeth C. Brew, M.D.
Resident in Surgery, University of Colorado Health Sciences Center, Denver, Colorado

James M. Brown, M.D.
Assistant Professor of Surgery, University of Colorado Health Sciences Center, Denver, Colorado

Jon M. Burch, M.D.
Professor of Surgery, University of Colorado Health Sciences Center; Chief of General Surgery, Denver General Hospital, Denver, Colorado

David N. Campbell, M.D.
Professor of Surgery, University of Colorado Health Sciences Center, Denver, Colorado

Sandra C. Carr, M.D.
Fellow in Vascular Surgery, Northwestern University Medical School, Chicago, Illinois

Jodi A. Chambers, M.D.
Assistant Clinical Professor, University of Colorado Health Sciences Center, St. Anthony's Hospital, Denver, Colorado

Joseph C. Cleveland, Jr., M.D.
Resident in Surgery, University of Colorado Health Sciences Center, Denver, Colorado

James R. Denton, M.D.
Chief Resident in Surgery, University of Colorado Health Sciences Center, Denver, Colorado

Adam Deutchman, M.D.
Assistant Clinical Professor of Surgery, University of Colorado Health Sciences Center, Denver, Colorado

James B. Downey, M.D.
Resident in Surgery, University of Colorado Health Sciences Center, Denver, Colorado

Ben Eiseman, M.D.
Professor Emeritus of Surgery, University of Colorado Health Sciences Center, Denver, Colorado

Christina A. Finlayson, M.D.
Fellow in Surgical Oncology, Fox Chase Cancer Center, Philadelphia, Pennsylvania

Reginald J. Franciose, M.D.
Assistant Professor of Surgery, University of Colorado Health Sciences Center, Denver, Colorado

Randall S. Friese, M.D.
Resident in Surgery, University of Colorado Health Sciences Center, Denver, Colorado

David A. Fullerton, M.D.
Associate Professor, University of Colorado Health Sciences Center, Denver, Colorado

Glenn W. Geelhoed, M.D.
Professor of Surgery and of International Medical Education, George Washington University Medical Center, Washington, D.C.

Michael J.V. Gordon, M.D.
Assistant Professor of Surgery; Director of Hand Surgery, University of Colorado Health Sciences Center, Denver, Colorado

Michael A. Grosso, M.D.
Assistant Professor of Surgery, Cooper Hospital, University Medical Center, UMDNJ/Robert Wood Johnson Medical School at Camden, Camden, New Jersey

Frederick L. Grover, M.D.
Professor of Surgery, University of Colorado Health Sciences Center, Denver, Colorado

James B. Haenel, RRT
Critical Care Respiratory Specialist, Denver General Hospital, Denver, Colorado

Brian G. Halloran, M.D.
Resident in Surgery, University of Nebraska Medical Center, Omaha, Nebraska

Alden H. Harken, M.D.
Professor and Chairman, Department of Surgery, University of Colorado Health Sciences Center, Denver, Colorado

C. Edward Hartford, M.D.
Professor of Surgery, University of Colorado Health Sciences Center; Director, Burn Unit, University Hospital, Denver, Colorado

Gilbert Hermann, M.D., F.A.C.S.
Clinical Professor of Surgery, University of Colorado Health Sciences Center, Denver, Colorado

W. Stuart Johnston, M.D.
Resident in Surgery, University of Colorado Health Sciences Center, Denver, Colorado

Darrell N. Jones, Ph.D.
Research Associate, University of Colorado Health Sciences Center, Denver, Colorado

Igal Kam, M.D.
Associate Professor of Surgery; Chief of Transplant Surgery, University of Colorado Health Sciences Center, Denver, Colorado

Frederick M. Karrer, M.D.
Associate Professor of Surgery, University of Colorado Health Sciences Center; Director of Pediatric Transplantation, Children's Hospital, Denver, Colorado

Glenn L. Kelly, M.D.
Associate Clinical Professor of Surgery, University of Colorado Health Sciences Center, Denver, Colorado

Lawrence L. Ketch, M.D.
Associate Professor of Surgery; Chief, Division of Plastic and Reconstructive Surgery, University of Colorado Health Sciences Center, Denver, Colorado

William C. Krupski, M.D.
Professor of Surgery; Chief of Vascular Surgery, University of Colorado Health Sciences Center, Denver, Colorado

R. Dale Liechty, M.D.
Professor of Surgery, University of Colorado Health Sciences Center, Denver, Colorado

Kathleen Liscum, M.D.
Assistant Professor of Surgery, Baylor University, Houston, Texas

Luis Alberto Martinez-Frontanilla, M.D.
Associate Clinical Professor of Surgery, University of Colorado Health Sciences Center and Children's Hospital, Denver, Colorado

Robert C. McIntyre, Jr., M.D.
Assistant Professor of Surgery, University of Colorado Health Sciences Center, Denver, Colorado

Daniel R. Meldrum, M.D.
Resident in Surgery, University of Colorado Health Sciences Center, Denver, Colorado

David J. Minion, M.D.
Fellow in Vascular Surgery, Case Western Reserve University, Cleveland, Ohio

Max B. Mitchell, M.D.
Fellow, Cardiothoracic Surgery, University of Colorado Health Sciences Center, Denver, Colorado

Roger E. Moe, M.D.
Professor of Surgery; Director, BioClinical Breast Cancer Unit, University of Washington, Seattle, Washington

Ernest E. Moore, M.D.
Professor and Vice-Chairman of Surgery, University of Colorado School of Medicine; Chief of Surgery, Denver General Hospital, Denver, Colorado

Frederick A. Moore, M.D.
Chief, General Surgery, Trauma and Critical Care, Department of Surgery, University of Texas, Houston, Texas

Jeanne H. Nozawa
Department of Surgery, University of Colorado Health Sciences Center, Denver, Colorado

William R. Nelson, M.D.
Clinical Professor of Surgery, University of Colorado Health Sciences Center, Denver, Colorado

John S. Nichols, M.D., Ph.D.
St. Anthony Hospital, Denver, Colorado

Lawrence W. Norton, M.D.
Professor and Vice-Chairman, Department of Surgery, University of Colorado Health Sciences Center, Denver, Colorado

John Ogunkeye, M.S.C.
Executive Administrator, Department of Surgery, University of Chicago Hospitals, Chicago, Illinois

Bruce Paton, M.D.
Clinical Professor of Surgery, University of Colorado Health Sciences Center, Denver, Colorado

William H. Pearce, M.D.
Professor of Surgery, Northwestern University Medical School, Chicago, Illinois

Nathan W. Pearlman, M.D.
Professor of Surgery, University of Colorado Health Sciences Center, Denver, Colorado

Norman E. Peterson, M.D.
Professor of Urology/Surgery, University of Colorado Health Sciences Center; Chief of Urology, Denver General Hospital, Denver, Colorado

Steven L. Peterson, M.D.
Resident in Surgery, University of Colorado Health Sciences Center, Denver, Colorado

Marvin Pomerantz, M.D.
Professor of Surgery; Chief, General Thoracic Surgery, University of Colorado Health Sciences Center, Denver, Colorado

J. Brad Ray, M.D.
Resident in Surgery, University of Colorado Health Sciences Center, Denver, Colorado

Robert A. Read, M.D., Ph.D.
Assistant Professor of Surgery, University of Colorado Health Sciences Center, Denver, Colorado

Thomas F. Rehring, M.D.
Resident in Surgery, University of Colorado Health Sciences Center, Denver, Colorado

John A. Ridge, M.D., Ph.D.
Chief, Head and Neck Surgery Section, Fox Chase Cancer Center, Philadelphia, Pennsylvania

Robert T. Rowland, M.D.
Resident in Surgery, University of Colorado Health Sciences Center, Denver, Colorado

Robert B. Rutherford, M.D.
Professor of Surgery, University of Colorado Health Sciences Center, Denver, Colorado

Kennith H. Sartorelli, M.D.
Assistant Professor of Pediatric Surgery, University of Vermont College of Medicine, Burlington, Vermont

Mark D. Stegall, M.D.
Associate Professor of Surgery; Director of Pancreas Transplantation, University of Colorado Health Sciences Center, Denver, Colorado

John H. Sun, M.D.
Resident in Surgery, University of Colorado Health Sciences Center, Denver, Colorado

Kathleen M. Teasley, M.S., R.Ph.
Associate Professor of Pharmacy; Co-Director, Nutritional Support Service, University of Colorado Health Sciences Center, Denver, Colorado

Greg Van Stiegmann, M.D.
Associate Professor of Surgery, University of Colorado Health Sciences Center, Denver, Colorado

Thomas A. Whitehill, M.D.
Assistant Professor of Surgery, University of Colorado Health Sciences Center; Chief of Vascular Surgery, Denver VA Medical Center, Denver, Colorado

Glenn J.R. Whitman, M.D.
Professor of Surgery and Chief of Cardiothoracic Surgery, Medical College of Pennsylvania, Philadelphia, Pennsylvania

Rebecca Wiebe, M.D.
Chief Resident, University of Colorado Health Sciences Center, Denver, Colorado

PREFACE TO THE FIRST EDITION

Surgical Secrets is not intended as a textbook in the traditional sense. It is a pathway of questions from diagnosis to recovery. We first discovered the need for this approach when our students were assigned chapters in a major surgical textbook and then on discussion could not "pull out" the key information. The way we solve this as surgeons is by a series of key questions.

The editors gave the contributing authors wide latitude in style (some are long, some are short) and encouraged them to duplicate the verbal teaching process they use on rounds, in the OR, and on oral exams.

We teach students by asking questions. Knowing "the right question" and its answer is the key to clinical surgery for both a student and the most experienced practitioner. Of the two components of learning surgery, one is experiential and the other didactic, the part that can be written. The only way to learn the experiential component is by long hours of watching, trying and trying again. It takes a *long* time.

But the other part of learning surgery, the "book knowledge," can and should be learned rapidly. A student should learn surgery 101, 202 . . . 606 all simultaneously, for a patient problem is almost always a complex constellation of decisions, questions, and judgments. To suggest that a student should not learn the ins and outs of aortic grafts, and instead be exposed only to fundamental wound healing concepts, is to belittle the student's ability to handle complicated concepts. Surgery, unlike calculus, is not abstract and can be learned (insofar as the didactic information is concerned) in full breadth at an early stage.

This volume is designed to be carried in a coat pocket. We hope it will also be carried in the coat pockets of many experienced surgeons as they ask the "questions of surgical practice" in their daily work.

Surgical Secrets is *not* intended only to be a guide to help pass an examination. Rather, the questions here teach the knowledge a surgeon must know in order to take care of a patient with a particular problem. The questions by themselves trace the thought process a surgeon uses when thinking about the problem.

Socrates was correct. The best way to teach is to question. We hope we have followed his precepts, perhaps providing even more help in finding answers.

Charles M. Abernathy, M.D.
Brett B. Abernathy, M.D.

PREFACE TO THE SECOND EDITION

We estimate that over one half of *all* medical students over the last five years have bought *Surgical Secrets* (we assume the other half either borrowed it or stole it!). This confirms our notion that learning medical information in a question-and-answer format is a preferred method for many students. Somehow, reading a chapter in *Surgical Secrets* seems to "set the glue" on the information in a different way from reading a similar chapter in a large textbook.

We were amazed as we reviewed and revised the book at how much information it contains. Although we editors and the authors have edited and read the chapters many times, we are frequently asked questions from *Surgical Secrets* that even we can't answer!

This edition features a new "Atlas of Technical Tips." Original line drawings depict methods of tying sutures, holding needles, and other basic techniques. This Atlas is not intended to be comprehensive, but instead represents a starting point for the use of surgical instruments. We also believe that it lends a sense of "completeness" to *Surgical Secrets*.

Enjoy the book and learn from it, and don't hesitate to send us notes about its content (a suggestion form is provided on page 318). Like all good surgeons, we are constantly striving for improvement.

Charles M. Abernathy, M.D.
Alden H. Harken, M.D.

PREFACE TO THE THIRD EDITION AND DEDICATION TO CHARLIE ABERNATHY

Charlie Abernathy never had a neutral effect on anyone. Charlie's effervescent enthusiasm for education, medicine, books, students, innovation, cattle, DNA, old cars, skiing, critical care, and his patients will sustain happy and rewarding memories for all of us lucky enough to have known him. Charlie challenged us all. Most of us feel pretty good if we have one or two good ideas each decade. Charlie sparked an idea a minute—and most of them were pretty good.

After medical school at Northwestern and surgical training in Boston and Colorado, Charlie joined Ted Dickinson to practice surgery in Montrose, Colorado. Charlie was a superb surgeon, gifted internist, sensitive psychiatrist, compassionate pediatrician, imaginative urologist/gynecologist, and practical family physician ("specialization" Charlie would have said "is for insects").

Charlie's loyalty and love for the University of Colorado prompted him to run for university Regent. The Regents are the nine folks who run our university, and in state-wide campaigns frequently pull more voters than the governor's race. Predictably, Charlie was elected. Soon thereafter, we successfully recruited Charlie and Martha back to the Department of Surgery at Denver General and the University Hospitals. With Charlie around, we "red-lined" excitement and the "fun-meter was always in the green zone." Charlie challenged everything and everyone.

While perusing a stand of black walnut trees (Charlie planned to make them into capnometers that could induce the "diving seal reflex" in trauma victims, thus redistributing limited blood flow toward metabolically downregulated vital organs), Charlie thought: "You know, medical education is all backwards. Medical students read textbooks to discover the answers. We faculty members don't fool with the answers—we simply change the questions. In order to conceptualize surgical biology (and to thrive on ward rounds), students need to know the right questions."

Thus originated the concept for *Surgical Secrets*, which later blossomed into *The Secrets Series®*, Q & A books in over 20 medical disciplines designed to make the subject interesting to medical students, residents, and even practitioners. Characteristically, Charlie identified a way to make medical education stimulating, rewarding, and fun.

In this third edition of *Surgical Secrets*, we hope to have captured some vintage Abernathy—his irreverence, challenge, humor, dignity, erudition, and "working model" doctor practicality. You will note that the questions have been thoroughly updated or completely changed. New authors have written a number of the chapters in order to give a new perspective on the material. Chapters new to this edition include tuberculosis, heart and lung transplantation, antibiotics, penetrating thoracic trauma, urinary tract trauma, and health care management.

If we have been able to impart even just a little Abernathy in the following pages, we are convinced that the "questions" of surgical biology will live for another group of surgical students and residents.

With affection, admiration, and respect, we dedicate this edition to Charlie's enduring memory.

Alden H. Harken, M.D.
Ernest E. Moore, M.D.
Linda C. Belfus

I. General

1. CARDIOPULMONARY RESUSCITATION AND INITIAL TREATMENT OF HEMORRHAGIC SHOCK

Michael Grosso, M.D., and Alden H. Harken, M.D.

AIRWAY AND BREATHING

1. The first and foremost priority! Why?
Blood oxygen saturation in the unventilated patient falls to approximately 85% with 40 to 90 seconds of apnea and decreases sharply from then on.

2. Is there an immediate need for an oral, nasopharyngeal, or S tube airway?
No. Although they serve a useful function to maintain a patent airway and also serve as bite block to facilitate suctioning, they may induce vomiting or vocal cord spasm in the stuporous or semiconscious patient.

3. What is the most effective method for removing a foreign body obstructing an airway?
Controversial
Many techniques are cited. For a completely obstructed airway in the unconscious patient, a back blow will deliver 35 mmHg of airway pressure, and an abdominal thrust will deliver 15 mmHg of airway pressure. The recommended technique is four successive back blows followed by four successive abdominal thrusts. For a partially obstructed airway (patient is able to phonate), an abdominal thrust will generate 2200 ml of flow/sec compared with 200 ml/sec for a back blow.

4. What is the most common cause of airway obstruction in the unconscious patient?
The base of the relaxed tongue against the posterior pharyngeal wall (relieved by head tilt, jaw thrust, or chin lift).

5. How do you establish an airway in the patient with a suspected neck injury?
Of the three basic maneuvers—head tilt, chin lift, and jaw thrust—the jaw thrust requires the least amount of cervical hyperextension.

6. Is endotracheal intubation required in all cases of respiratory arrest?
No. With minimal skill and training, mouth-to-mouth resuscitation can deliver 16–18% inspired oxygen with adequate tidal volumes. The use of bag and mask along with an oxygen supply can deliver 95–100% oxygen. These are relatively safe and effective techniques for ventilatory support. Airway control by endotracheal intubation can be attempted once additional skilled personnel arrive.

7. What are the disadvantages of ventilatory support without endotracheal intubation?
Positive-pressure breathing (mouth-to-mouth or bag and mask) can be associated with significant delivery of air to the stomach. Gastric distention can impair diaphragmatic movement and therefore limit ventilation. In addition, increased pressure may cause regurgitation and, worse, aspiration. These can be prevented by proper airway positioning and by avoiding excessive tidal volume with ventilation.

1

8. How do you deal with gastric distention?

Do not attempt direct abdominal pressure. This can actually promote regurgitation and aspiration and cause gastric rupture. Normal intragastric pressure is 7 cm H_2O. Regurgitation is likely with pressure greater than 20 cm H_2O. Gastric distention is quickly alleviated by placing a nasogastric tube and by applying suction.

9. You decide to intubate the patient. What size tube?

For a 70-kg adult, an endotracheal tube with an internal diameter of 8.0 or 8.5 mm is recommended. A guideline often used: select a tube with an internal diameter approximately equal to the width of the patient's thumbnail.

10. Is the endotracheal tube in proper position?

It is imperative that proper tube placement be confirmed. Four quick and relatively reliable techniques can confirm proper tracheal position of the tube: (1) auscultation of both lung fields should yield equal breath sounds, (2) observation of symmetric chest rise with each ventilation, (3) absence of auscultated air sounds over the epigastrium during ventilation, and (4) observation of pink rather than cyanotic mucous membranes and extremities. Even if all of these criteria are met, tube placement should be confirmed by chest radiograph as soon as possible.

11. Oral or nasal intubation?

Oral intubation is the preferred method. The tube is directly visualized through the vocal cords, ensuring proper placement. Nasal intubation is a "blind technique" relatively contraindicated in patients with maxillofacial trauma (risk of intracranial placement of the tube through an anterior fossa fracture) and in patients with known or suspected coagulopathy (because nasal mucosa is well vascularized, intubation can cause major epistaxis). However, in the patient with suspected cervical spine injury, nasal intubation can be accomplished while maintaining cervical immobilization and therefore is the preferred method in this setting (unless the patient is apneic).

12. What is the role of esophageal obturator airway (EOA)?

None. The EOA was adopted to eliminate the problem of gastric dilatation as well as to provide a reliable technique for regulation of ventilation. The tube can be placed quickly. Successful attempts range from 96–99%. The major drawbacks are risk of esophageal perforation (low, 0.2–2%) and inadvertent tracheal placement preventing ventilation. No data indicate that the device is safe in patients with cervical spine injury; therefore, at present, it is not recommended in the trauma patient. In addition, the technique probably has no role in in-hospital resuscitation because other methods of airway control are accessible. At present, the EOA is falling into disfavor because alternative techniques (mask or endotracheal tube) are both safer and more effective.

CIRCULATION

13. What is the proper method of external chest compression?

The rescuer should be positioned beside the patient's chest. The compression point is located by identifying the xiphoid-sternal junction and measuring two fingerbreadths toward the head. The heel of one hand is placed here. The heel of the second hand is placed over the first. The fingers may be interlocked. Keep the arms straight and the shoulders directly over the victim's sternum. The compression depth should be 4–5 cm. Maintain hand position on the sternum at all times. With one rescuer: 15 compressions followed by 2 ventilations, repeat cycle. With two rescuers: 5 compressions, 1 ventilation. Compression rates: one rescuer, 80/minute; two rescuers, 60/minute. Monitor the carotid pulse for effectiveness of CPR and to assess return of spontaneous pulses.

14. What are the essentials of external chest compressions?

The key to effective CPR is to produce blood flow. Typically, one can produce a pulse and a systolic blood pressure with any adequate chest compressions. However, to produce blood flow and, in turn, tissue perfusion requires prolonging the compression phase. Increasing the compression phase from 30–50% more than *doubles* the flow. Compression rate is relatively unimportant. Rates between 40 and 80/minute all produce comparable flows.

15. What are the complications of external chest compressions?
Complications of CPR are multiple and frequent. Rib and sternal fractures range from 40–80%. Major cardiac or pericardial injuries are rare but may occur (lacerations). Bone marrow and fat emboli are common—80% in one series. In addition, damage to intraabdominal organs has been reported, including lacerations, contusions, and rupture of liver, spleen, kidneys, colon, stomach, and diaphragm. Strict attention to details of hand placement and compression depth will minimize complications.

16. Is a "central line" the best access to the venous systemic circulation? *Controversial*
The "central line," i.e., internal jugular or subclavian vein catheter, appears, at first glance, to be part of any successful resuscitation. It is a technique that is mastered relatively early in one's surgical career. Its role in resuscitation, however, is somewhat dubious. Contrary to popular belief, large volumes of fluid can be delivered to the venous system more quickly via large-bore peripheral venous catheters. A 14-gauge, 5-cm catheter (peripheral) can deliver twice the flow of a 16-gauge, 20-cm catheter (central). In addition, central-line placement is associated with significant complications, including pneumothorax, air embolus, and puncture of large arteries. Finally, the placement of a central line may require interruption of CPR. Adequate venous access, therefore, can be easily achieved by the placement of peripheral catheters via the percutaneous or cutdown approach. However, central venous catheters offer the ability to obtain a central venous pressure (CVP) once a rhythm is restored and can identify the presence of cardiac tamponade. Moreover, in shock, especially hypovolemia, the peripheral venous system may be collapsed, making cannulation extremely difficult.

17. When should/should not the MAST suit be used? *Controversial*
The military antishock trouser (MAST) suit is an inflatable, three-component garment that surrounds the abdomen and both lower extremities. When inflated, the suit provides an increase in total peripheral resistance (TPR). This combination leads to increased central blood pressure (increased venous return, increased stroke volume, increased cardiac output; BP = CO × TPR, i.e., both CO and TPR are increased with the MAST suit). Indications for use include trauma arrest, systolic blood pressure less than 80 mmHg secondary to hypovolemic shock, continued retroperitoneal hemorrhage from pelvic fractures, hemorrhage requiring direct pressure for control, and femoral shaft fractures requiring immobilization. *Contraindications:* pulmonary edema, evisceration of abdominal contents, pregnancy, and decreased pulmonary function, i.e., pneumothorax. The controversy concerns the patient in deep shock after trauma in the field. Application of the MAST suit is theoretically sensible in this setting. However, these patients are often losing blood at very rapid rates and are possibly suffering from tension pneumothorax or pericardial tamponade. The time spent to apply the suit may be better spent rapidly transporting the patient to an emergency facility where appropriate, definitive, life-saving measures can be applied.

18. Colloid or crystalloid resuscitation fluid? *Controversial*
There are data to support both sides. Colloid advocates claim the solutions remain primarily in the intravascular space and thereby are more effective in elevating blood volume. Crystalloid advocates state that capillaries will leak albumin in the shock state. Many studies have shown that resuscitation with crystalloid is safe, especially with respect to pulmonary complications. Given its availability, low cost, and safety, crystalloid solution (lactated Ringer's) is at present the choice for initial fluid resuscitation.

19. When is blood needed?
For the patient in hemorrhagic shock, if hypotension remains after infusion of 2 L of crystalloid fluid, a blood transfusion should be started. Type-specific blood is appropriate while waiting for

complete cross-match. Whole blood is preferable to packed cells because it provides additional volume. Keep in mind that banked blood is low in factors V and VIII and platelets. Most authors recommend fresh frozen plasma for every 5–10 units of transfused blood to avoid dilutional coagulopathy. In addition, the citrate in banked blood will bind the circulating calcium. Give 500 mg calcium chloride (or gluconate) for every 4 units of transfused blood. Cold (4°C) banked blood should pass through blood warmers/filters to avoid acidosis and prevent microcirculatory clogging secondary to platelet microaggregates.

20. Open or closed chest cardiac compression? *Controversial*
In the nontraumatic cardiac arrest victim, closed-chest cardiac compression can be instituted immediately, is relatively safe, and, if performed correctly, can provide adequate tissue perfusion. Open, direct cardiac compression requires training and experience in performing thoracotomy and open massage. With the chest open, respiratory support is mandatory. Complications are many, including laceration of the lung, myocardium, or coronary arteries, phrenic nerve damage, and sepsis. In most instances, open-chest cardiac massage *will not* succeed when closed-chest compression, combined with drug therapy and ventilation, has failed. Indications for thoracotomy are presented in question 26.

21. What are the common causes of electromechanical dissociation (EMD)? How are they best treated?
EMD is typified by an orderly electrical rhythm in the absence of detectable blood pressure. In the setting of cardiac arrest, initial treatment consists of intravenous calcium chloride (see question 24). Keep in mind the potentially correctable situations that commonly cause EMD: (1) tension pneumothorax (diagnosis: hyperresonant chest, decreased breath sounds, chest radiograph), which is alleviated rapidly by placement of a large-bore needle into the pleural space on the side of the collapsed lung, and (2) pericardial tamponade (diagnosis: Beck's triad—distant heart sounds, distended neck veins/elevated CVP, and hypotension), which is relieved by pericardiocentesis or thoracotomy with pericardiotomy (controversial; see question 26). EMD also is associated with hypovolemia (which already should have been corrected), ventricular rupture (traumatic or secondary to myocardial infarction), pulmonary embolism, and pump failure secondary to massive MI.

22. Can one assist failing circulation mechanically? *Controversial*
At present, mechanical assistance of circulatory failure consists of intraaortic balloon counterpulsation (IABP) and left ventricular assist devices (LVADs). The latter are currently undergoing clinical trials. IABP is a technique to assist circulation in patients with cardiogenic shock not responsive to fluid therapy or pressors. The device increases coronary perfusion during diastole (with balloon inflated [40 ml], aortic diastolic pressure and coronary perfusion pressure increase) and decreases left ventricular work during systole (the balloon is actively deflated, thus leaving a 40 ml empty space in the aorta, which dramatically decreases "afterload"). IABP has been widely used following coronary artery or valve surgery. Its role in cardiogenic shock after acute arrest is still under investigation. In this setting its use is considered experimental. LVADs, of which there are many types, provide a means of either partially or totally bypassing the heart on a temporary basis. A tremendous amount of research is currently being conducted on this subject. The role in arrest situations is not yet known.

MONITORING

23. What is the role of end-tidal CO_2 in monitoring cardiac arrest?
Carbon dioxide is excreted by the lungs in amounts approximately equal to the oxygen that is consumed (defined by the respiratory quotient). When the lungs are connected to a beating heart, CO_2 efflux (sensed as end-tidal CO_2) denotes a functioning cardiopulmonary system and a happy patient. If the CO_2 sensor detects no CO_2, then either no CO_2 is being transported to the lungs

(poor circulation) or the sensor is in the wrong location (e.g., the esophagus). Thus, end-tidal CO_2 can be used to indicate whether the endotracheal tube is in fact in the trachea. Second, end-tidal CO_2 is *circulation-dependent* in low-flow states and can be used to evaluate the effectiveness of internal/external cardiac massage. Portable devices using CO_2-sensitive dye are available for this purpose.

DRUG THERAPY

24. List the drugs commonly used during resuscitation and the appropriate dosages.

Oxygen—to reverse hypoxia, 100%; measurable pulmonary toxicity has not been detected in less than 36 hours.

Sodium bicarbonate ($NaHCO_3$)—to reverse acidosis (hypoxia-induced anaerobic metabolism leads to acid accumulation; ventilatory failure leads to carbon dioxide retention—acidosis). Initial dose is 1 mEq/kg. One ampule (50 ml) contains 50 mEq of sodium bicarbonate. Bicarbonate combines with hydrogen ions to form carbon dioxide and water; thus, adequate ventilation is required for bicarbonate therapy to be fully effective. Overzealous use may result in hypokalemia (alkalosis shifts potassium ions intracellularly) and hypernatremia/hyperosmolality (each HCO_3^- is accompanied by a sodium ion).

Epinephrine—alpha, beta agonist. Intravenous dosage is 5–10 ml of 1:10,000 solution. Short duration; repeat dose may be necessary after 5 minutes. Inactivated by alkali; do not mix with bicarbonate solutions. Although enhancing myocardial performance, epinephrine greatly increases myocardial oxygen demand (ventilate!).

Atropine—parasympatholytic (vagolytic), thereby increasing the discharge rate of the sinus node. Useful in treating sinus bradycardia associated with hemodynamic compromise. Dose of 0.5 mg IV is repeated at 5-minute intervals until a desirable rate is achieved (60 beats/minute). Supplied as a 0.1 mg/ml solution—5 nl or 0.5 ng/ml solution—1 ml. Increased heart rate increases myocardial oxygen demand; atropine should be used only if the bradycardia causes hemodynamic compromise (heart rate less then 60 beats/minute).

Lidocaine—a local anesthetic, known to suppress ventricular arrhythmias (automatic and re-entrant). An IV bolus of 1 mg/kg is followed by IV infusion at 2–4 mg/min. An additional IV bolus can be given at 10 minutes after initial dose if arrhythmias persist. Toxicity is limited to the CNS and does not occur with a total dose less than 500 mg. Serious side effects include focal and grand mal seizures (treat with diazepam, 5 mg IV).

Bretylium tosylate—a postganglionic adrenergic blocker with positive inotropic and antiarrhythmic effects. Elevates ventricular fibrillation threshold (as does lidocaine), but, as it is an alpha blocker, the blood pressure will drop. For ventricular tachycardia, 500 mg over 8–10 minutes. Controversy surrounds its most effective use (see question 25).

Verapamil—a slow-channel (calcium) blocking agent used to block the AV node and to treat paroxysmal supraventricular tachycardia that is causing hemodynamic compromise. Dose: 0.1 mg/kg; dilute dose with 10 ml saline and infuse 1 ml/min until the supraventricular tachycardia either breaks or blocks. Repeat dose after 30 minutes if not effective. The drug reduces systemic vascular resistance; therefore, blood pressure should be monitored closely during its use. A well-known property of verapamil is its direct depression of cardiac contractility, yet *cardiac output* usually remains unchanged secondary to reflex sympathetic response.

Calcium chloride—positive inotropic agent. Calcium ions bind to regulatory proteins, which inhibit the formation of cross-bridges between muscle contractile filaments. Release of this inhibition by calcium binding allows cross-bridge formation, tension generation, and finally fiber shortening. Used when electrical rhythm is present but effective ejection of blood is absent (electromechanical dissociation; see question 21). Dose: calcium chloride (or gluconate), 250–500 mg IV push. Do not mix with bicarbonate—will precipitate.

Adenosine—a naturally occurring vasodilating hormone synthesized by vascular endothelial cells. Adenosine also dramatically slows AV nodal conduction. It is therefore useful in the therapy of supraventricular tachyarrhythmias. The dose is 6 mg injected in a rapid intravenous bolus (may be repeated several times). The half-life of intravenous adenosine is only 12 seconds. Measurable systemic hypotension occurs in less than 2% of patients because adenosine is metabolized before it hits the systemic vessels.

25. Lidocaine or bretylium for ventricular arrhythmias? *Controversial*
For treatment of ventricular fibrillation or ventricular tachycardia, lidocaine combined with electroshock therapy has long been the gold standard. Bretylium has a prolonged onset of action in the treatment of ventricular tachycardia, approximately 20 minutes or more. Lidocaine is the initial drug of choice for ventricular tachycardia; for refractory or recurrent ventricular tachycardia, bretylium may then be tried. Data indicate, however, that bretylium is as effective as lidocaine in the treatment of ventricular fibrillation. For ventricular fibrillation, its apparent onset of action is within a few minutes; 5 mg/kg may be given in IV bolus, followed by electrical defibrillation. More data are presently being compiled.

EMERGENCY SURGICAL PROCEDURES

26. When should emergency thoracotomy be performed?
Emergency thoracotomy is a dramatic, life-saving technique; however, strict guidelines should govern its use. It is indicated in patients with *trauma* who: (1) present in cardiac arrest, (2) remain hypotensive despite adequate fluid therapy, and (3) exhibit signs of massive intraabdominal bleeding without response to blood or fluid challenge. It is also indicated to perform cardiac massage on patients in whom chest wall deformities preclude external chest compressions. The open chest allows direct cardiac compression, direct defibrillation, control of cardiac or thoracic hemorrhage, repair of exsanguinating hemorrhage sites, direct relief of cardiac tamponade and tension pneumothorax, and aortic cross-clamping to control extrathoracic hemorrhage. Despite anecdotal reports on small series of survivors, judicious use is required in trauma patients arriving at the emergency department in extremis. In a large consecutive series of 400 patients with *blunt* trauma, there were no survivors, despite thoracotomy, in patients with absent vital signs or absent signs of life in the field.

BIBLIOGRAPHY

1. American College of Surgeons: Textbook of Advanced Trauma Life Support. Chicago, American College of Surgeons, 1993.
2. Brown CG, Werman HA: Adrenergic agonists during cardiopulmonary resuscitation. Resuscitation 19:1, 1990.
3. Emergency Cardiac Care Committee: Guidelines for cardiopulmonary resuscitation and emergency cardiac care. JAMA 268:2171–2274, 1992.
4. Girardi LN, Barie PS: Improved survival after intraoperative cardiac arrest in non-cardiac surgical patients. Arch Surg 130:15–18, 1995.
5. Lowenstein SR: Cardiopulmonary resuscitation in noninjured patients. In Wilmore DW, Cheung L, Harken AH, et al (eds): Scientific American Surgery, vol 1. New York, Scientific American, 1995, pp 1–24.

2. SHOCK

Alden H. Harken, M.D.

1. What is shock?

Shock is: Not just low blood pressure

Not just decreased peripheral perfusion

Not just limited systemic oxygen delivery

Ultimately, shock is decreased tissue respiration. Shock is suboptimal consumption of oxygen and excretion of carbon dioxide at the cellular level.

2. Is shock related to cardiac output?

Of course. However, a healthy medical student can redistribute blood flow preferentially to vital organs. Many of us have seen the 21-year-old, gun-slinging Harley Road Hog with a bullet in his liver, blood pressure of 60/–, and sufficient persistent cerebral perfusion to recount how "four dudes jumped me." That is classy utilization of limited cardiac output.

3. Is organ perfusion democratic?

Absolutely not. Limited blood flow is always redirected toward the carotid and coronary arteries. Peripheral vasoconstriction steals blood initially from the mesentery, then skeletal muscle, then kidneys and liver.

4. Is this vascular autoregulatory capacity uniform in all patients?

No. With age and atherosclerosis, patients lose their ability to redistribute limited blood flow. Thus, a 20% decrease in cardiac output (or a fall in blood pressure to 90 mmHg) can be life-threatening to a Supreme Court justice, whereas it may be undetectable in a triathlete. Fortunately, Darwin evolved us so that handguns and motorcycles are used only by young males.

5. For diagnostic and therapeutic purposes, can shock be usefully classified?

Yes.

1. **Hypovolemic shock** mandates volume resuscitation.

2. **Cardiogenic shock** mandates cardiac stimulation (both pharmacologic and eventually mechanical).

3. **Peripheral vascular collapse shock** mandates pharmacologic manipulation of the peripheral vascular tone (and direct attention to the etiology of the vasodilation—typically sepsis).

6. Is it advisable to treat all shock in the same sequential fashion?

Ultimately, yes. Whether a cigar-chomping banker presents with a big GI bleed (hypovolemic shock) or crushing substernal chest pain (cardiogenic shock), the surgeon should take, in order, the following steps:

1. Optimize volume status; give volume until further increase in right-sided (central venous pressure) and left-sided (pulmonary capillary wedge pressure) preload confers no additional benefit for cardiac output or blood pressure. (This step is pure Starling's law—place the patient's heart at the top of the Starling curve.)

2. If cardiac output, blood pressure, and tissue perfusion remain inadequate despite adequate preload, the patient has a pump (cardiogenic shock) problem. Infuse cardiac inotropic drugs (beta agonist) to the point of toxicity (typically cardiac ectopy—lots of frightening, premature ventricular contractions). For pharmacologically refractory cardiogenic shock, insert an intraaortic balloon pump (IABP).

3. If the patient exhibits a surprisingly high cardiac output and a paradoxically low blood pressure (such unusual loss of vascular autoregulatory control is associated typically—but not always—with sepsis), the surgeon may infuse a peripheral vasoconstrictor drug (alpha agonist).

7. What is the preferred access route for volume infusion?
Flow depends on catheter length and radius. Volume may be infused at twice the rate through a 5-cm, 14-gauge peripheral catheter as through a 20-cm, 16-gauge central line (see chapter 1). Assessment of central venous pressure (and left-sided filling pressure) may be necessary if the patient fails to respond to initial volume resuscitation.

8. Should one infuse crystalloid, colloid, or blood?
If the goal is only to improve preload and thus to repair cardiac output and blood pressure, crystalloid solution should be sufficient. It is controversial whether infused colloid remains in the vascular compartment. If the goal is to augment systemic oxygen delivery, red cells bind **much more** oxygen than plasma (see chapter 4).

9. When cardiac preload is adequate, what inotropic agents are useful?
The array of agents is mind-boggling. Pick several and get comfortable with them. Dobutamine, epinephrine, and norepinephrine are the chocolate, vanilla, and strawberry of the 32 flavors of cardiogenic drugs. These three drugs are all that the surgeon needs.

10. Is dopamine the same as dobutamine?
No. Dopamine stimulates renal dopaminergic receptors and may be quite useful in low doses (2 μg/kg/min) to counteract the renal arteriolar vasoconstriction that accompanies shock. Dopamine has no place as a primary cardiac inotropic agent.

11. Discuss the use of dobutamine, epinephrine, and norepinephrine.
Dobutamine is a beta-1 agonist (cardiac inotrope), but also has some beta-2 effects (peripheral vasodilation).
> *Start at:* 5 μg/kg/min and increase to point of toxicity (cardiac ectopy).
> *Note:*   Infuse to desired effect (do not stick rigidly to a preconceived dose). Because dobutamine has some vasodilating effects, it may be difficult to infuse into typically hypotensive patients in shock.

Epinephrine is a combined beta- and alpha-adrenergic agonist, with the beta effects predominating at lower doses.
> *Start at:* 0.05 μg/kg/min and increase to point of toxicity (cardiac ectopy).
> *Note:*   As with dobutamine, infuse to desired effect.

Norepinephrine is a combined alpha- and beta-adrenergic agonist, with the alpha effects predominating at all doses.
> *Start at:* 0.5 μg/kg/min and increase to point of toxicity (cardiac ectopy).
> *Note:*   Relatively pure peripheral vasoconstriction is uncommonly indicated and should be used only to modulate the peripheral vascular tone in peripheral vascular collapse shock.

12. When is an intraaortic balloon pump (IABP) indicated?
Mechanical circulatory support is indicated when the preload to both ventricles (CVP and PCWP) has been optimized and further cardiac stimulatory drugs are limited by frightening runs of premature ventricular contractions.

13. What does an IABP do?
Diastolic augmentation and systolic unloading.

14. What is diastolic augmentation?
A soft 40-ml balloon is inserted percutaneously through the common femoral artery into the descending thoracic aorta. The balloon is not occlusive, and it should not touch the walls of the aorta. When it is inflated, it is exactly like acutely transfusing 40 ml of blood into the aorta, thus augmenting each left ventricular stroke volume by 40 ml. Balloon infusion is triggered off the QRS complex from a surface ECG (any lead). The balloon is always inflated during diastole to increase diastolic blood pressure and thus augment coronary blood flow (CBF). Eighty percent of CBF occurs during diastole.

15. What is systolic unloading?
Balloon deflation is an active (not a passive) process. Helium is abruptly sucked out of the balloon, leaving a 40-ml empty space in the aorta. The left ventricle can eject the first 40 ml of its stroke volume into this empty space—at dramatically reduced workload. An intraaortic balloon, therefore, increases coronary oxygen delivery (CBF) while decreasing cardiac oxygen consumption.

16. What are the contraindications to IABP?
Aortic insufficiency: diastolic augmentation distends and injures the left ventricle.
Atrial fibrillation: balloon inflation and deflation cannot be appropriately timed.

BIBLIOGRAPHY

1. Abrams JH, Cerra F, Holcroft JW: Cardiopulmonary monitoring. In Wilmore DW, Brennan MF, Harken AH, et al (eds): Scientific American Surgery. New York, Scientific American, 1995.
2. Holcroft JW, Robinson MK: Shock. In Wilmore DW, Cheung L, Harken AH, et al (eds): Scientific American Surgery. New York, Scientific American, 1995.

3. PULMONARY INSUFFICIENCY

Alden H. Harken, M.D.

1. What is pulmonary insufficiency?
The huge alveolar-capillary surface of the lung (the size of a singles tennis court) is not working efficiently if the patient's arterial oxygen tension (PaO_2) is less than 50 mmHg and the arterial carbon dioxide tension ($PaCO_2$) is greater than 50 mmHg. This is the 50:50 rule. Furthermore, the patient who works hard to stay on the correct side of the 50:50 rule may soon run out of energy.

2. How much energy is expended in work of breathing?
A healthy medical student expends about 3% of total oxygen consumption (energy utilization) on work of breathing. After injury, particularly a big burn, patients may increase fractional energy expenditure of breathing up to 20%.

3. What surgical incisions most significantly compromise a patient's vital capacity?
Intuitively, an extremity incision or injury influences vital capacity least, followed sequentially by a lower abdominal incision, median sternotomy, thoracotomy, and upper abdominal incision. An upper abdominal incision is **worse than** a thoracotomy.

4. Is a chest radiograph helpful in assessing respiratory failure?
Of course it is. But the radiograph must be interpreted carefully.

5. What should one look for on the chest radiograph of a patient with impending respiratory failure?
1. Are both lungs fully expanded?
2. Are there **localized** areas of infiltrate, atelectasis, or consolidation?
3. Are there **generalized** areas of infiltrate, atelectasis, or consolidation?

6. Why is the local vs. generalized distinction important in assessing respiratory failure?
A local process may be assessed by aspiration or bronchoscopy to diagnose pneumonia or tumor. Generalized multilobar infiltrates are more likely to represent a diffuse alveolar-capillary leak syndrome.

7. What is ARDS?
Adult respiratory distress syndrome (ARDS) is a diffuse, multilobar capillary transudation of fluid into the pulmonary interstitium that dissociates the normal concordance of alveolar ventilation (Va) with lung perfusion ($\dot{Q}$).

8. What governs fluid influx across pulmonary capillaries?
Starling initially described the balance between intravascular hydrostatic pressure (Pc), which tends to push fluid out, and colloid oncotic pressure (COP), which sucks fluid in across the capillary endothelial barrier (K). Thus:

$$\text{Fluid flux} = K(Pc - COP)$$

9. What causes ARDS?
Anything that increases lung dysfunction by promoting wet lung. Thus:
1. **Heart failure** backs up pulmonary intravascular hydrostatic pressure (Pc), forcing fluid into the pulmonary interstitium.
2. **Malnutrition and liver failure** decrease plasma protein and thus COP. Fluid is not sucked back out of the lung.
3. **Sepsis** may break down the capillary endothelial barrier (K), thus permitting water and protein to leak into the lung.

10. What is high- vs. low-pressure ARDS?
Purists appropriately note that lung congestion due to high intravascular hydrostatic pressure secondary to heart failure is really not primary respiratory distress syndrome. Thus, if the pulmonary capillary wedge pressure (PCWP) is greater than 18 mmHg, the diagnosis is high-pressure pulmonary edema (not ARDS).

11. What is a normal colloid osmotic pressure?
COP is normally 20–22 mmHg.

12. How is COP calculated?
75% of COP is normally created by serum albumin along with globulins and fibrinogen. Thus:

$$COP = 2.1 \text{ (total protein)}$$

If an osmotically active, moleculelike hetastarch is infused, this calculation is fouled up.

13. What is low-pressure ARDS?
Low-pressure ARDS is a redundant term. To make the diagnosis of ARDS, the PCWP must be less than 18 mmHg; better yet, pure ARDS exists only if the PCWP is more than 4 mmHg less than the COP.

14. How can the pulmonary capillaries leak if the COP exceeds the PCWP?
The current concept invokes a septic expression of neutrophil CD11 and CD18 adhesion receptors, which stick to pulmonary vascular endothelial intercellular adhesion molecules (ICAM). Furthermore, septic stimuli provoke the adherent neutrophils to release intravascular proteases

and oxygen radicals. Resultant endovascular damage breaks down the capillary endothelial barrier (K), permitting lung leak—even at low hydrostatic pressure.

15. What is a Lasix sandwich?

Most surgeons, when their backs are against the wall, give 25 gm of albumin followed in 20 minutes by 20 mg Lasix IV. They reason that the albumin pulls fluid out of the water-logged lung and that the Lasix promotes a diuresis to rid the patient of extra water. This therapeutic concept probably works only in patients who are not very sick. The sicker the patient, the faster the infused albumin leaks and equilibrates across the damaged endovascular endothelial barrier. Thus, little water is sucked out of the sick lung in preparation for the diuresis. Watch—you will see surgeons try this approach. Some people believe in miracles; critical care surgeons tend to rely on them.

16. What are the goals of the therapy for ARDS?
1. Reduce lung edema.
2. Reduce oxygen toxicity (inspired O_2 concentration < 60% is safe).
3. Limit lung barotrauma (avoid peak inspiratory pressure in excess of 40 cm H_2O).
4. Promote matching of ventilation (Va) and perfusion ($\dot{Q}$)
5. Maintain systemic oxygen delivery.

17. What governs the distribution of lung perfusion ($\dot{Q}$)?

Mostly gravity. Thus the dependent portions of lung are always better perfused.

18. What is hypoxic pulmonary vasoconstriction (HPV)?

Most students believe that after dedicating the entire second year of medical school to pheochromocytoma and HPV, both entities may be safely forgotten. At least in the case of HPV, this is not true. A patient who has just undergone carotid endarterectomy illustrates the relevance of HPV. As the patient awakens from anesthesia, the blood pressure is 220/120 mmHg. Arterial PO_2 with 100% oxygen is 500 mmHg. So that the patient will not blow the carotid anastomosis, the surgeon urgently infuses nitroprusside. In 20 minutes the blood pressure is 120/80, but PO_2 (still with 100% oxygen) has dropped to 125 mmHg!

Did the lab technician screw up the blood gas analysis? No—this is an example of the clinical significance of HPV, which controls pulmonary arteriolar delivery of deoxygenated blood toward ventilated alveoli and away from poorly ventilated lung regions. The patient was using HPV to attain a PO_2 of 500 mmHg. But all antihypertensive agents (such as nitroprusside) and most general anesthetics block HPV. Thus the PO_2 increment from 125 to 500 mmHg is all due to HPV. HPV beautifully steered perfusion toward ventilated areas of lung.

19. What governs the distribution of ventilation (Va) in lung?

A large pleural pressure gradient (more negative at the top of the lung by 20 cm H_2O) squeezes gas primarily out of the dependent lung during each exhaled breath. Thus the regional compliance of dependent lung is much better than that of the lung apex, which is still distended with gas at end exhalation. Therefore, the usual approach is to perfuse **and** ventilate dependent lung preferentially. God was smart when he built us. He provided us with a V/$\dot{Q}$ close to 1.

20. How does ARDS compromise lung function?

The trachea is held open with cartilaginous rings, but terminal bronchioles are not. Wet lung collapses the terminal bronchioles, thus trapping distal alveolar gas.

21. How long does it take for pulmonary arterial (deoxygenated) blood to equilibrate completely with trapped alveolar gas?

About ¾ of a second. After that, no more oxygen is added and no more carbon dioxide is eliminated from the perfusing blood.

22. What term is used when pulmonary blood traverses the lung without oxygen or carbon dioxide gas exchange?
A shunt—or ($Va/\dot{Q} = 0$).

23. What is the therapy for terminal airways closure and resultant shunt secondary to the wet lung of ARDS?
Positive end-expiratory pressure (PEEP) should hold open terminal bronchioles, thus promoting ventilation of previously trapped alveoli and minimizing the shunt.

24. When may the patient come off mechanical ventilation and be extubated safely?
The patient should be sufficiently alert to protect the airway, require an inspired oxygen concentration no greater than $FiO_2 = 0.4$, and be comfortable breathing on a T-piece (without the mechanical ventilation) for 60 minutes at a respiratory rate less than 20 and a minute ventilation less than 10 L/min. The patient should be able to generate a negative inspiratory force greater than –20 cm H_2O. Finally, after 1 hour on the T-piece oxygenation should provide a hemoglobin saturation greater than 85% without respiratory acidosis (see chapter 4).

BIBLIOGRAPHY

1. Baue PS, Hudo LJ, Fischer E: Comparison of Apache II and Apache III scoring systems for mortality prediction in critical surgical illness. Arch Surg 130:77–82, 1995.
2. Demling RH, Goodwin CW: Pulmonary dysfunction. In Wilmore DW, Cheung L, Harken AH, et al (eds): Scientific American Surgery. New York, Scientific American, 1995.
3. Holcroft JW, Robinson MK: Shock. In Wilmore DW, Cheung L, Harken AH, et al (eds): Scientific American Surgery. New York, Scientific American, 1995.
4. Ishaaya AM, Nathan SD, Belman MJ: Work of breathing after extubation. Chest 107:204–209, 1995.
5. Shapiro BA, Peruzzi WT: Changing practices in ventilator management: A review of the literature and suggested clinical correlations. Surgery 117:121–133, 1995.

4. ARTERIAL BLOOD GASES

Alden H. Harken, M.D.

1. Mr. O'Flaherty has just undergone an inguinal herniorrhaphy under local anesthesia. The recovery room nurse asks permission to sedate him. She says that he is confused and unruly and keeps trying to get out of bed. Is it safe to sedate Mr. O'Flaherty?
Absolutely not. A confused, agitated patient in the recovery room or surgical intensive care unit (SICU) **must** be recognized as acutely hypoxemic until proved otherwise.

2. Mr. O'Flaherty is moved to the SICU. At 2:00 AM the SICU calls to report that Mr. O'Flaherty has a PO_2 of 148 mmHg on face mask oxygen. Is it okay to roll over and go back to sleep?
Absolutely not. More information is needed.

3. You glance at the abandoned cup of coffee sitting on your well-worn copy of *Surgical Secrets*. What is the PO_2 of that cup of coffee?
148 mmHg.

4. How can Mr. O'Flaherty and the coffee have the same PO_2?
The abandoned coffee has presumably had ample time to equilibrate completely with atmospheric gas. At sea level the barometric pressure is 760 mmHg. To obtain the partial pressure of

oxygen in the coffee, subtract water vapor pressure (47 mmHg) and multiply by the concentration of oxygen (20.8%) in the atmosphere. Thus:

$$PO_2 = (760 - 47) \times 20.8\% = 148 \text{ mmHg}$$

5. What is the difference between Mr. O'Flaherty's and the coffee's PO_2?
Nothing. Both represent the partial pressure of oxygen in fluid. A complete set of blood gases is necessary.

6. What is a complete set of blood gases?
  PO_2
  PCO_2
  pH
  Hemoglobin saturation
  Hemoglobin concentration

7. If Mr. O'Flaherty and the coffee have the same PO_2, how would Mr. O'Flaherty do if he were exchange-transfused with coffee?
Badly.

8. Why?
Although the oxygen tensions are the same, the **amount** of oxygen in blood is vastly greater.

9. How does one quantitate the amount of oxygen in blood?
Arterial oxygen content (CaO_2) is quantitated as ml of oxygen/100 ml of blood. (**Watch out:** almost all other concentrations are traditionally provided per ml or per liter—**not** per 100 ml.) Because ml of oxygen is a volume in 100 ml of blood, these units are frequently abbreviated as vol. %.

10. Why is blood thicker than coffee (or wine)?
Because hemoglobin binds a huge amount of oxygen. Ten grams of fully saturated hemoglobin (hematocrit about 30%) binds 13.4 ml of oxygen, whereas 100 ml of plasma at a PO_2 of 100 mmHg contains only 0.3 ml of oxygen.

11. Does the position of the oxyhemoglobin dissociation curve make any difference?
  • Increase in PCO_2.
  • Increase in hydrogen ion concentrations (**not** pH).
  • Increase in temperature.
  All shift the oxyhemoglobin curve to the right; that is, oxygen is released more easily in the tissues. Within physiologic limits, however, Mae West probably said it best: "There is less to this than meets the eye."

12. If arterial oxygen content (CaO_2) or ultimately systemic oxygen delivery (cardiac output $\times$ CaO_2) is what the surgeon really wants to know, why does the nurse report Mr. O'Flaherty's PO_2 instead of his CaO_2 at 2:00 AM?
No one knows.

13. What is the fastest and most practical method of increasing Mr. O'Flaherty's arterial oxygen content?
Transfusion of red blood cells. The patient's arterial oxygen content is increased by 25% with transfusion from a hemoglobin concentration of 8 to 10 gm%. The patient's arterial oxygen content is affected negligibly by an increase in arterial PO_2 from 100 to 200 mmHg (hemoglobin is fully saturated in both instances).

14. What is a transfusion trigger?
The hematocrit at which a patient is automatically transfused. This is **not** a useful concept. The NIH Consensus Conference, drawing data from Jehovah's Witnesses, patients with renal failure, and monkeys concluded that it is not necessary to transfuse a patient until the hematocrit reaches 21%. Traditional surgical dogma mandates a hematocrit above 30%. When the patient is in trouble, however, authorities in surgical critical care encourage transfusion to a hematocrit of 45% to optimize systemic oxygen delivery.

15. What governs respiratory drive?
PCO_2 and pH are inextricably intertwined by the Henderson-Hasselbach equation. By juggling this equation in the cerebrospinal fluid (CSF) of goats, it is clear that CSF hydrogen ion concentration (not PCO_2) controls respiratory drive. However, this distinction is not clinically important. What is important is that if a person becomes acidotic either with diabetic ketoacidosis or by running up a flight of stairs, minute ventilation ($\dot{V}_E$) is increased.

16. How tight is respiratory control? Or, if you hold your breath for 1 minute, how much do you want to breathe?
A lot.

17. After 60 seconds of apnea, what happens to $PaCO_2$?
It increases only from 40 to 47 mmHg. Thus, tiny changes in PCO_2 (and pH) translate into a huge respiratory stimulus. Normally, respiratory compensation for metabolic acidosis is very tight.

18. What is base excess?
Base excess is a poor man's indicator of the metabolic component of acid-base disorders. After correcting the PCO_2 to 40 mmHg, the base excess or base deficit is touted as an indirect measure of serum lactate. Although many parameters directing volume resuscitation in shock are more practical, expeditious, and direct (see chapter 2), base deficit has been advertised as helpful. The base excess or deficit is calculated from the Sigaard-Anderson nomogram in the blood gas laboratory. Normally, of course, there is no base excess or deficit. Acid-base status is "just right."

BIBLIOGRAPHY
1. Bartlett RH: Critical Care Handbook, 13th ed. Ann Arbor, MI, University of Michigan Press, 1995.
2. Davis JW, Shackford SR, Mackensie RC, Hoyt DB: Base deficit as a guide to volume resuscitation. J Trauma 28:1464–1467, 1988.
3. Messmer KFW: Acceptable hematocrit levels in surgical patients. World J Surg 11:41–46, 1987.
4. Perioperative red cell transfusion. National Institutes of Health Consensus Conference Statement, vol 7, no 4. Bethesda, MD, U.S. Department of Health and Human Services, 1988.

5. FLUIDS AND ELECTROLYTES

Alden H. Harken, M.D.

1. How does one convert 1 mg of sodium into milliequivalents (mEq)?
Divide by the atomic weight of sodium. Thus, 1 gm (1000 mg) of sodium divided by 23 equals 43.5 mEq.

2. How many mEq of sodium are in 1 teaspoon of salt?
One teaspoon of salt contains 2400 mg or 104 mEq of sodium.

3. How much does a 40-pound block of salt cost?
$3.40 at the feed store.

4. What is the electrolyte content of intravenous fluids?

Electrolyte Content of Intravenous Fluids

SOLUTIONS (mEq/L)	SODIUM	POTASSIUM	CHLORIDE	BICARBONATE/ LACTATE
Normal saline (0.9% NaCl)	154		154	
Ringer's lactate solution	130	4	109	28*
D5/$\frac{1}{2}$ normal saline	77		77	

* Lactate is immediately converted to bicarbonate.

5. How do these concentrations relate to body fluid and electrolyte compartments?

Electrolyte Concentrations in Body Fluids

COMPARTMENTS (mEq/L)	SODIUM	POTASSIUM	CHLORIDE	BICARBONATE
Plasma	142	4	103	27
Interstitial fluid	144	4	114	30
Intracellular fluid	10	150		10

6. What are the daily volumes (ml/24 hr) and electrolyte contents (mEq/L) of body secretions for a 70-kg medical student?

Daily Volumes and Electrolyte Contents of Body Secretions

	ml/24 hr	SODIUM	POTASSIUM	CHLORIDE	BICARBONATE
Saliva	+1500	10	25	10	30
Stomach	+1500	50	10	130	
Duodenum	+1000	140	5	80	
Ileum	+3000	140	5	104	30
Colon	−6000	60	30	40	
Pancreas	+ 500	140	5	75	100
Biliary	+ 500	140	5	100	30
Sweat*	+1000	50			
Gatorade		21		21	

* See question 7.

7. Are sweat glands responsive to aldosterone? Can they be trained?
Yes and yes. Thus Archie Bunker's sweat contains 100 mEq/L sodium, whereas an Olympic marathon runner retains sodium (sweat sodium may be as low as 20–30 mEq/L).

8. Is Gatorade really just flavored athlete's sweat?
Yes.

9. What are the daily maintenance fluid and electrolyte requirements for a 70-kg student?

Total fluid volume	2500 ml
Sodium	70 mEq (1 mEq/kg)
Potassium	35 mEq (½ mEq/kg)

10. Does the routine postoperative patient require intravenous sodium or potassium supplementation? Routine serum electrolyte testing?
No and no.

11. Can a patient with a good heart and kidneys overcome all but the most woefully incompetent fluid and electrolyte management?
Yes.

12. Can one throw a healthy medical student into congestive failure by intravenous infusion of 100 ml of D_5/S per kg per hour?
No. One will simply be ankle-deep in urine.

13. What is a subtraction alkalosis?
Vigorous nasogastric suction of a patient with a lot of gastric acid eliminates hydrochloric acid, leaving the patient alkalotic.

14. Which electrolyte is most useful in repairing a hypokalemic metabolic alkalosis?
Chloride.

15. What are the best indicators of a patient's status?
   • Heart rate
   • Blood pressure
   • Urine output
   • Big-toe temperature

16. Is a warm big toe indicative of a hemodynamically stable patient?
Most likely. The vascular autoregulatory ability of a young healthy patient is huge. The carotid and coronary circulations are maintained until the bitter end. Conversely, if the patient's big toe is warm and perfused, the patient is stable.

17. What is the minimal adequate postoperative urine output?
½ ml/kg/hr.

18. What is a typical postoperative urine sodium?
Less than 20 mEq/L.

19. Why?
Surgical stress prompts mineralocorticoid (aldosterone) secretion so that the normal kidney retains sodium.

20. What is paradoxical aciduria?
Postoperative patients, by virtue of nasogastric suction (loss of gastric acid), blood transfusions (the citrate in blood is converted to bicarbonate), and hyperventilation (decreased PCO_2) are typically alkalotic. Patients are also stressed, and their kidneys retain sodium and water. The renal tubules must exchange some other cations for the retained sodium. The kidney chooses to exchange potassium and hydrogen ions. Thus, even in the face of systemic alkalosis, the postoperative kidney absorbs sodium and excretes hydrogen ions, producing a paradoxical aciduria.

21. What is third-spacing?
Both hypotension and infection prime neutrophils (CD11 and CD18 receptor complexes), promoting adherence to vascular endothelial cells. Subsequent activation of adherent neutrophils spews out proteases and toxic superoxide radicals, blowing big holes in the vascular lining. Water and plasma albumin leak through the holes. The volume pulled out of the vascular space into the

third space of the interstitial and hollow viscus (gut) creates relative hypovolemia and requires additional fluid replacement.

22. What is a Lasix sandwich?
Twenty-five percent albumin followed by 20 mg Lasix IV. If the patient is edematous, the intravenous albumin theoretically sucks water osmotically out of the interstitial third space. As the excessive water enters the vascular compartment, furosemide (Lasix) produces a healthy diuresis. In most intensive care patients, however, the infused albumin rapidly equilibrates across the damaged vascular endothelium. Thus, no additional water is pulled into the blood volume. Although surgeons often order Lasix sandwiches, they probably work only in healthy patients who do not need them.

BIBLIOGRAPHY

1. Hanson AS, Linas S: Hypokalemia and hyperkalemia. In Parsons PE, Wiener-Kronish JP (eds): Critical Care Secrets. Philadelphia, Hanley & Belfus, 1992.
2. Lowry SF, Brennan MF: Life-threatening electrolyte abnormalities. In Wilmore DW, Brennan MF, Harken AH, et al (eds): Scientific American Surgery. New York, Scientific American, 1995.
3. Sahn SA, Heffner JE: Critical Care Pearls. Philadelphia, Hanley & Belfus, 1989.
4. Shires GT, Canizaro PC: Fluid and electrolyte management of the surgical patient. In Sabiston DC Jr (ed): Textbook of Surgery. Philadelphia, W.B. Saunders, 1991.

6. NUTRITIONAL ASSESSMENT AND ENTERAL NUTRITION

Kathleen M. Teasley, M.S., R.Ph., and Frederick A. Moore, M.D.

NUTRITIONAL ASSESSMENT

1. What are the indications for nutritional support?
Factors influencing the need for nutritional support include the age of the patient, the presence of critical illness, and the presence and severity of malnutrition. In general, infants and young children are more susceptible to nutritional complications than adults because of their limited reserves and their need to support growth and development. The previously well-nourished patient also benefits from early nutritional support. The hypermetabolic, hypercatabolic response inherent to critical illness, if not supported by exogenous nutrients, results in acute protein malnutrition, which compromises immunologic function and leads to subclinical multiple organ dysfunction. In noncritically ill patients, brief periods (e.g., 5–7 days) can be tolerated without aggressive intervention. However, in severe malnutrition, there is a greater need to initiate nutritional support to reverse malnutrition before it further affects other outcomes.

2. What is nutritional assessment?
Clinical evaluation should include a **medical history** to determine the presence of factors that may predispose the patient to malnutrition, such as weight loss, anorexia, vomiting, diarrhea, and decreased or unusual intake. The **physical examination** focuses on an assessment of lean body mass (presence of muscle wasting), loss of subcutaneous fat, and the physical findings of micronutrient deficiencies (e.g., dermatitis, glossitis, cheilosis). **Laboratory data** should include visceral protein concentrations (see question 4) and micronutrient concentrations (if clinical evaluation suggests possible deficiencies). Data may also include measures of immune function (e.g, total lymphocyte count, delayed cutaneous hypersensitivity). The creatinine-height index has

been used to determine lean body mass by comparing actual creatinine excreted to a predicted value based on the sex and height of a patient. Anthropometric measurements are gross measures of body cell mass (see question 5) and, therefore, reflect somatic protein (muscle mass) and adipose stores.

3. How is malnutrition classified?
Three terms are used to describe protein-calorie malnutrition (PCM). **Marasmus** is a chronic condition resulting from a deficiency in total energy intake. There is wasting of both somatic protein and adipose stores, but visceral protein production is preserved. Immune function and muscle function are usually impaired. Cancer patients commonly have marasmus. **Kwashiorkor** results from adequate calorie intake but a relative protein deficiency. There is depletion of visceral protein pools with a relative preservation of adipose tissue. This condition may develop rapidly in the setting of metabolic stress (e.g., trauma, infection, burns) and may be accompanied by impaired immune function. **Mixed kwashiorkor-marasmus** is a form of severe PCM manifested by reduced visceral protein synthesis superimposed on wasting of somatic protein and adipose stores. Immunocompetence is impaired, and there is poor wound healing. It can occur in chronically ill, starved patients who are undergoing hypermetabolic stress.

4. How is visceral protein status assessed?
Visceral protein status is assessed by measuring serum concentrations of selected hepatically synthesized transport proteins that have been shown to correlate with nutritional status. These include albumin, transferrin, prealbumin, and retinol-binding protein. Depletion of visceral proteins may be categorized as mild, moderate, or severe.

PROTEIN	NORMAL VALUE	MILD	MODERATE	SEVERE
Albumin, gm/dl	3.5–5.0	2.8–3.5	2.1–2.7	< 2.1
Transferrin, mg/dl	200–400	150–200	100–150	< 100
Prealbumin, mg/dl	10–40	10–15	5–10	< 5
Retinol-binding protein, mg/dl	2.7–7.6	*	*	*

* Not determined.

Other factors that may affect the serum concentration of these proteins include fluid status, hepatic function, and abnormal losses via the GI tract or kidneys. It also must be emphasized that the liver reprioritizes protein synthesis in response to stress by decreasing production of these normal constitutive proteins so as to produce more acute phase proteins.

5. What are anthropometric measurements? How are they used?
Height, weight, limb size. They are relatively insensitive to acute changes in nutritional status; therefore, they are mostly useful in monitoring patients requiring long-term nutritional support, such as home parenteral nutrition. Body weight is the most commonly used of these measures. Actual body weight should be interpreted in view of fluid status and relative to ideal weight for height or usual (e.g., pre-illness or pre-weight loss) weight. Measures of limb size include mid-arm muscle circumference (MAMC), which correlates with skeletal muscle mass, and triceps skin-fold thickness (TSF), which estimates the subcutaneous fat.

6. Why is urinary nitrogen measured? How are results interpreted?
Urinary urea nitrogen (UUN) is measured as an indicator of the protein catabolic rate. It is also used to determine a nitrogen balance (see question 7). UUN represents 60–90% of the nitrogen excreted in the urine and, therefore, is a rough approximation of total urinary nitrogen (TUN). As the stress level increases, the concomitant increase in protein catabolism results in an increase in urinary nitrogen. Quantitatively this can be interpreted as follows:

CLINICAL CONDITION	URINARY NITROGEN LOSS (GM/DAY)
Nonstressed, starvation	< 8
Low stress (e.g., elective surgery)	8–12
Moderate stress (e.g., polytrauma)	13–18
High stress (e.g., sepsis)	> 18

7. What is nitrogen balance?

Nitrogen balance is the difference between nitrogen intake and nitrogen output. Nitrogen intake is determined from dietary protein intake per day (grams of nitrogen = grams of protein ÷ 6.25). Nitrogen output per day is determined by measuring urine urea nitrogen in a 24-hour urine collection and adding 4 gm/day to approximate non-urea nitrogen loss in the urine plus other insensible N_2 losses. Nitrogen balance = (protein intake, gm/day ÷ 6.25) – (UUN, gm/day) – 4 gm/day. Traditionally a prime goal in nutritional support has been to place the patient in positive nitrogen balance.

8. What is a metabolic cart study?

A metabolic cart study (also called indirect calorimetry) measures inspired gas concentrations, expired gas concentrations, and minute volume (VE) to determine oxygen consumption (VO_2, L/min) and carbon dioxide production (VCO_2, L/min). Resting energy expenditure (REE) can be calculated using the Weir equation:

$$REE = [(3.9 \times VO_2) + (1.1 \times VCO_2)]1.44 - (2.8 \times UUN)$$

Other derived variables include respiratory quotient (see question 9) and the ventilatory equivalent ($VEco_2$). $VEco_2$ is simply the amount VE required to excrete 1 liter of CO_2 produced ($VEco_2 = VE/CO_2$). When faced with a high minute ventilation requirement, it is helpful in differentiating hypermetabolism from pulmonary dysfunction.

9. What is a respiratory quotient? How is it interpreted?

The respiratory quotient (RQ) is an indicator of net substrate oxidation and, hence, provides insight into substrate utilization. The mathematical expression for RQ is carbon dioxide production (VCO_2, L/min) divided by oxygen consumption (VO_2, L/min). In general, an RQ of < 0.7 reflects net fat oxidation, and an RQ of > 1.0 reflects lipogenesis. Values in-between reflect proportional utilization of substrates or mixed fuel oxidation.

10. How are nutritional requirements determined?

The U.S. Recommended Dietary Allowances (RDAs) can be used as a guide for most people who are not critically ill or in need of nutritional repletion. In general, the critically ill patient has increased protein and energy requirements. Traditionally the Harris-Benedict equation is used to give an estimate of resting energy expenditure. This is multiplied by a stress factor (1.3–2.0) to calculate the initial target nutritional goal. Subsequent needs are then titrated by UUN and metabolic cart determinations. At higher levels of intake, monitoring substrate tolerance is needed to avoid complications (e.g., glucose intolerance exacerbated by excess carbohydrate intake). Additionally, requirements for nutritional repletion are generally greater than those for maintenance.

ENTERAL NUTRITION

11. What is enteral nutrition? When should it be used?

Enteral nutrition is the nonvolitional administration of nutrients into the gastrointestinal tract that can be achieved through one of several accesses: the nasoenteric route (e.g., nasogastric, nasoduodenal, nasojejunal) or a feeding enterostomy (e.g., gastrostomy, needle catheter jejunostomy), which may be placed surgically or nonsurgically (e.g., percutaneously via endoscopy). In general, enteral nutrition is indicated in patients in whom oral intake is inadequate, who are at risk for nutrition-related complications, and who have a functional, accessible GI tract. Examples of clinical conditions in which enteral nutrition has been used include severe dysphagia, burns, low-output enterocutaneous fistulas, and anorexia, as well as in critically ill patients who have adequate intestinal function.

12. What products are available for enteral nutrition?
A wide variety of products is available. The products may be categorized into **polymeric formulas** (which contain nutrients in high molecular weight forms and require normal digestive and absorptive ability), **predigested formulas** (which contain one or more partially digested macronutrients or combinations of nutrients and can be absorbed in patients with compromised GI tracts), and **modular formulas** (which are composed of individual nutrients or combinations of nutrients but are nutritionally incomplete and intended for use as supplements or in combination with other products). The choice of formula depends on many factors, including the patient's nutritional requirements, substrate tolerance, placement of the feeding access, disease state, and clinical condition. In addition, the cost of these products varies; in general, products that are disease-specific or contain nutrients in an elemental form are more expensive.

13. How should enteral feedings be administered?
Several methods may be used for enteral feeding. The choice of method depends on the characteristics of the product to be used, the patient's GI status, and location of the feeding catheter tip. Options include bolus, intermittent, continuous, and cyclic feeding. **Bolus feeding** is rapid administration (≤10 minutes) with a feeding syringe. It is associated with a high incidence of complications such as nausea, pain, and vomiting. **Intermittent feeding** is the administration of the enteral formula (usually by gravity flow) over a period of 30–40 minutes every 3–4 hours. This method may result in complications similar to those of bolus feeding. Bolus and intermittent administration should be used only for gastric feedings. **Continuous feeding** usually involves pump-assisted feeding over 24 hours a day. It is well tolerated by most patients and necessary for jejunal feedings. **Cyclic feeding**, which is also pump-assisted, is continuous administration over a limited period, usually at night. It is used to facilitate ambulation during the day or to supplement oral intake. When enteral feeding is first initiated, hyperosmolar formulas, when administered into the small bowel, should be diluted by ½ or ¼ strength and infused at a slow rate (e.g., 25 ml/hr). The formula can be advanced by rate at intervals of 6–24 hours, depending on patient tolerance, and then by strength at intervals of 6–24 hours.

14. What complications are associated with enteral nutrition?
Complications may be classified into three general categories: mechanical, gastrointestinal, and metabolic. **Mechanical complications** are associated with the feeding access and include pharyngeal irritation and mucosal damage, obstruction of the feeding tube lumen, and tube displacement. **Gastrointestinal complications** include nausea, vomiting, distention, cramping, hypermotility, diarrhea, gastric retention, and constipation. These complications may be due to inappropriate administration of the enteral feeding or inappropriate selection of feeding formula; they also may be independent of enteral feeding and indicative of a problem with gastrointestinal function. **Metabolic complications** include glucose intolerance, electrolyte imbalances, and nutrient excesses or deficiencies.

15. What guidelines should be followed for monitoring patients receiving enteral nutrition?
Monitoring should assess efficacy of the nutritional regimen as well as detect complications. Laboratory data should include measurements of nutritional status (see questions 2, 4, and 5), urinary urea nitrogen, electrolytes, blood glucose, and renal and hepatic function; the frequency of obtaining such data depends on the clinical status of the patient, but generally once weekly is appropriate. Monitoring also should include frequent evaluation of the feeding tube's position and patency, and with gastric feedings gastric residuals should be checked. The patient also should be evaluated for signs and symptoms of gastrointestinal complications.

CONTROVERSIES

16. Which is better—enteral or parenteral nutrition?
The optimal route of substrate delivery continues to be debated. Safety, convenience, and cost have traditionally favored the enteral route, but an inappropriate fear of gastrointestinal intolerance has discouraged its use in the postoperative stressed patient. Now, however, basic research indicates compelling physiologic benefits for enteral feeding. Substrates delivered by the enteral route are better utilized than those administered parenterally. In addition, total enteral nutrition (TEN), compared with current total parenteral nutrition (TPN), prevents gastrointestinal mucosal atrophy, attenuates the stress response to injury, maintains immunocompetence, and preserves normal gut flora. Prospective, randomized, controlled trials in patients sustaining major trauma have consistently shown that early TEN is associated with reduced septic morbidity compared with TPN.

17. Do new "immune-enhancing" formulas offer additional clinical benefits?
Recent basic and clinical research suggests that the beneficial effects of enteral nutrition can be amplified by supplementing specific nutrients that exert pharmacologic immune-enhancing effects beyond the prevention of acute protein malnutrition. Such nutrients include glutamine, arginine, omega-3 polyunsaturated fatty acids (PUFA), and nucleotides. At present, at least three immune-enhancing enteral formulas (i.e., enriched with various combinations of the above nutrients) are commercially available. In addition, five prospective randomized trials suggest that this strategy of nutritional immunomodulation may offer clinical benefit to stressed surgical patients. Additional studies are needed to confirms such observations.

BIBLIOGRAPHY

1. American Society of Parenteral and Enteral Nutrition, Board of Directors: Guidelines for use of parenteral and enteral nutrition in adult and pediatric patients. J Parent Ent Nutr 17(4):1SA–52SA, 1993.
2. Cerra FB, Shronts EP, Raup S, Konstantinides N: Enteral nutrition in hypermetabolic surgical patients. Crit Care Med 17:619–622, 1989.
3. Dempsey DT, Mullen JL, Buzby GP: The link between nutritional status and clinical outcome: Can nutritional intervention modify it? Am J Clin Nutr 47:352–356, 1988.
4. Feurer I, Mullen JL: Bedside measurement of resting energy expenditure and respiratory quotient via indirect calorimetry. Nutr Clin Pract 1:43–49, 1986.
5. Moore FA, Feliciano DV, Andressy RJ, et al: Early enteral feeding, compared to parenteral, reduced postoperative septic complications. Ann Surg 216:172–184, 1992.
6. Moore FA, Moore EE, Kudsk KA, et al: Clinical benefits of an immune-enhancing diet for early postinjury enteral feeding. J Trauma 37:607–615, 1994.
7. Teasley KM: Assessment, prevalence and significance of malnutrition. In DiPiro, Talbert, Hayes, et al (eds): Pharmacotherapy: A Pathophysiologic Approach. New York, Elsevier, 1989.
8. Zaloga GP: Nutrition. In Zaloga GP (ed): Critical Care. St. Louis, Mosby, 1994.

7. PARENTERAL NUTRITION

Kathleen M. Teasley, M.S., R.Ph., and Frederick A. Moore, M.D.

1. What is parenteral nutrition?
Parenteral nutrition (PN) is a form of nutritional support in which nutrients (e.g., protein, carbohydrates, fats, electrolytes, vitamins, trace minerals, and fluids) are supplied via an intravenous delivery system. When used as the sole means of providing nutrition, this therapy is referred to as total parenteral nutrition (TPN).

2. What are the indications for PN?

Clinical settings in which PN is indicated as a part of routine care include patients with an inability to absorb nutrients via the gastrointestinal tract, such as those with massive bowel resection, radiation enteritis, severe inflammatory bowel disease, severe diarrhea, and intractable vomiting; patients undergoing high-dose chemotherapy, radiation, and bone marrow transplantation; patients with moderate to severe pancreatitis; severely catabolic patients; and patients with severe malnutrition in the face of a nonfunctional gastrointestinal tract. Other settings in which PN may be useful include major surgery accompanied by moderate stress, enterocutaneous fistulas, bowel obstruction, and hyperemesis gravidarum. PN should not be used in patients whose prognosis does not warrant aggressive nutritional support.

3. How is PN delivered?

PN may be infused via a peripheral or central venous access. The factors that determine route of infusion are nutritional requirements, anticipated length of PN therapy, viability of peripheral veins, risk of central venous catheterization, and fluid status. PN solutions that are administered via a peripheral venous access should have an osmolarity ≤ 600 mOsm in order to avoid damage to the vein; therefore, peripheral PN formulas are relatively dilute (e.g., 40 gm of amino acids per liter and 50 gm of dextrose per liter with restricted electrolyte concentrations). Because of a low caloric density, large volumes are required to meet total nutritional requirements. Short-term (less than 10 days) or supplemental PN may be achieved via peripheral venous access if the patient can tolerate ≥ 2000 ml of fluid per day. Patients who need long-term PN, are fluid restricted, and have high nutritional requirements should have a central venous access for PN.

4. What are the usual nutritional components of a PN regimen?

Nonprotein calories, protein, essential fatty acids, electrolytes, vitamins, trace minerals, and fluids. Nonprotein calories are provided as a balance of carbohydrate and fat. Dextrose monohydrate (caloric density 3.4 kcal/gm) is the carbohydrate. Fat emulsions (caloric density 9 kcal/gm) made from either soybean oil (e.g., Intralipid) or a mixture of soybean oil and safflower oil (e.g., Liposyn II) provide fat calories and are the source of essential fatty acids (linoleic, linolenic, and arachidonic acids). Protein (calorie density 4 kcal/gm) is provided as crystalline amino acids. A standard amino acid solution contains a balance of essential and nonessential amino acids (e.g., Freamine III, Travasol, Novamine, Aminosyn). Specialty amino acid solutions are available for use in specific disease states (see question 5). The electrolyte cations, which include sodium, potassium, magnesium, phosphorus, and calcium, are admixed into the PN solution using one of several anions. Acid-base status may be affected by the amount of chloride or acetate used in providing sodium and potassium. The concentrations of calcium and phosphorus are limited to avoid precipitation of a calcium phosphate salt. Multivitamin products that meet AMA recommendations contain vitamins A, C, D, and E as well as the B vitamins, including folate but not vitamin K, which must be added separately. A multitrace mineral product is added to provide copper, chromium, manganese, zinc, and selenium.

5. What are speciality amino acid solutions? When are they indicated?

Specialty amino acid formulas designed to meet age- or disease-specific requirements include stress (high branched-chain [HBC] AA), hepatic failure (low aromatic AA), renal failure (high essential AA), and pediatric formulas. Although the efficacy of pediatric formulas has ben documented, the use of other specialty formulas remains controversial. Studies comparing high branched-chain AA solutions with standard AA formulas in stressed patients have shown improvements in nitrogen retention, visceral protein levels, and immune function but have failed to demonstrate reduced morbidity or mortality. The use of specific organ failure formulas (hepatic and renal) has not been shown to improve nutritional status or outcome compared with standard AA solutions.

6. What is "mixed-fuel" stress formula PN?

PN has been modified to match the altered substrate utilization observed in stressed patients. Critical illness induces a hypercatabolic state. Endogenous protein stores are mobilized to provide amino acids for gluconeogenesis, protein synthesis, and substrate for production of adenosine triphosphate. To blunt autocannibalism of endogenous protein stores, PN provides increased amounts of exogenous amino acids. Solutions with branched chain-enriched amino acids have been promoted to amplify nitrogen retention; however, the increased expense does not justify their routine use in stressed patients. Glucose intolerance is manifested by hyperglycemia and insulin resistance. Similarly, lipid intolerance may exist with high serum triglyceride levels. As a result, the ratio of nonprotein calories (NPC) to nitrogen (N) is reduced to 80–100:1 in severely stressed patients and 100–120:1 in moderately stressed patients. Nonprotein calories are provided as a balance of carbohydrate and fat (e.g., 60–80% of NPC as carbohydrates and 20–40% of NPC as fat).

7. What are the objectives for monitoring PN therapy?

The objectives are three-fold: (1) to determine the efficacy of the PN therapy; (2) to determine changes in metabolic status (stress level); and (3) to detect complications associated with PN. Measurements of efficacy (see chapter 2) in the acute care setting include weight, visceral protein status (e.g., albumin, transferrin, prealbumin, and retinol-binding protein), nitrogen balance, and wound healing. Metabolic status should be viewed first from the clinical perspective. Are there signs of sepsis? Is the patient hyperdynamic? (For example, what is the minute ventilation requirement?) Metabolic status can be further assessed by laboratory variables that evaluate substrate tolerance (e.g., blood glucose and serum triglycerides) as well as protein catabolic rate (24-hour urine urea nitrogen). A metabolic cart study can document energy expenditure, respiratory quotient, and ventilatory equivalent (see question 8 in chapter 6).

8. What potential complications are associated with PN therapy?

The three categories of complications are (1) nutritional (e.g., overfeeding, underfeeding, specific nutrient deficiencies or toxicities); (2) metabolic (e.g., hyperglycemia, electrolyte, fluid, and acid-base imbalances, liver function abnormalities); and (3) infectious (e.g., bacteremia). Detection of complications includes monitoring blood glucose, electrolytes (including calcium, magnesium, and phosphorus), renal function, hepatic function, fluid status, and serum triglycerides. Central-line infections are best prevented by establishing policies that ensure sterile technique and periodic changing of lines. Temperature, white cell count, and the catheter site should also be monitored.

9. Why do patients on PN often develop hyperglycemia? How should it be managed?

Patients on PN develop hyperglycemia for various reasons, including stress-induced glucose intolerance, concurrent use of corticosteroids, pancreatitis, preexisting diabetes mellitus, and excessive glucose administration. Intravenous glucose should be administered at a rate of 1–5 mg/kg/min. Higher rates exceed glucose oxidation capabilities; therefore, hyperglycemia and hepatic steatosis occur. In patients predisposed to hyperglycemia, the glucose intake should be initiated at a rate of 2 mg/kg/min and advanced slowly (e.g., increase by 0.5–1.0 mg/kg/min every 24 hours) to maintain a blood glucose in the range of 200–250 mg/dl, not to exceed 5 mg/kg/min. Insulin may be necessary. In addition, fat should be used to balance nonprotein calories and in the severely glucose intolerant patient may represent up to 60% of calories.

10. What is the cost of PN?

The cost is highly variable and depends on the specific products and amounts used. For example, the specialty amino acids solutions are 1.5–5 times more expensive than standard amino acid solutions. Lipid emulsions are more expensive than dextrose monohydrate; therefore, regimens with a higher proportion of calories as fat will be more expensive. The cost of PN also includes the cost of laboratory monitoring, insertion, and maintenance of a vascular access, and an infusion device. The estimated total daily cost of PN therapy ranges from $150–500. It has been argued, however, that when used for the appropriate indication, PN is cost-effective because it reduces the morbidity and mortality associated with malnutrition.

CONTROVERSIES

11. Preoperative PN

For: Advocates of preoperative nutritional support cite the relationship between malnutrition and postoperative outcome. Malnourished patients have an increased risk for septic complications, problems with wound healing, longer hospital stays, and increased mortality. The unproved contention is that by improving nutritional status preoperative PN will reduce postoperative morbidity and mortality.

Against: Results of studies evaluating preoperative PN and outcome are variable; therefore, providing preoperative PN remains controversial. In addition, two recent trials suggest that perioperative TPN in fact may promote postoperative septic complications.

12. PN in patients with cancer

For: Malnutrition is a frequent complication of cancer as well as of the therapies used to treat it. In patients who cannot be fed enterally, PN should be used as an adjunct to chemotherapy, radiation therapy, and surgery. Patients who are better nourished may tolerate chemotherapy and radiation therapy with fewer complications, and patients undergoing surgery may have fewer postoperative complications. In addition, quality of life may be improved because of the sense of well-being and increased strength associated with an improvement in nutritional status.

Against: Animal data show enhanced tumor growth with selected types of cancer when the animal is parenterally fed. Therefore, concern exists that in feeding the patient, the tumor is also fed and will have an accelerated rate of growth. In addition, the complications associated with PN are a potential source of morbidity. In particular, immunosuppressed patients with cancer may have an increased risk for infectious complications due to PN.

13. Use of lipids in critically ill, especially septic, patients

For: The metabolic changes that occur in critically ill patients include glucose intolerance and insulin resistance. Consequently, meeting caloric needs with carbohydrate calories is difficult and may further exacerbate the complications associated with poor blood glucose control. Providing a proportion of the nonprotein calories as lipid facilitates attaining the desired caloric intake without "stressing" carbohydrate metabolism and meets essential fatty acid requirements.

Against: Lipid particles are taken up by the reticuloendothelial system (RES) in a dose-dependent fashion. When lipid is given in high doses (> 2.5 gm/kg/day) or infused over a short period (< 10 hours), the RES may become saturated with lipid and, hence, unable to scavenge microbes and other particulate matter. This may result in an increased susceptibility to sepsis. Furthermore, the currently available lipid emulsions are composed of long-chain fatty acids. Of these, linoleic acid (representing 49–66% by weight of the fatty acids) is the precursor for prostaglandin synthesis as well as other mediators of the inflammatory response and may be immunosuppressive. It has been proposed that an excessive intake of linoleic acid may inhibit the immune system, facilitate the inflammatory response, and compromise the patient's ability to fight infection. Currently, the clinical significance of these concerns is under investigation.

BIBLIOGRAPHY

1. American Society of Parenteral and Enteral Nutrition, Board of Directors: Guidelines for use of total parenteral nutrition in the hospitalized adult patient. J Parent Ent Nutr 17(4):1SA–52SA, 1993.
2. Brennan WF, Pisters PW, Posner M, et al: A prospective randomized trial of total parenteral nutrition after major pancreatic resection for malignancy. Ann Surg 220:436–444, 1994.
3. Buzby GP, Williford WD, Peterson OL, et al: A randomized clinical trial for total parenteral nutrition in malnourished surgical patients: The rationale and impact of previous clinical trials and pilot study on protocol design. Am J Clin Nutr 47:357–365, 1988.
4. Cerra FB, Alden PA, Negro F, et al: Sepsis and exogenous lipid modulation. J Parent Ent Nutr 12(Suppl):63S–68S, 1988.
5. Cerra FB, Mazuski JE, Chuter E, et al: Branched chain metabolic support: A prospective randomized double blind trial in surgical stress. Ann Surg 199:286–294, 1984.

6. Fan ST, Lo C, Lai E, et al: Perioperative nutritional support in patients undergoing hepatectomy for hepatocellular carcinoma. N Engl J Med 331:1547–1552, 1994.
7. Jensen G, Seidner D, Mascioli E, et al: Fat emulsion infusion and reticuloendothelial system (RES) function in man [abstract]. J Parent Ent Nutr 12:4S, 1988.
8. Venus B, Smith RA, Patel CB, et al: Hemodynamic and gas exchange alterations during Intralipid infusions in patients with adult respiratory distress syndrome. Chest 95:1278–1281, 1989.
9. Veterans Affair Total Parenteral Nutrition Cooperative Study Group: Perioperative total parenteral nutrition in surgical patients. N Engl J Med 325:525–532, 1991.
10. Wolfe RR, Allsop JR, Burke JF: Glucose metabolism in man: Response to intravenous glucose infusion. Metabolism 28:210–218, 1979.
11. Zaloga GP: Nutrition. In Zaloga GP (ed): Critical Care. St. Louis, Mosby, 1994.

8. POSTOPERATIVE FEVER

Alden H. Harken, M.D.

1. What is a fever?

Normal core temperature varies between 36°C and 38°C. Because we hibernate a little at night, we are cool (36°C) just before rising in the morning; after revving our engines all day, we are hot at night (up to 38°C). A fever is a pathologic state reflecting a systemic inflammatory process. The core temperature is above 38°C, but rarely above 40°C.

2. What is malignant hyperthermia?

Malignant hyperthermia is a rare, life-threatening response to inhaled anesthetics or some muscle relaxants. Core temperature rises above 40°C. Abnormal calcium metabolism in skeletal muscle produces heat, acidosis, hypokalemia, muscle rigidity, coagulopathy, and circulatory collapse.

3. How is malignant hyperthermia treated?

- Stop the anesthetic.
- Give sodium bicarbonate (2 mEq/kg IV).
- Give dantrolene (calcium channel blocker at 2.5 mg/kg IV).
- Continue dantrolene (1 mg/kg every 6 hr for 48 hr).
- Cool patient with alcohol sponges and ice.

4. What causes fever?

Macrophages are activated by bacteria and endotoxin. Activated macrophages release interleukin-1, tumor necrosis factor, and interferon, which reset the hypothalamic thermoregulatory center.

5. Can fever be treated?

Aspirin, acetaminophen, and ibuprofen are cyclooxygenase inhibitors that block the formation of prostaglandins (PGE_2) in the hypothalamus and effectively treat fever.

6. Should fever be treated?

Treatment of fever is controversial. No evidence suggests that suppression of fever improves patient outcome. Patients are more comfortable, however, and the surgeon receives fewer calls from the nurses.

7. Should fever be investigated?

Absolutely. Fever indicates that something (frequently treatable) is going on. The threshold for inquiry depends on the patient. A transplant patient with a temperature of 38°C requires scrutiny, whereas a healthy medical student with an identical temperature of 38°C 24 hours after an appendectomy can be cheerfully ignored.

8. What is a fever work-up?
- Order blood cultures, urine Gram stain and culture, and sputum Gram stain and culture.
- Look at the surgical incision(s).
- Look at old and current IV sites for evidence of septic thrombophlebitis.
- If breath sounds are worrisome, order a chest radiograph.

9. What is the most common cause of fever during the early postoperative period (1–3 days)?
The traditional answer is atelectasis. A total pneumothorax, however, does not cause fever. How is it that a little atelectasis causes fever and a lot of atelectasis (pneumothorax) does not? The most likely explanation is that sterile atelectasis (and early postoperative lung collapse is typically not infected) has nothing to do with fever.

10. Do surgical incisions compromise spontaneous breathing patterns?
Absolutely. Vital capacity has been measured in a large group of patients 24 hours after various surgical procedures. An upper abdominal incision is the worst, followed by lower abdomen incision and then (counterintuitively) by thoracotomy, median sternotomy, and extremity incision.

11. Should atelectasis be treated with incentive spirometry?
Yes—but not to avoid fever.

12. What is a wound infection?
By definition, an infected wound contains more than 10^5 organisms per gram of tissue.

13. Are certain wounds prone to infections?
Each milliliter of human saliva contains up to 10^8 aerobic and anaerobic, gram-positive and gram-negative bacteria. Thus, all human bite wounds must be considered as contaminated. Surprisingly, animal bite wounds are typically less contaminated. (It is safer to kiss your dog than your fiancé[e]).

14. Do incisions become infected early after surgery?
The incision must be examined in a patient with a brisk fever (39°C) less than 12 hours after surgery. Look for a foul-smelling, serous discharge in a particularly painful wound (all incisions hurt) with or without crepitus. Gram stain of the serous discharge for gram-positive rods confirms or excludes the diagnosis of clostridial infection.

15. What is the therapy for clostridial gas gangrene?
- The wound should be opened immediately, with fluid resuscitation of the patient. The mainstay of therapy is aggressive surgical debridement of necrotic tissue (skin, muscle, fascia). Make a big hole, and do not worry about closing it.
- Give penicillin, 12 million U/day IV for 1 week.
- Hyperbaric oxygen is not convincingly helpful.

16. Are nonclostridial necrotizing wound infections a cause of concern?
Hemolytic streptococcal gangrene, idiopathic scrotal gangrene, and gram-negative synergistic necrotizing cellulitis are distinct entities but have been lumped into the single category of necrotizing fasciitis. They all require the same initial approach:
1. Fluid and electrolyte resuscitation
2. Broad-spectrum antibiotics ("triples")
3. Aggressive surgical debridement of all necrotic tissue (stuff that does not bleed)

17. What are triple antibiotics?
Triple antibiotics are a shotgun approach to potentially life-threatening infections when the patient is seriously ill and the surgeon is seriously concerned:
  1. Gram-positive coverage (e.g., ampicillin)
  2. Gram-negative coverage (e.g., gentamicin)
  3. Anaerobic coverage (e.g., flagyl)
To avoid overgrowth of yeast and resistant bacteria, one should focus on the culprit bacteria as soon as the cultures come back.

18. What types of surgical procedures predispose to wound infections?
Gastrointestinal procedures, especially when the colon is opened.

19. When do wound infections typically occur?
5–7 days after surgery.

20. How is a wound infection treated?
The wound should be opened and completely drained.

21. Is it necessary to irrigate an infected wound?
Tap water irrigation decreases the bacterial load and promotes healing. Alcohol is toxic to tissues. Sodium hydrochlorite (Dakin's solution) and hydrogen peroxide kill fibroblasts and slow epithelialization. As a rule of thumb, put nothing into a wound that you would not put in your eye.

22. When do urinary tract infections occur?
The longer the urethral (Foley) catheter is in place, the more likely the infection. Urologic instrumentation at the time of surgery may accelerate the process considerably. Bugs crawl up the outside of the urethral catheter, and by 5–7 days after surgery the majority of patients harbor infected urine.

23. How is as urinary tract infection (UTI) diagnosed?
Urine culture with more than 10^5 bacteria/ml defines a UTI. White cells on urinalysis are highly suspect.

24. What are the most common late causes of postoperative fever?
Septic thrombophlebitis (from an IV line) and occult (usually intraabdominal) abscess tend to present even 2 weeks or more after surgery.

BIBLIOGRAPHY

1. Lawrence WT, Bevin AG, Sheldon GF: Acute wound care. In Wilmore DW, Cheung LY, Harken AH, et al (eds): Scientific American Surgery. New York, Scientific American, 1993.
2. Lewis RT: Soft tissue infection. In Wilmore DW, Cheung LY, Harken AH, et al (eds): Scientific American Surgery. New York, Scientific American, 1993.
3. Rodeheaver G: Controversies in wound management. Wounds 1:19, 1989.
4. Wilmore DW: Fever hyperpyrexia and hyperthermia. In Wilmore DW, Cheung LY, Harken AH, et al (eds): Scientific American Surgery. New York, Scientific American, 1994.

9. OXYGEN DELIVERY AND CONTINUOUS OXYGEN MONITORING

Frederick A. Moore, M.D., and James Haenel, R.R.T.

1. How does a pulse oximeter work?
The principles of oximetry are relatively simple. Light-absorption characteristics differ for reduced hemoglobin (RHb), oxygenated hemoglobin (O_2Hb), methemoglobin (Met Hb), and carboxyhemoglobin (CO Hb). A conventional laboratory cooximeter transmits multiple narrow wavebands of light through a blood sample and measures the relative attenuation of the different wavelengths to determine the relative concentration of different hemoglobin moieties. For oxyhemoglobin, this is referred to as "fractional" hemoglobin saturation:

$$\text{Fractional} = [(O_2Hb/RHb + O_2Hb + \text{Met Hb} + \text{CO Hb})] \times 100$$

In contrast, the pulse oximeter measures "functional" hemoglobin saturation:

$$\text{Functional} = [O_2Hb/(RHb + O_2Hb)] \times 100$$

Current pulse oximeters transmit only two wavelengths of light, red (680 nm) and infrared (940 nm), which best differentiate oxyhemoglobin from reduced hemoglobin. The probe contains two light-emitting diodes on one side and a photodetector on the other. By using optical plethysmography, the pulse oximeter looks at hemoglobin saturation during arterial pulsation.

2. What is the reported accuracy of pulse oximetry?
The device is highly accurate over a hemoglobin saturation range of 70–95%.

3. How accurate are clinicians in determining arterial desaturation by "visual oximetry"?
Clinicians are not very good at it. In 1947 Comroe and Botello, using a newly developed oximeter, documented that cyanosis was not consistently detected by visual examination (regardless of level of clinical skill) until hemoglobin saturation fell below 75%. Pulse and respiratory rate, time-honored monitoring variables, were also found to be insensitive indicators of hypoxemia. When in doubt, use the oximeter.

4. What are the four most common circulating species of hemoglobin in the adult? How does the pulse oximeter respond to an abnormal species of hemoglobin?
1. Reduced hemoglobin (RHb)
2. Oxygenated hemoglobin (O_2Hb)
3. Methemoglobin (Met Hb)
4. Carboxyhemoglobin (CO Hb)

As discussed in question 1, a pulse oximeter was designed to detect the relative amounts of RHb and O_2Hb and does not distinguish the presence of Met Hb and CO Hb (each has a unique light-absorption pattern). In carbon monoxide or cyanide poisoning, the oximeter interprets an abnormal hemoglobin as a combination of oxygenated and reduced hemoglobin, which results in an erroneously high saturation. This is referred to as a spectral artifact. Suspicion of an abnormal circulating hemoglobin species (carboxyhemoglobin or methemoglobin) should be ruled out with a conventional lab cooximeter.

5. Are there any other environmental or clinical conditions that may result in inaccurate pulse oximetry values?
Reliability depends on a strong arterial pulsation plus good light transmission. Therefore, inaccuracy occurs with hypotension (MAP < 50 mmHg), hypothermia (< 35°C), vascular disease, and

vasopressor therapy. In addition, bright lights, intravenous dyes, and excessive motion produce an artifact in signal transmission.

6. What is the relationship between oxygen saturation (SaO_2) and partial pressure of oxygen (PaO_2)?

Proper use of pulse oximetry requires recall of the relationship of SaO_2 to PaO_2 as expressed in the oxyhemoglobin dissociation curve. A leftward shift in this curve caused by hypothermia, alkalosis, or blood transfusion results in a lower PaO_2 for a given SaO_2. For example, in a hyperventilated person with head trauma with a $PaCO_2$ of 22 mmHg and pH of 7.50, SaO_2 will remain greater than 90% until PaO_2 drops below 50 mmHg. When the PaO_2 exceeds 100 mmHg, the curve is virtually flat. It is common practice in initial resuscitation and transport of critically injured patients to place them on 100% oxygen to ensure a high PaO_2. Consequently, a large drop in PaO_2 may occur with no discernible change in SaO_2. Although this drop does not adversely affect peripheral delivery of oxygen, the clinician is lulled into a false sense of security.

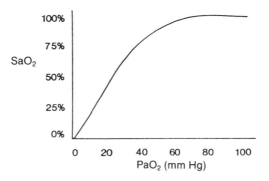

Oxyhemoglobin dissociation curve.

7. What are the indications for continuous pulse oximetry?

Pulse oximetry has achieved widespread acceptance and will soon be considered standard monitoring in critical care units. At present, pulse oximetry is reserved for high-risk patients—postoperative, posttransportation, or newly ventilated patients and patients with high FiO_2 (> 60%) or PEEP (> 8 cm H_2O)—and for use during weaning and major ventilator changes. Liberal use of intermittent pulse oximetry is encouraged. Critically ill patients who are not in the ICU (emergency department or radiology suite) are at high risk for developing hypoxemia. The acutely ill patient who is subjected to a prolonged diagnostic evaluation is at high risk for unrecognized hypoxemia. In this setting, logistics limit the application of standard monitoring techniques, and rarely is one-to-one nursing feasible. By monitoring blood oxygenation, pulse oximetry signals inadequate FiO_2, hypoventilation, and deterioration in alveolar gas exchange. A mechanically ventilated patient who is manually ventilated with an Ambu bag during transportation frequently experiences a change in FiO_2. Patients with high requirements of FiO_2, minute ventilation, or positive end-expiratory pressure are also at substantial risk for developing hypoxemia and require continuous O_2 monitoring.

8. How does a continuous mixed venous oximeter work?

Mixed venous oximetry uses the principles of reflective spectrophotometry. Narrow wavebands of light are transmitted via a fiberoptic bundle to the blood flowing past the tip of the catheter and are reflected by a separate fiberoptic bundle to a photodetector that determines relative absorption of the specific wavelength. A microprocessor then calculates mixed venous hemoglobin saturation (SvO_2). Physio-Control Corporation (Redmond, WA) first marketed a two-wavelength system in a pulmonary artery catheter. It was not accepted clinically because of difficulties with calibration, drift, vessel wall artifact, catheter stiffness, and clot formation. Oximetrix, Inc.

(Mountain View, CA) developed a three-wavelength system to minimize these problems. This system is incorporated into a 7.5-French, 5-lumen, balloon-tipped, thermodilution pulmonary artery catheter, the insertion of which is as easy as a standard pulmonary artery catheter.

9. What is the normal value for mixed venous O_2 saturation?
The average oxygen tension in mixed venous blood (PvO_2) is 40 mmHg. Under standard conditions this is equivalent to an SvO_2 of 75%, which corresponds to the steep portion of the oxyhemoglobin dissociation curve. Therefore, variations in peripheral oxygenation causing small changes in PvO_2 result in significant changes in SvO_2; that is, SvO_2 is a sensitive marker of the adequacy of peripheral oxygen delivery to meet oxygen needs.

10. Using a pulmonary arterial catheter, how can oxygen delivery and consumption be determined?
The Fick equation shows the relationship between oxygen delivery (DO_2) and oxygen consumption (VO_2):

$$VO_2 = CO \times (CaO_2 - CvO_2)$$

where CaO_2 is arterial oxygen content, CvO_2 is mixed venous oxygen content, and CO is cardiac output. Oxygen delivery is determined by the following equation:

$$DO_2 = CaO_2 \times CO$$

where CaO_2 is $(1.36 \times$ [hemoglobin concentration] $\times$ [arterial saturation]) $+ (PaO_2 \times 0.003)$.

11. Describe the four primary causes responsible for a sudden fall in SvO_2.
Rearrangement of the Fick equation to solve for SvO_2 gives the following:

$$SvO_2 = SaO_2 - (VO_2)/(1.34)(CO)(Hb)$$

where SaO_2 is arterial oxygen saturation, VO_2 is oxygen consumption, CO is cardiac output, and Hb is hemoglobin concentration. A stable, normal SvO_2 ensures a balance of DO_2 and VO_2, whereas a sudden fall in SvO_2 provides an early warning of (1) low CO, (2) arterial oxygen desaturation, (3) a drop in hemoglobin, or (4) an increased VO_2.

12. Why does SvO_2 rise during delivery of a general anesthetic? Why does it rise with septic shock?
Commonly SvO_2 will be either normal or elevated during delivery of a general anesthetic because of suppression of metabolic demands, i.e., decreased VO_2. During sepsis, large peripheral shunts in the face of high cardiac outputs and poor oxygen extraction may be responsible for elevating the SvO_2.

13. What are the advantages of continuous monitoring of venous oxygen saturation?
Continuous tracking of SvO_2 eliminates the need for frequent, time-consuming hemodynamic profiling. It also provides prompt feedback about interventions. For example, in a severely traumatized patient requiring massive transfusion, a persistently low SvO_2 suggests active bleeding that requires operative intervention, whereas a rising SvO_2 indicates an effective resuscitative maneuver. The monitoring system also facilitates the clinical use of oxygen transport variables, such as DO_2, VO_2, O_2 extraction ratio, and intrapulmonary shunt fraction. With insertion of appropriate data (height, weight, SaO_2, Hb, and standard hemodynamic parameters), a computer does the calculation and provides a printout of these derived variables. Unfortunately, such calculations have a potential for inherent errors. Most notably, measurements of cardiac output may vary as much as 10%. The oximetric monitoring system displays each cardiac output thermodilution curve on a video screen, which permits elimination of poor injections, thus improving determinations of cardiac output. In addition, the SvO_2 value used in the calculations is measured directly rather than calculated from blood gas analysis data. Given the simplicity of this system, repeating the measurements and calculation can reduce error.

14. What is transcutaneous oxygen monitoring (TCM)?

TCM is a method of continuously recording skin PO_2 ($P_{tc}O_2$), which is not necessarily equal to arterial PO_2. The sensor is a modified Clark, polarographic electrode applied to the stratum corneum of the skin. This layer is composed of keratinized, dead epithelial cells in a lipid/protein matrix that normally limits O_2 diffusion. In 1975 Van Duzee observed that the lipid component of the stratum corneum melts as skin temperature increases. As a result, gas diffusion increases by as much as 1,000-fold. The $P_{tc}O_2$ electrode is therefore designed to heat the skin to 44–45°C. The elevated temperature also increases dermal blood flow and "arterializes the capillary blood."

15. If the skin beneath the sensor is "arterialized," why is the $Pa_{tc}O_2$ not equal to the PaO_2?

Four factors contribute to the difference between the $P_{tc}O_2$ and PaO_2: (1) the rightward shift of the oxygen-hemoglobin dissociation curve with heating, (2) stratum corneum O_2 permeability, (3) metabolic consumption of oxygen by the dermal tissue, and (4) cutaneous blood flow. Factors 1 and 3 tend to cancel each other, so the relationship between $P_{tc}O_2$ and PaO_2 is effectively linear and dependent only on O_2 permeability and skin blood flow.

16. What is the $P_{tc}O_2$ index?

The relationship between $P_{tc}O_2$ and PaO_2 is expressed by the $P_{tc}O_2$ and PaO_2 index:

$$P_{tc}O_2 \text{ index} = P_{tc}O_2/PaO_2$$

For healthy people, this index changes with age: 1.0 in newborns, 0.84 in children, and 0.79 in adults.

17. How does skin PO_2 relate to the arterial PO_2 and perfusion?

A number of clinical studies have examined the utility of $P_{tc}O_2$ in predicting PaO_2. In healthy people the correlation is excellent, but $P_{tc}O_2$ does not equal PaO_2. The two variables differ for many physiologic and pathologic reasons. $P_{tc}O_2$ should be viewed as a separate PO_2 variable that is affected by two major factors: PaO_2 and cardiac output. Tremper and Shoemaker showed that in hemodynamically stable adults (CI > 2.2 L/min/m²), $P_{tc}O_2$ correlates well (r = 0.89) with PaO_2 over a wide range of PaO_2 (23–495 mmHg). In their study, the $P_{tc}O_2$ index was 0.79 ± 0.12. But with progressive shock, the correlation of $P_{tc}O_2$ to PaO_2 deteriorated. In patients with severe shock (CI < 1.5 L/min/m²), $P_{tc}O_2$ correlated with cardiac output. Therefore, when there is a sudden unexplained drop in $P_{tc}O_2$, arterial blood gases (ABGs) are invaluable in differentiating a decrease in PaO_2 from a decrease in CO.

18. How should a hypoxic event be managed?

Once a hypoxic event has been identified, supplemental oxygen is applied. The first maneuver is to hand-ventilate patients with an artificial airway. A ruptured tube cuff is self-evident, whereas difficult bagging implies airway obstruction, bronchospasm, or tension pneumothorax. Inability to pass a suction catheter confirms obstruction. If this is not reversible by changing head position or by cuff deflation, the endotracheal tube is immediately replaced. If there is difficult bagging and no evidence of airway obstruction, a quick chest examination is done to exclude a tension pneumothorax. The mechanical ventilator and breathing circuit are inspected, vital signs obtained, and the chest systematically evaluated. ABGs are measured to confirm hypoxia and rule out hypoventilation.

Additional work-up generally includes urgent portable anteroposterior chest roentgenograms. ECGs are obtained selectively. Recent medications, interventions (suctioning, position changes, nursing care), and changes in clinical status are carefully reviewed. In patients with a pulmonary artery catheter, pulmonary capillary wedge pressure (PCWP), cardiac index, and oxygen transport variables are determined. A scintigraphic lung (V/Q) scan is used to evaluate clinical suspicion of pulmonary embolism.

ICU HYPOXIC EVENTS

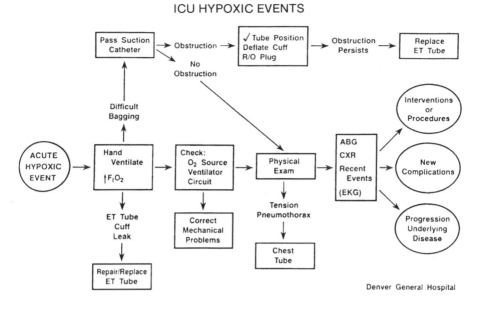

Denver General Hospital

BIBLIOGRAPHY

1. Comroe JH, Botello S: Unreliability of cyanosis in recognition of arterial anoxemia. Am J Surg 214:1 1947.
2. Haenel JH, Moore FA, Moore EE: Advance in continuous oxygen monitoring in trauma patients. In Mattox KL (ed): Perspectives in Trauma. Forum Medicum, Vol 1, No IV, 1990.
3. Nelson LD: Continuous venous oximetry in surgical patients. Ann Surg 203:329, 1986.
4. Tremper KK, Barker SJ: Pulse oximetry. Anesthesiology 70:98–108, 1989.
5. Tremper KK, Shoemaker WC: Transcutaneous oxygen monitoring for critically ill adults, with and without low flow shock. Crit Care Med 9:706, 1981.

10. ARTERIAL PRESSURE MONITORING AND CENTRAL VENOUS PRESSURE MONITORING

Thomas A. Whitehill, M.D., and Glenn J.R. Whitman, M.D.

ARTERIAL PRESSURE MONITORING

1. What are the indications for intraarterial cannulation?

Indications include continuous blood pressure monitoring of the unstable patient (especially when cuff pressures are unreliable at very high or very low systemic blood pressure); multiple or frequent blood sampling, including arterial blood gas determinations, chemistries, and hematology profile (particularly in respirator-dependent patients); and induced hypotension (particularly with vasodilating drugs such as sodium nitroprusside).

2. What are the preferred sites for arterial cannulation?

The radial artery is the vessel of choice because of accessibility, ease of cannulation, and good collateral circulation through the palmar arch that can readily be confirmed. The next most common cannulation site is either the dorsal pedal artery or the femoral artery, each of which also has the advantage of collateral flow. However, there is a higher incidence of complications, especially site infection or line sepsis, for these latter sites.

3. What is the Allen test?
A physical diagnostic exam used to determine the adequacy of collateral circulation in the hand and whether the radial or the ulnar artery is dominant.

4. How do you perform a modified Allen test?
Using both hands, compress the patient's radial and ulnar arteries at the wrist so as to occlude all flow to the hand. Raise the patient's hand over the head and have him or her clench the fist several times to force all venous blood from the hand. This should result in a pale, cool hand. Let the patient relax and lower the hand, and then take the pressure off the ulnar artery; the hand should become pink immediately. If it stays pale but becomes pink *only* when the radial artery is released, there is insufficient collateralization throughout the hand from the ulnar artery to permit cannulation of the radial artery.

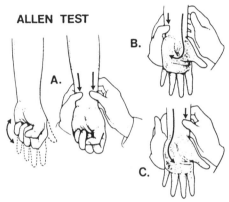

ALLEN TEST

(From James EC, Corry RJ, Perry JF Jr (eds): Basic Surgical Practice. Philadelphia, Hanley and Belfus, 1987, p 474.)

5. What is an alternative method to determine adequate collateralization of the palmar arterial arch prior to radial arterial cannulation?
Doppler ultrasound (9-mHz pencil probe or 5.2-mHz "flat" probe) can be used at the bedside to confirm completeness of collateral flow. If a complete arch is present and patent, then compression of the ulnar artery alone should not eliminate any Doppler signal obtainable from any of the five digits; the same should be demonstrable when the radial artery is compressed. If there is incomplete collateralization from either the radial or ulnar artery, one should use the other wrist for arterial cannulation.

Hint: Try the nondominant wrist/hand first; if it is usable, then the catheter and its tubing system will be less in the patient's way.

6. How do you place a radial arterial catheter?
The forearm, wrist, and hand are immobilized on a padded arm board with a rolled towel placed under the dorsum of the wrist. The skin is cleansed with an iodine solution, and infiltrative lidocaine (1% without epinephrine) is used to anesthetize the intended puncture site. A 20-gauge over-the-needle Teflon catheter is used to cannulate the artery using sterile technique. After the artery is entered by both the needle and its overlying catheter, the needle is slowly withdrawn and the catheter threaded up to the artery. The catheter is then attached to a short piece of high-pressure extension tubing that is equipped with a three-way stopcock, and then to a pressure transducer system. The system is secured to the patient with both a suture at the catheter puncture site and tape. A sterile dressing is then applied.

7. What is the most common complication of arterial cannulation? How can it be prevented?

Major complications of radial arterial cannulation include partial or complete vessel obstruction with resultant distal ischemia emboli, massive hemorrhage, ecchymosis, loss of pulse, and local infection; the most common of these is transient arterial thrombosis (up to 88%). It can best be prevented by decreasing the duration of catheterization and using the smallest-gauge catheter applicable (usually a 20-gauge).

CENTRAL VENOUS PRESSURE
MONITORING

8. What is central venous pressure (CVP)?

Central venous or right atrial pressure is the blood pressure that "pushes" blood into the right ventricle during the period of diastolic filling. The higher the CVP, the more the blood will flow into the right ventricle. Starling's law indicates that with increasing end-diastolic volume (to a point), more blood will be ejected during systole; thus, increased CVP usually leads to an increased stroke volume. Normally, the right ventricle can fill adequately with an astonishingly low CVP (3–5 mmHg).

9. What are the indications for placement of a CVP monitoring catheter?

Indications include shock or cardiopulmonary arrest requiring rapid administration of blood and fluid, facilitation of fluid administration and management, emergency insertion of a transvenous pacemaker, lack of adequate peripheral veins, and administration of long-term hypertonic solutions (total parenteral nutrition) or antibiotics.

10. How do you measure CVP?

A catheter must be placed in the superior vena cava (SVC) or right atrium. Because there is negligible pressure drop between the SVC and the right atrium, either one of these locations is acceptable, as all intrathoracic veins have nearly the same pressure. The catheter can be threaded into the intrathoracic position from either an antecubital vein cutdown site or a percutaneous "central" subclavian/internal jugular approach. Either fluid column manometric or electronic transducer systems can be used to interpret the resultant transmitted pressure wave.

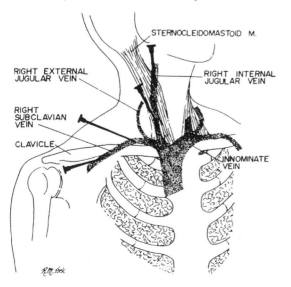

Sites for percutaneous CVP catheter placement into the jugular vein medial and lateral to sternocleidomastoid muscle, as well as into the subclavian vein above and below the clavicle. (From Shoemaker WC, Thomson WL, Holbrook PR (eds): Textbook of Critical Care. Philadelphia, W.B. Saunders, 1984, p 111, with permission.)

11. What are the contraindications to percutaneous subclavian or internal jugular venous catheterization?
The risk of bleeding during subclavian or jugular access in a patient with coagulopathy is low but not zero. In a patient with an abnormal coagulation state (for whatever reason) or in a patient who is profoundly thrombocytopenic (< 20,000), it may be safer to access the central venous compartment by peripheral cutdown and placement of a "long line." Similarly, a patient with chronic obstructive pulmonary disease and hyperinflated lungs and some respiratory distress might not tolerate an inadvertent pneumothorax very well. Inadvertent arterial puncture is generally not a problem unless the patient has a coagulopathy or platelet deficit.

12. How do you place a CVP catheter by direct subclavian vein puncture?
With the patient in a mild head-down (Trendelenburg) position, the infraclavicular area is widely prepared with an antiseptic solution, and sterile drapes/towels are placed. Using sterile technique, the operator infiltrates an area near the midclavicular area with 1% lidocaine using a 21-gauge needle; this infiltrative "local" is then extended beneath the clavicle directed toward the suprasternal notch, always maintaining suction with the syringe unless lidocaine is being injected. It is extremely important to hug the undersurface of the clavicle with the needle—never direct the needle toward the underlying lung and its pleurae, or a pneumothorax will most certainly result. When the subclavian vein is entered with the "finder" needle, dark blood is easily withdrawn and flushed back into the vein. The small finder needle is then removed, and a 16- or 18-gauge needle, again attached to a 10-ml syringe, is inserted along the same infraclavicular track. Presumably, if the subclavian vein was found with the small needle, it should be easy to reenter it with the larger needle. When this occurs, dark blood is again easily withdrawn. The syringe is then removed from the needle, taking care not to move the needle tip from its intravascular position. A gloved finger is placed over the needle hub to prevent both aspiration of air and exsanguination. A plastic catheter is then passed through the access needle and its tip positioned in the SVC/right atrium. The appropriate intravascular catheter length should be based on whether the right or left subclavian is used (10–15 cm, respectively).

13. How do you place an internal jugular catheter for central venous access and CVP measurement?
With the patient in the Trendelenburg position, turn the head away from the side to be catheterized. Under sterile conditions and a wide preparation and drape, locally infiltrate an area about the lateral borer of the sternocleidomastoid (SCM) muscle just above the confluence of the sternal and clavicular components of the muscle (about 2–3 cm above the clavicular head). Direct the "finder" needle under the muscle toward the ipsilateral hip, palpating the carotid artery so as not to puncture it. Again, the catheter is passed once the needle's location is ensured.

14. What is the Seldinger technique?
It is an easier, more reliable, and safer technique for gaining vascular access after the subclavian or jugular vein is localized with an 18-gauge "thin-wall" needle. With the needle held securely in the intravascular location, a guide wire is passed through the needle and into the vein. Once the needle is removed over the guide stylet, the 16- or 18-gauge central venous catheter is passed over the wire to establish intravascular cannulation; the guide wire is then removed from the catheter.

15. How is a CVP catheter secured?
After placing any catheter of this type, it is imperative to suture it well at both the skin puncture site and also at a second point along the catheter to guard against accidental dislodgment. When a valuable line like this is placed, it is always nice to know that you can pick the patient up by his catheter.

16. How do you confirm the position of the CVP catheter?
After placement of a central catheter of any type, it is mandatory to obtain a chest radiograph to confirm the location of the catheter tip and to guarantee that there is not a pneumothorax. If the

catheter tip is shown to be within the right ventricle or to extend into the contralateral subclavian vein, it must be withdrawn appropriately.

17. What is the most common complication of CVP catheter placement?

Bacterial contamination of a CVP catheter has a variable occurrence rate of 8–88%. The majority of studies indicate that most catheters are initially contaminated by bacteria during insertion. Contamination rates significantly increase if the catheters are left in place for longer than 72 hours. A fibrin sheath surround these catheters and can become contaminated from distant infected sites from hematogenous spread. Systemic antibiotics have little effect on the frequency of positive cannula cultures. Obviously, rigid adherence to aseptic and sterile insertion techniques will decrease the high rate of infection. Regimented catheter change routines are also quite important. The incidence of pneumothorax is probably slightly higher with subclavian vein cannulation (4%) than with internal jugular cannulation; the incidence of inadvertent carotid artery puncture is slightly higher for the latter, as one would suspect.

BIBLIOGRAPHY

1. Beford RF, Wollman H: Complications of percutaneous radial artery cannulation. Anesthesiology 38:228, 1973.
2. Brieges BB, Carden E, Takacs FA: Introduction of central venous catheters through arm veins with a high success rate. Can Anesth Soc J 26:128, 1979.
3. Davis FM, Stewart JM: Radial artery cannulation. Br J Anaesth 52:41, 1980.
4. Jones RM: Percutaneous radial artery cannulation. Anesthesiol Rev 8:41, 1981.
5. Mitchell SE, Clark RA: Complications of central venous catheterization. AJR 133:467, 1979.
6. Rosen M, Latto IP, Ng WS: Percutaneous central venous cannulation. BMJ 281:372, 1980.
7. Ross AHM, Andersen JR, Walls ADF: Central venous catheterization. Ann Roy Coll Surg (London) 62:454, 1980.
8. Ryan J, Raines J, Dalton BC: Arterial dynamics of radial artery cannulation. Anesth Analg 52:1017, 1973.

11. PULMONARY ARTERY PRESSURE MONITORING

Glenn J.R. Whitman, M.D., and Thomas A.Whitehill, M.D.

1. What is a Swan-Ganz catheter?

It is a long catheter (80 cm) that is marked every 10 cm throughout its length. It has at least two lumens and sometimes three. One lumen extends to its end and is referred to as the "distal port." A second lumen extends to 20 cm proximal to the end and is called the "proximal port." Some catheters have a third lumen that exits even more proximally (30 cm proximally to the distal port) and is called the infusion port; it is used for the delivery of drugs, not pressure monitoring. All Swan-Ganz catheters have an inflatable balloon tip (1.5 cc). The Swan-Ganz catheter is in place when the distal port is in the pulmonary artery (but not beyond the mediastinal shadow on chest radiograph). The distal lumen, then, enables one to assess pulmonary artery pressure. The proximal port reflects right atrial pressure. Furthermore, by gently blowing up the balloon, the pulmonary artery in which the catheter lies can be occluded. In this case, the distal port will reflect pulmonary venous pressure (rather than arterial pressure), which is an accurate assessment of the mean left atrial pressure and, by inference, the left ventricular end-diastolic pressure.

2. Describe placement of a Swan-Ganz catheter.

After placement of a 7-French introducer into the subclavian vein, the internal jugular vein, or the femoral vein, the catheter is passed through the introducer to 20 cm. Then, with or without fluoroscopic guidance, the balloon is inflated, and, while distal port pressure is being monitored, the catheter is "floated," i.e., with the balloon inflated. The tip of the catheter will be directed by blood flow into the right atrium, through the tricuspid valve into the right ventricle, and then out the right ventricular outflow tract into the pulmonary artery. A few tricks may help: (1) Fluoroscopy is helpful but usually totally unnecessary. (2) Once the balloon is inflated, feed the catheter through the introducer rather quickly so that it can, in fact, "float" and follow the blood flow into the heart. (3) As soon as the right ventricle is entered, stop and record the intraventricular pressure "for the chart" while mentally recording the length of catheter necessary to reach the right ventricle at the level of the tricuspid valve. Then, again with the balloon inflated and with your eyes on the monitor (registering distal port pressure), pass the catheter quickly into the pulmonary artery. At this point, the right ventricle trace changes such that a dicrotic notch is seen during diastole with an end-diastolic pressure higher than that seen in the right ventricle. (4) If confused about placement, remember that the pulmonary artery trace has a negative slope during diastole; in contrast, a positive diastolic slope is seen in the right ventricle. (5) Once in the pulmonary artery, continue to slowly pass the catheter (balloon inflated) until the systolic-diastolic curve changes into a straight line with only rounded peaks (generally associated with breathing). This new pressure (read off the "mean" mode) is the pulmonary capillary wedge pressure (PCWP). Deflate the balloon, and the pulmonary artery pulsatile trace should reappear. If not, withdraw the catheter slowly until it does. Then reinflate the balloon (always slowly) until the PCWP trace reappears. (6) Order an immediate chest radiograph to confirm placement. Remember, always inflate the balloon slowly, and stop when the PCWP trace appears. One can rupture the pulmonary artery with overinflation, a potentially lethal situation. Furthermore, for similar reasons, never withdraw the catheter with the balloon up.

3. When is it worth placing a Swan-Ganz catheter?

Whenever one wishes to assess accurately cardiac performance and pulmonary hemodynamics, the measurement of cardiac output and ventricular filling pressures (left ventricular end-diastolic pressure is indirectly reflected by the PCWP) is essential and involves the placement of a Swan-Ganz catheter. Clinical situations include (1) shock, (2) preoperative evaluation for lung resection, (3) management of acute myocardial infarction with hypotension, (4) intraoperative management of (a) aortic surgery, (b) any surgery involving severe fluid shifts, and (c) the cardiac patient, and (5) the management of acute renal failure.

4. What are normal cardiac intracavitary pressures?

RA	RV		PA		LA	LV	
	Dias.	Sys.	Dias.	Sys.	PCWP	Dias.	Sys.
0–8 mmHg	0–8	15–30	3–12	15–30	1–10	3–12	100–140

5. How is cardiac output measured with a Swan-Ganz catheter?

A thermodilution cardiac output is measured by injecting a known amount of fluid at a known temperature (e.g., 100 cc at 12°C) into the proximal port of the Swan-Ganz catheter. At the distal tip of the catheter, a temperature-sensitive probe reads a change in the temperature of the blood passing it. By electronically integrating this change in blood temperature over time, a computer attached to the Swan-Ganz catheter can evaluate the flow across the probe, which it reports in liters per minute. In an effort to diminish variability, injection should always be made at a specific time within the respiratory cycle (e.g., end-expiration), and the value used should be the mean of three outputs. Even so, expect variability of 15%.

6. When is a thermodilution cardiac output inaccurate?

A left-to-right shunt will add shunted blood to the cold saline bolus, giving a falsely elevated cardiac output. Similarly, tricuspid regurgitation generates an abnormal curve with a falsely elevated reading. The higher the cardiac output, the less accurate the computation. At best, a thermodilution cardiac output is accurate to within 15–20% of true output.

7. How do you determine the systemic (peripheral) vascular resistance (SVR)?
By the formula:

$$\text{SVR} = \frac{\overline{\text{BP}} - \overline{\text{CVP}} \times 80}{\text{CO}}$$

where   SVR   =   systemic vascular resistance (dynes/sec/cm^{-5});
             BP   =   mean arterial blood pressure (mmHg);
            CVP   =   central venous pressure (mmHg);
             CO   =   cardiac output (L/min).

One should not regard SVR as a measure of afterload to which the heart is exposed. The mean blood pressure is a better number on which to focus, attempting to keep it in the 65–75 mmHg range (when trying to optimize cardiac output). Regardless of how high the SVR, when the mean blood pressure is 60, it is unwise to lower it further. In such a situation, cardiac output must be increased to lower SVR further.

8. How are right- or left-sided filling pressures used to evaluate shock?
Management of the patient in shock requires knowledge of the arterial pressure as well as right atrial pressure, pulmonary artery pressure, pulmonary capillary wedge pressure (PCWP), and cardiac output. Prompt characterization of the hemodynamic pattern allows an etiologic diagnosis and points the way to therapy.

Hypovolemic shock. Right and left filling pressures are low, as is cardiac output. Peripheral vascular resistance is high. Because of severe vasoconstriction, the measured cuff blood pressure may be normal. (In patients with heart disease, central venous pressure is frequently a poor reflection of left ventricular filling.) The diagnosis is confirmed, as volume repletion with rising filling pressures is associated with increased cardiac output, normalization of systemic pressure, and decreased peripheral vascular resistance.

Cardiogenic shock. Elevation of right ventricular filling pressures without an elevated PCWP in the face of shock is characteristic of cor pulmonale, right ventricular infarction, pulmonary embolus, or tamponade. Therapy is directed toward minimizing pulmonary vascular resistance, improving myocardial contractility in cor pulmonale, and possibly performing pulmonary arterial thrombectomy in pulmonary embolism. Surgery, or, at least, catheter drainage, is required for the relief of tamponade. Augmented left ventricular filling pressure is characteristic of cardiogenic shock and is associated with cardiomegaly and pulmonary edema (PCWP > 18–20). Therapy for pulmonary edema is directed toward ensuring adequate but not excessive preload, minimizing afterload, and improving myocardial contractility. Remember "MOST DAMP":

M	— Morphine	**D**	— Digoxin
O	— Oxygen	**A**	— Aminophylline
S	— Sitting up	**M**	— Micturition (Lasix)
T	— Tourniquets (rotating)	**P**	— Phlebotomy

Septic shock. The hallmark of septic shock is normal or low-normal filling pressure, supranormal cardiac output, and very low peripheral vascular resistance (< 600). Treatment requires fluid resuscitation and possibly systemic vasoconstriction while the underlying cause (e.g., abdominal abscess) is treated.

9. What is an oximetric Swan-Ganz catheter?
It is a Swan-Ganz catheter that has a fiberoptic monitor at its distal tip that continuously measures HbO$_2$ saturation [SO$_2$(%)]. When properly positioned, the distal catheter tip will be in the pulmonary artery, and the O$_2$ saturation will reflect that of mixed venous blood (SvO$_2$).

10. What is the importance of SvO_2?

To answer this question, certain fundamental principles must be understood:

    1. **Blood oxygen content (cO_2)**

        O_2 dissolved in blood + O_2 combined with hemoglobin

        O_2 dissolved = $0.003 \times PO_2$

        O_2 combined with hemoglobin = $1.38 \times Hb \times SO_2$

    Example: Hb = 12 gm, PO_2 = 60 torr, SaO_2 = 90%

$$C_aO_2 = (0.003 \times 60) + (1.38 \times 12 \times 0.90)$$
$$= 0.18 + 14.9$$
$$= 15.08 \text{ cc } O_2/100 \text{ cc blood or } 15.08 \text{ vol.\%}$$

As is usually the case, the dissolved O_2 makes up only a small percentage of the CO_2 (in this example, 1%). Therefore, its contribution to CO_2 is omitted in further discussion.

    2. **The A-VO_2 difference.** Understanding how to determine the oxygen content of blood permits determination of the difference in arterial vs. mixed venous O_2 content, or the A-VO_2 difference. By knowing the pulmonary artery or mixed venous HbO_2 saturation (SvO_2), the computation is straightforward:

    A-VO_2 difference $(C_aO_2 - C_vO_2)$

        = Hb 1.38 SaO_2 – Hb 1.38 SvO_2

        = Hb 1.38 $(SaO_2 - SvO_2)$

    The typical situation where:

        Hb = 15 (mg)% SaO_2 = 96% SvO_2 = 75%

    The A-VO_2 diff = $15 \cdot 1.38 \cdot (SaO_2 - SvO_2)$

        = $15 \cdot 1.38 \cdot (97\text{--}75)$

        = 20.7 (0.21)

        = 4.35 vol.%

That is, every 100 cc of blood that travels around the body gives up 4.35 cc of O_2. The normal range for the A-VO_2 diff is 3–5 vol.%.

    3. **The Fick principle.** In a steady-state situation, the body uses O_2 at the rate of 125 cc O_2/min/m². Therefore, given a known body surface area (BSA) of a patient, one can roughly determine the minute O_2 consumption. Furthermore, by measuring the A-VO_2 difference, one can determine the contribution of each 100 cc of blood that travels around the patient's body to the total minute O_2 consumption ($\dot{V}O_2$). Thus, in a man with a BSA = 2 m², his minute O_2 consumption ($\dot{V}O_2$) = 250 cc. If his measured A-VO_2 diff = 4.35 cc, as in the example above, then one may conclude that every 100 cc of blood contributes 4.35 cc to his $\dot{V}O_2$ of 250 cc. Thus 4.75 liters of blood must travel around this patient's body each minute to meet his requisite O_2 requirement. Thus, by assuming a known $\dot{V}O_2$ and by measuring the A-VO_2 difference, one can determine the cardiac output, i.e., CO = ($\dot{V}O_2$ ÷ A-VO_2 diff) × 10.

11. What, then, is the significance of SvO_2?

If one assumes a steady state in which the Hb and PO_2 remain constant, then C_aO_2 remains constant. In this situation, CvO_2 will be totally dependent on cardiac output and $\dot{V}O_2$. However, CvO_2 = Hb · 1.38 · SvO_2. Thus, the only variable is SvO_2. An oximetric Swan-Ganz catheter that gives a continuous digital readout of SvO_2 is the equivalent of a continuous online measure of cardiac output and minute oxygen consumption. In a steady state in which $\dot{V}O_2$ remains constant, the higher the SvO_2, the higher the cardiac output. The caveat is that one must be assured of a constant PO_2, Hb, and $\dot{V}O_2$. Determining cardiac output by the Fick principle assumes $\dot{V}O_2$. In fact, $\dot{V}O_2$ can be measured with a "metabolic cart," and a very accurate cardiac output can thus be determined. Clinically, however, this is unnecessary. In the ICU patient we are far less interested in absolutes than in trends. Thus, as long as the Hb, $\dot{V}O_2$, and PO_2 remain constant, a rising SvO_2 indicates an increase in cardiac output.

    By providing continuous measurement of the SvO_2, the oximetric Swan-Ganz catheter permits immediate hemodynamic assessment of interventions such as increasing preload, decreasing afterload, or adding inotropic support. The effect of positive end-expiratory pressure (PEEP) in the ventilated patient can be determined within minutes, and a "best PEEP" trial becomes a trivial matter. The effect of arrhythmias and pacing on cardiac output can be determined. Thus, in critically ill patients requiring constant attention and intervention, a continuous on-line SvO_2 monitor is an invaluable tool.

12. When is the oximetric Swan-Ganz catheter inaccurate or misleading?
When the catheter has been in place for prolonged periods (24–72 hours), the fiberoptic tip may become covered with fibrin. The transmitted light intensity then diminishes, and the readings become inaccurate. The new oximetric Swan-Ganz catheters have a light-intensity measurement that alerts the clinician as to when the device is not accurate because of this problem. A drop in hematocrit may also lower the SvO_2. This is a real phenomenon and not an artifact. If the A-VO_2 difference is 5 vol.% and the Hb is 15 gm%, then the $SvO_2 = 75\%$. However, if the Hb is 7.25, then the $SvO_2 = 50\%$. On the basis of Hb alone, with no change in cardiac output, the SvO_2 can change.

BIBLIOGRAPHY

1. Benumof JL, Sandman LJ, Arkin DB, Diamont M: Where pulmonary arterial catheters go. Anesthesiology 46:336, 1977.
2. Buchbinder N, Ganz W: Hemodynamic monitoring—invasive techniques. Anesthesiology 45:146, 1976.
3. Caerus JA, Holder D: Ventricular fibrillation due to passage of a Swan-Ganz catheter. Am J Cardiol 35:589, 1975.
4. Dalen JE: Bedside hemodynamic monitoring. N Engl J Med 301:1176, 1979.
5. Elliott CG, Zimmerman GA, Glemmer TP: Complications of pulmonary artery catheterization in the care of critically ill patients: A prospective study. Chest 76:647, 1979.
6. Gardner RM: Direct blood pressure measurement—dynamic response requirements. Anesthesiology 54:227, 1981.
7. O'Quinn R, Marini JJ: Pulmonary artery occlusion pressure: Clinical physiology, measurement, and interpretation. Am Rev Respir Dis 128:319, 1983.
8. Pace NL: A critique of the flow-directed pulmonary arterial catheterization. Anesthesiology 47:455, 1977.
9. Stevens JH, Raffin TA, Mihm FG, et al: Thermodilution cardiac output measurement. Effects of the respiratory cycle on its reproducibility. JAMA 253:2240, 1985.
10. Swan HJC, Ganz W: Complications of flow-directed balloon-tipped catheters. Ann Intern Med 91:494, 1979.
11. Swan HJC, Ganz W: Use of balloon flotation catheters in critically ill patients. Surg Clin North Am 55:501, 1975.

12. WOUND INFECTION AND WOUND DEHISCENCE

Steven L. Peterson, D.V.M., M.D., and Ben Eiseman, M.D.

1. What is the definition of surgical wound infection?
The National Nosocomial Infections Surveillance System (NNISS) advocates the uniform use of the term **surgical site infections** (SSIs) in describing wound infections and lists rigid criteria for defining extent of tissue involvement. This classification system facilitates communication and surveillance. By these criteria, SSIs present within 30 days of surgery unless a foreign body is left in situ, in which case 1 year must elapse before a surgical wound infection can be excluded. Infections are divided into incisional SSIs and organ/space SSIs. Incisional SSIs are further classified as involving only the skin and subcutaneous tissues (superficial incisional SSIs) or involving deep soft tissues (e.g., fascial and muscle layers) of the incision (deep incisional SSIs). Organ/space SSIs involve any part of the anatomy other than the incision opened or manipulated during the operative procedure.

2. Can wounds be classified in a way that predicts their risk of infection?
Yes. The wound classification system first advocated in 1964 is based on degree of gross contamination and stratifies wounds into one of four categories: clean, clean-contaminated, contaminated, and dirty-infected. It is still considered to be highly predictive. **Clean wounds** are nontraumatic wounds in which no inflammation is encountered, no breaks in sterile technique occur, and no hollow viscus is entered. **Clean-contaminated wounds** are identical except that a hollow viscus is entered. **Contaminated wounds** are caused by trauma from a clean source or by minor spillage of infected materials. **Dirty-infected wounds** are caused by trauma from a contaminated source or gross spillage of infected material into an incision. Recent data for the NNISS revealed infection rates of 2.1%, 3.3%, 6.4%, and 7.1% for clean, clean-contaminated, contaminated, and dirty-infected wounds, respectively.

3. What local wound factors affects the probability of infection?
The degree of contamination of the wound (e.g., wound class) and the amount of nonviable tissue are the most important predictive factors. Dead space, foreign material, coagulated blood, undrained serum, and excessive suture are also important. Adequacy of local blood supply is also important, as evidenced by the low infection rate in wounds of the face.

4. What other factors are important in predicting probable wound infection?
In addition to wound class, physical status as classified by the American Society of Anesthesiologists, duration of surgery, results of intraoperative cultures, and duration of preoperative hospital stay are significant predictors of postoperative surgical site infections.

5. Does prophylaxis with systemic antibiotics decrease the probability of infection?
The use of antibiotics in contaminated and dirty-infected wounds is clearly indicated and represents therapy rather than prophylaxis. In clean-contaminated wounds consensus supports their routine use as prophylaxis. The routine use of prophylactic antibiotics in clean wounds is controversial; however, two recent reports involving 1,218 and 3,202 patients undergoing clean procedures demonstrated a 48% and 41% reduction in wound infection, respectively, with their use. Criticism of the studies focuses on the extrapolation of limited types of operations (herniorrhaphy and breast surgery) to the extremely broad scope of operations encompassed by the clean category. What is clear with regard to prophylactic antibiotics is that maximal benefit is obtained when tissue concentrations are therapeutic at the time of contamination. Efficacy, therefore, is enhanced when prophylactic antibiotics are administered immediately before surgical incision; late administration is similar to no administration. One or two doses after the end of the operation are sufficient; additional doses only promote the emergence of resistant organisms. Topical antimicrobials applied directly to the wound add nothing to appropriate use of systemic antibiotics and in fact may compromise healing by delaying epithelialization.

6. What nonpharmacologic means are available to minimize postoperative wound infection?
Prophylactic antibiotics cannot compensate for poor surgical technique. Good surgical technique minimizes contamination when the gastrointestinal, genitourinary, or respiratory tracts are opened during clean-contaminated procedures. Good technique further demands that all blood and dead tissue be removed or minimized in a surgical wound before closure. Irrigation of wounds also assists in control of infection by reducing absolute bacterial counts. Appropriate use of electrocautery does not increase wound infection rates.

7. Is primary closure appropriate for obviously dirty or contaminated wounds?
Primary closure is a difficult surgical decision. On the one hand, it is always tempting, because, if one can avoid infection, the morbidity is less and the cosmetic appearance is better. However, if infection develops, the consequences are serious and the wound must be reopened. Factors that affect the decision include degree of contamination, amount of dead tissue or empty space that

must be left in the wound, adequacy of blood supply, efficacy of drains, time since wounding, and presence of foreign bodies. It is always safer to leave a dirty wound open and to allow it to heal secondarily or perhaps to use delayed primary closure 3–5 days after the injury. Delayed primary closure is a compromise that often differentiates the experienced surgeon from the enthusiastic amateur.

8. What are the most common organisms involved in wound infections?
Staphylococci are by far the most common organisms, just as they are the most common skin flora. Otherwise, the infection depends on the nature of the contaminating agent. If the gut was violated, *Enterobacteriaceae* and anaerobes are common; biliary tract and esophagus incisions yield these organisms plus enterococci. Other areas, such as the urinary tract or vagina, contain specific organisms such as group D streptococci, *Pseudomonas* sp., and *Proteus* sp.

9. What is the wound infection rate after commonly performed operations?
Cholecystectomy	3%	Inguinal herniorrhaphy	2%
Appendectomy	5% (25% if ruptured)	Thoracotomy	6%
Colectomy	12%		

10. What are the classic signs of wound infection?
Calor (heat)	Tumor (swelling)
Rubor (redness)	Dolor (pain)

11. How is a wound infection best treated?
Open the wound and drain the pus (ubi pus ibi evacua). The role of antibiotics is limited to containing associated cellulitis or to minimizing associated generalized sepsis.

12. Which organism should be suspected if, early in the postoperative course, rapidly progressive erythema and tenderness develop in the wound edges?
Group B streptococci.

13. What organism produces a reddish brown exudate early in the postoperative course?
Clostridium.

14. When does wound infection typically develop? What are the systemic and local consequences if the infection is left untreated?
The characteristic wound infection occurs 5–7 days postoperatively. Clostridium infection resulting from an abundance of devitalized tissue in a closed space may become manifest within hours. If left untreated, the patient with a wound infection develops signs of generalized sepsis. Locally, the wound breaks down, and the infection dissects through tissue planes and continues to advance. If the infection progresses rapidly, especially in a compromised host, necrotizing fasciitis may develop. Finally, the strength layers of the wound closure may break open (dehisce).

15. What is wound dehiscence?
Wound dehiscence is the partial or total disruption of any or all layers of the operative wound. Evisceration is rupture of all layers of the abdominal wall and extrusion of the abdominal viscera.

16. What factors predispose to dehiscence?
Factors that are injurious to the chemical and/or cellular processes involved in wound healing may contribute to wound dehiscence. Infection is identified in over one-half of wounds that undergo dehiscence. Age greater than 60 years, obesity and increased intraabdominal pressure, malnutrition, renal or hepatic insufficiency, diabetes mellitus, use of corticosteroids or cytotoxic drugs, and radiation have been implicated in wound dehiscence. The single most important factor, however, is adequacy of closure. Fascial edges should not be devitalized. Linea alba

sutures should be placed lateral to the transition zone between the linea alba and rectus abdominis sheath; sutures should be tied correctly without excessive tension; and suture material of adequate tensile strength should be chosen.

17. When does wound deshiscence occur?
Wound dehiscence may occur at any time after surgery; however, it is most common between the fifth and tenth postoperative days when wound strength is at a minimum.

18. What are the signs and symptoms of wound dehiscence?
Normally a ridge of palpable thickening (healing ridge) extends about 0.5 cm on each side of the incision within 1 week. Absence of this ridge may be a strong predictor of impending wound breakdown. More commonly, leakage of serosanguinous fluid from the wound is the first sign noted. In some instances, sudden evisceration may be the first indication of abdominal wound dehiscence. The patient also may describe a sensation of tearing or popping associated with coughing or retching.

19. What is the proper management of wound dehiscence?
Wound deshiscence without evisceration is best managed by immediate elective reclosure of the incision. If the patient is an unacceptable candidate for surgery, it may be acceptable to allow the incisional hernia to persist until a later date. If partial wound dehiscence is noted during treatment of a wound infection, the repair should be delayed until complete resolution of the infection is firmly established. Dehiscence of a laparotomy wound with evisceration represents a surgical emergency with a 10–20% mortality rate. Initial treatment in this instance consists of appropriate resuscitation while protecting the eviscerated organs with moist towels; the next step is prompt surgical closure. Exposed bowel and/or omentum should be thoroughly lavaged and returned to the abdomen; the abdominal wall should be closed with retention sutures; and the skin wound should be packed open.

BIBLIOGRAPHY

1. Classen DC, Evans RS, Pestotnik SL, et al: The timing of prophylactic administration of antibiotics and the risk of surgical-wound infection. N Engl J Med 326:281–286, 1992.
2. Culver DH, Horan TC, Gaynes RP, et al: Surgical wound infection rates by wound class, operative procedure and patient risk index. Am J Med 91(Suppl 3B):152S–163S, 1991.
3. Groot G, Chappell EW: Electrocautery used to create incisions does not increase wound infection rates. Am J Surg 167:601–603, 1994.
4. Leaper DJ: Prophylactic and therapeutic role of antibiotics in wound care. Am J Surg 167(Suppl 1A):15S–20S, 1994.
5. Mulvihill SJ, Pellegrini CA: Postoperative complications. In Way LW (ed): Current Surgical Diagnosis and Treatment, 10th ed. Norwalk, CT, Appleton & Lange, 1994, pp 24–39.
6. Platt R, Zaleznik DF, Hopkins CC, et al: Perioperative antibiotic prophylaxis for herniorrhaphy and breast surgery. N Engl J Med 322:153–160, 1990.
7. Platt R, Zucker JR, Zaleznik DF, et al: Prophylaxis against wound infection following herniorrhaphy and breast surgery. J Infect Dis 166:556–560, 1992.
8. Sheridan RL, Tompkins RG, Burke JF: Prophylactic antibiotics and their role in the prevention of surgical wound infection. Adv Surg 27:43–65, 1994.

13. ACUTE ABDOMEN

Alden H. Harken, M.D.

1. What is the surgeon's responsibility when confronted by a patient with an acute abdomen?
(1) To identify how sick the patient is and (2) to determine whether the patient needs to go directly to the operating room, needs to be admitted for resuscitation or observation, or can safely be sent home.

2. What is the most dangerous course?
To send the patient home.

3. Is it important to make the diagnosis in the emergency department?
No. Frequently time spent confirming a diagnosis in the emergency department is lost to in-hospital resuscitation and/or treatment in the operating room. The only patient who needs a relatively firm diagnosis is a patient who is to be sent home.

4. If the essential goal is not to make the diagnosis, what should the surgeon do?
   1. Resuscitate the patient. Most patients do not eat or drink while they are getting sick. Thus, most patients are depleted of at least several liters of fluid. Depletion is worse in patients with diarrhea or vomiting.
   2. Start a big IV line.
   3. Replace lost electrolytes (see chapter 5).
   4. Insert a Foley catheter (this approach does not hurt the patient, and it is a real crowd pleaser).
   5. Examine the patient.

5. Are symptoms and signs uniquely misleading in any groups of patients?
Yes. Watch out for the following groups:
   1. The very young, who cannot talk.
   2. Diabetics, because of visceral neuropathy.
   3. The very old, in whom, much as in diabetics, abdominal innervation is dulled.
   4. Steroids, which depress inflammation and mask everything.
   5. Immunosuppression (a heart transplant patient may act cheerfully even with dead or gangrenous bowel).

6. What history is needed?
   1. **The patient's age.** Neonates present with intussusception; young women present with ectopic pregnancy, pelvic inflammatory disease, and appendicitis; the elderly present with colon cancer, diverticulitis, and appendicitis.
   2. **Associated problems.** Previous hospitalizations, prior abdominal surgery, medications, heart and lung disease? An extensive gynecologic history is valuable; however, it is probably safer to assume that all women between 12 and 40 years old are pregnant.
   3. **Location of abdominal pain.** *Right upper quadrant:* gallbladder or biliary disease, duodenal ulcer. *Right flank:* pyelonephritis, hepatitis. *Midepigastrium:* duodenal or gastric ulcer, pancreatitis, gastritis. *Left upper quadrant:* ruptured spleen, subdiaphragmatic abscess. *Right lower quadrant:* appendicitis (see chapter 31), ectopic pregnancy, incarcerated hernia, rectus hematoma. *Left lower quadrant:* diverticulitis, incarcerated hernia, rectus hematoma. **Note:** Cancer, unless it obstructs (colon cancer), and bleeding (diverticulosis) typically do not hurt.

4. **Duration of pain.** The pain of a perforated duodenal ulcer or perforated sigmoid diverticulum is sudden, whereas the pain of pyelonephritis is gradual and persistent. The pain of intestinal obstruction is intermittent and crampy. **Note:** Although the surgeon is rotating through a GI service, the patient may not know this and may present with urologic, gynecologic, or vascular pathology.

PHYSICAL EXAMINATION

7. Are vital signs important?
Yes. They are vital. If both heart rate and blood pressure are on the wrong side of 100 (heart rate > 100; systolic BP < 100), watch out! Tachypnea (respiratory rate > 16) reflects either pain or systemic acidosis. Fever may develop late, particularly in an immunosuppressed patient who may be afebrile in the face of florid peritonitis.

8. What is rebound?
The peritoneum is well innervated and exquisitely sensitive. It is not necessary to hurt the patient to elicit peritoneal signs. Depress the abdomen gently and release. If the patient winces, the peritoneum is inflamed (rebound tenderness).

9. What is mittelschmerz?
Mittelschmerz is pain in the middle of the menstrual cycle. Ovulation is frequently associated with intraperitoneal bleeding. Blood irritates the sensitive peritoneum and hurts.

10. What do bowel sounds mean?
If something hurts (like a sprained ankle), the patient tends not to use it. Thus, inflamed bowel is quiet. Bowel contents squeezed through a partial obstruction produce high-pitched tinkles. Bowel sounds are notoriously unreliable, however.

11. What is the significance of abdominal distention?
Distention may derive from either intra- or extraenteric gas or fluid (worst of all, blood). Abdominal distention is always both significant and bad.

12. Is abdominal palpation important?
Yes. But remember, the patient is (or should be) the surgeon's friend; there is no need to cause pain. Palpation guides the surgeon to the anatomic zone of most tenderness (usually the diseased area). It is best to start palpation in an area that does not hurt. Rectal (test stool for blood) and pelvic examinations further localize pathology.

13. What is Kehr's sign?
The diaphragm and the back of the left shoulder enjoy parallel innervation. Thus, concurrent left upper quadrant and left shoulder pain indicate diaphragmatic irritation from a ruptured spleen or subdiaphragmatic abscess.

14. What is a psoas sign?
Irritation of the retroperitoneal psoas muscle by an inflamed retrocecal appendix causes pain on flexion of the right hip or extension of the thigh.

LABORATORY STUDIES

15. How is a complete blood count helpful?
1. **Hematocrit.** If high (> 45%), the patient is most likely very dry and/or may have chronic obstructive lung disease (COPD). If low (< 30%), the patient probably has a more chronic blood disease.

2. **White blood cell count.** It takes time (hours) for inflammation to release cytokines and elevate the white cell count. A normal white blood cell count is entirely consistent with significant abdominal trouble.

16. Is urinalysis necessary?

Absolutely. White cells in the urine may redirect attention to the diagnosis of pyelonephritis or cystitis. Hematuria points to renal or ureteral stones. Because an inflamed appendix may lie directly on the right ureter, both red and white blood cells may be found in the urine of patients with appendicitis.

17. What is a "three-way of the abdomen"?

1. **Upright chest radiograph.** Look for free air under the diaphragm (perforated viscus) and pneumonia or pneumothorax.

2. **Upright abdomen.** Look for free air under the diaphragm and air-fluid levels (intestinal obstruction). Remember to look for sigmoid or rectal air (partial obstruction).

3. **Supine abdomen.** This radiograph tells nothing.

Most ureteral stones can be visualized; only 10% of gallstones are radiopaque, and appendiceal fecaliths are rarely noted. **Honors:** Air in the biliary system indicates a biliary-enteric fistula. In association with intestinal air-fluid levels, the diagnosis is gallstone ileus.

18. What is a sentinel loop?

Except in children (who swallow everything, including air), small bowel gas is always pathologic. A single loop of small bowel gas adjacent to an inflamed organ (e.g., the pancreas) may point to the disease.

19. Is ultrasound valuable?

Yes—if the working diagnosis is cholecystitis, gallstones, ectopic pregnancy, or ovarian cyst.

20. Is abdominal CT scanning valuable?

Yes—if the working diagnosis is an intraabdominal abscess (sigmoid diverticulitis), pancreatitis, retroperitoneal bleeding (leaking abdominal aortic aneurysm; this patient should have gone straight to the operating room), or intrahepatic or splenic pathology.

21. What is a double-contrast CT scan?

The bowel is delineated with barium or gastrograffin. The blood vessels are delineated with an iodinated vascular dye. Thus the CT scan precisely displays the abdominal contents relative to vascular and intestinal landmarks. Contrast CT imaging of pancreatitis is valuable to assess zones of perfusion and/or necrosis.

SURGICAL TREATMENT

22. If the patient is sick (and not getting better), what should be done?

After fluid resuscitation the patient's abdomen should be explored. An exploratory laparotomy has been touted as the logical conclusion of a complete physical examination.

23. Is a negative laparotomy harmful?

Yes. But patients can uncomfortably survive a negative laparotomy, whereas missed bowel infarction (or even appendicitis) can be life-threatening.

24. What is the most challenging problem in all of medicine?

An acute abdomen.

BIBLIOGRAPHY

1. Abernathy CM, Hamm RM: Surgical Scripts. Philadelphia, Hanley & Belfus, 1994.
2. Gordon LA: Gordon's Guide to the Surgical Morbidity and Mortality Conference. Philadelphia, Hanley & Belfus, 1994.
3. Hiatt JR: Management of the acute abdomen: A test of judgement. Postgrad Med 87:38–42, 1990.
4. Silen W: Cope's Early Diagnosis of the Acute Abdomen. New York, Oxford University Press, 1987.
5. Velanovich V: Pre-operative laboratory screening based on age, gender and concomitant medical diseases. Surgery 115:56–61, 1994.

14. SURGICAL SEPSIS: PREVENTION AND MANAGEMENT

Glenn W. Geelhoed, M.D., MPH

ANTIBIOTICS AND SURGERY

1. Antibiotics cure infections—right?
No. If you believe that antibiotics are the answer to infections—particularly surgical infection—give them by the kilogram to a patient without intact host defenses and see how well they work. Impaired host defenses are seen in radiation sickness, bone marrow failure from cancer, and antimetabolite treatment. If nothing else, AIDS has taught us that antibiotics alone cannot rescue the immune-impaired patient from infection.

2. But antibiotics inhibit the growth of sensitive bacteria in petri dishes, do they not?
Yes. Culture and sensitivity determination are made by streaking out isolates of one infecting organism on plates of culture media on which are placed discs impregnated by antibiotic. The examiner notes zones of inhibition around the discs marked "s." But the petri dish contains no phagocytes, opsonins, globulins, cytokines, or complement—none of the factors of host defense that ultimately must resolve the infection. Such host factors are necessary—and frequently sufficient to control the infectious process. Without them, even an antibiotic marked "s" is insufficient for clinical control of the infectious process.

3. What, then, is the role of antibiotics in the management of surgical infection?
Antibiotics are adjuncts in the control of infection. In the case of surgical infection, they are adjunctive to a surgical procedure—principally drainage of pus or debridement of devitalized tissue. And in the case of all infection, whether classed as medical or surgical, antibiotics and drainage procedures are adjuncts to the primary host defense response.

4. What are the adjunctive uses of antibiotics in infected surgical patients?
Antibiotics have three principal uses in medicine, the first two of which predominate in surgical patients: (1) prophylactic, (2) presumptive, and (3) precise. **Prophylaxis** is, by definition, preinoculous treatment with an antibiotic in anticipation of contamination in patients at risk. **Presumptive treatment** is the initiation of antibiotic therapy in a patient already contaminated, but with microorganism(s) unknown or at least unidentified at the start of treatment. **Precise therapy** is antibiotic treatment directed at the control of an organism identified by culture with treatment indicated by drug sensitivity.

All three of these indications are useful in medical management. Examples include (1) penicillin prophylaxis of a prosthetic heart valve, (2) antibiotic treatment of community-acquired pneumonia based on Gram stain, and (3) treatment of *Streptococcus viridans* subacute bacterial endocarditis.

5. For what reasons may an infection persist despite treatment with antibiotics for which the cultured organism has a demonstrated sensitivity?

1. Where is the pus? The patient may have an undrained collection such as a leak in an anastomosis. An antibiotic is rarely the appropriate single treatment for abscess or undrained collection.

2. Something is wrong with the patient. This is the time to assess the appropriateness of stopping chemotherapy, radiation, or immunosuppressive drugs such as steroids—or even the antibiotic itself.

3. Finally (and least likely), the laboratory may have erred in assessing the microbe(s) as sensitive to the drug.

6. Why is antibiotic treatment inappropriate for an abscess?

A focal abscess is treated by a *local* procedure. Because no blood circulates into an abscess, a blood-borne antibiotic cannot be delivered. Only the inflammatory outer margin of the abscess (a reflection of the intact host's effort to wall off the inoculum) can harbor viable organisms and white blood cells in the dynamic competition between host and invader. If the antibiotic were injected directly into the center of an abscess, it still would be ineffective; pK and pH are such that the drug cannot work, and organisms there are either dead or not reproducing.

The role of adjunctive antibiotics in the management of abscess is to protect the tissue planes through which the abscess is drained by a surgically invasive procedure—whether by needle or by knife.

ANTIBIOTIC PROPHYLAXIS IN SURGERY

7. To avoid overlooking the patient who may benefit and to prevent litigation by the patient who develops a postoperative wound infection, why not give prophylactic antibiotics to all patients undergoing operations?

Bad idea. First, this defensive practice does not work. More importantly, many patients have elective operations that entail very low incidence of infection and minimal risk from the rare infections that may ensue. Drug therapy of any kind is seldom without risk, never without cost, and often without demonstrated benefit. Therefore, the knee-jerk defensive response is wrong; in some series of low-risk patients, antibiotic prophylaxis actually increases the infection rate.

8. How is it possible both to administer antibiotics and to increase infection rates?

Certainly the selective process of antibiotic use may increase the virulence of infection in a group of host-impaired patients in the surgical intensive care unit. But how can profligate abuse of antibiotic prophylaxis cause harm to the patient undergoing routine elective operation?

The most potent immunosuppressive drugs currently used in transplantation started out as antibiotics. Cyclosporine is no longer used for its effect against microbes, but it is used to impair host resistance and to induce tolerance to an invading foreign tissue. In experimental transplantation, colonies of animals maintain functioning kidney grafts supported only by antibiotics such as ampicillin.

Perhaps for this reason prophylaxis trials comparing placebo with an effective antibiotic reveal a surprising result. If the prophylactic drug fails to prevent infection, the infection rates should be equal to placebo. In many reported series, however, the antibiotic-treated group exhibits a higher infection rate than the placebo group. Clearly not every patient undergoing elective operation should receive a prophylactic antibiotic.

9. When should prophylactic antibiotics be used in elective surgical procedures?

A patient at risk anticipates either (1) a significant incidence of infection from the operation or (2) a potentially lethal risk from an infrequent infection. An example of the first indication may be the patient undergoing elective colostomy closure; the rate of infection is high, although the associated danger is low. An example of the second indication may be the patient with an aortic aneurysm resection. The incidence of aortic vascular graft infection is low, but once an intraabdominal vascular graft is infected, the mortality rate escalates to 50%. The product of the rate and risk of infection should help to guide indications for prophylaxis. Another important determinant is the patient's immune status, as based on age, underlying disease (e.g., diabetes or AIDS), and factors of impaired local resistance such as fields of radiation fibrosis or prosthetic implantation. Thus, implantation of prosthetic material is a mandatory indication for antibiotic prophylaxis.

10. Is any clean, elective surgical procedure an indication for antibiotic prophylaxis?
No. The justification for prophylactic antibiotics in clean, elective surgery must be founded on compromised host immune status. The surgeon who can provide a rationale for prophylactic antibiotics in a patient undergoing a clean, elective operation (without prosthesis implantation) has just supplied a persuasive contraindication to the operation itself.

11. What is the primary criterion in the selection of a prophylactic antibiotic?
Low toxicity. Prophylactic antibiotics are given to vast numbers of patients who will not become infected with or without the drug. If the infection rate without prophylaxis is 5%, 95% of patients would not be infected even without the drug. If the drug were so miraculously effective that the infection rate were cut in half (to 2.5%), 95% still would not become infected, and 2.5% still would become infected even with prophylaxis. Thus the benefit is a 2.5% decrement in the rate of infection—and this decrement must exceed the toxicity of the drug. If the prophylactic antibiotic reduces infection by 2.5% yet carries a 10% toxicity rate, the harm-to-benefit ratio would be 4:1—and it would be better to skip the prophylaxis. Additional criteria for an effective prophylactic agent include the following:
　　1. It should have broad-spectrum efficacy against anticipated organisms.
　　2. It should not generate resistance.
　　3. It should not cross-react with other antibiotic classes.
　　4. Oddly enough, it should not be the optimal first-line therapy for any of the anticipated bacteria.

12. Does any current antibiotic meet the ideal criteria?
To an amazing extent, many familiar drugs qualify, principally those of the first-generation beta-lactam class, such as penicillin and cephalosporins.

13. What prophylaxis should be used in trauma?
Seat belts. The principle of antibiotic prophylaxis is that the drug must circulate before the bugs attack. Unless surgeons extend their practice to the barroom before the injury takes place, the inoculation has occurred before the patient arrives. Antibiotic management in trauma should be governed by the principles of presumptive treatment—or surgeons should wait until they know what they are shooting at (unless the bullet went through the colon).

SURGICAL INFECTION

14. What constitutes a surgical infection?
An *Escherichia coli* bacillus does not know whether it is on the "medical" or "surgical" service (neither do some of the patients). But there are several reasons to distinguish surgical infections:

Medical vs. Surgical Infections

DISTINCTION	MEDICAL	SURGICAL
Pathogenesis	Pathogens	Commensal flora
Number of organisms	Monobacterial	Polymicrobial
Culture	Organism known	Organism unknown (but suspected)
Therapy	Sensitivity-guided	Empirically initiated
Primary treatment	Antibiotic	Operation/drainage
Goal of treatment	Eradication	Containment

A surgical infection is a polymicrobial inoculum of commensal microbes that invade through a barrier breach. Primary therapy is an operation designed to drain or contain the localized infections, supported empirically by presumptive antibiotics and anticipating rather than proving the flora for which the patient is at risk.

15. Is the goal of antibiotic treatment of the surgical patient to sterilize all microbial flora?
No. In the first place, such a goal would not be possible, short of extraordinary "life-island" isolation, which has been attempted only occasionally for patients with bone marrow failure. Nor would sterilization be desirable, because commensal bacteria crowd out pathogens, synthesize vitamin K, and help to metabolize bile salts. Surgical treatment is designed to reconstitute barriers (e.g., skin, gut mucosa) containing resident flora and to prevent access by invasion through containment breeches such as traumatic, ischemic, or inflammatory routes. Incision and drainage (I and D) of walled-off pus and debridement of infected devitalized tissue can be gratifyingly effective and require negligible assistance from fancy antibiotics.

16. What flora-associated risks are commonly seen in surgical infections?

Flora-associated Risks in Surgical Infections

RISK	FLORA	TYPE	SOURCE
Cellulitis Febrile response Superficial abscess	Gram-positive aerobes	Staphylococci Streptococci	Skin
Endotoxic shock	Gram-negative aerobes	Coliforms	GI, GU, biliary tracts
Intraabdominal abscess, multiple organ failure	Gram-negative anaerobes	Bacteroides	GI tract

TREATMENT OF SURGICAL INFECTIONS

17. What are the principles of surgical infection control?
The "Big Ds": (1) drainage, (2) debridement, (3) diversion, (4) diet, and (5) drugs.

18. What are the primary and secondary criteria in selecting antibiotics for presumptive therapy?
The primary criterion is effectiveness; the antibiotic must work. Ideally, agents should not generate resistance against themselves. But in the first and final analysis, the effectiveness of treatment dwarfs all other factors, such as cost, toxicity, and generation of resistance.

19. If the surgeon knows or suspects the bug but does not yet know its sensitivities, what antibiotic should be initiated?

Antibiotics for Flora of Unknown Sensitivities

FLORA	ANTIBIOTIC
Gram-positive aerobes	Beta-lactam Penicillins Penicillin Pencillinase-resistant penicillins Ampicillin Piperacillin Cephalosporins First-generation cefazolin Second-generation cefoxitin Third-generation cefotaxime

(Continued on facing page)

Antibiotics for Flora of Unknown Sensitivities (Continued)

FLORA	ANTIBIOTIC
Gram-negative aerobes	Aminoglycosides, gentamicin, aztreonam
	Ampicillin
Gram-negative anaerobes	Clindamycin
	Cefoxitin
	Chloramphenicol
	Metronidazole
Full spectrum	Imipenem

20. What are triple antibiotics or "triples"?

If the patient is in big trouble, the surgeon may wish to start triple antibiotics until culture results permit more focused therapy:

1. Gram-positive aerobes   Ampicillin
2. Gram-negative aerobes   Gentamicin
3. Gram-negative anaerobes   Metronidazole (Flagyl)

If one drug covers more than one risk (e.g., clindamycin covers both gram-positive skin flora and gram-negative anaerobic bacteroides species), an aminoglycoside, such as gentamicin, should reduce triple therapy to dual therapy. More recently, monotherapy with imipenem has proved comparable to the gold-standard dual therapy in covering major infections. Monotherapy with imipenem is actually comparable to combination therapy, but the benefit is provable and cost-effective only in patients with more severe septic illness.

BACTEREMIA, SEPTICEMIA, AND PATIENT FAILURES

21. Is there a temporal pattern in patient mortality after polymicrobial inoculation?

Yes. Mortality in septic surgical patients is biphasic. The two peaks occur 1 week apart. If early control of gram-positive aerobes and clostridia is achieved, the two subsequent mortality peaks are associated with gram-negative aerobes and gram-negative anaerobes, respectively.

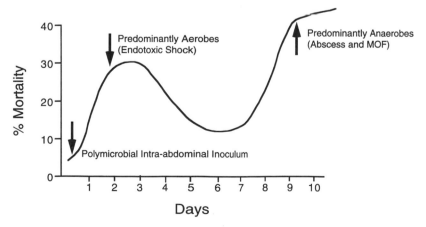

Biphasic mortality of combined infectious risks in polymicrobial inoculum.

22. What is the difference between bacteremia and septicemia?

Bacteremia is an **infectious** disease that sometimes is treated successfully with antibiotics. Septicemia is a systemic **inflammatory** process in which the local inflammatory response becomes generalized. Systemic circulation of activated inflammatory mediators (cytokines such as tumor necrosis factor, interleukins 1, 6, and 8) provokes a neutrophil-mediated, generalized vascular leak syndrome termed multiple systems organ failure. The prognosis is horrible.

23. If septicemia is an inflammatory disease, why not use antiinflammatory therapy?
Antiinflammatory therapy is a great idea, but it does not work. Focal control of the inoculum and tissue healing require local inflammation to contain infections. Antiinflammatory drugs, such as corticosteroids, may initially decrease systemic inflammatory damage but simultaneously fan the flames of local infection and a continuation of the inoculum.

CONTROVERSY

24. Can antibiotic usage compensate for shortcomings in surgical technique or judgment?
Do not count on it. Antibiotics are unnecessary in many patients, necessary and sufficient in few (usually medical) patients, and insufficient in most surgical patients. Remember the Big D's (see question 17). Wangensteen summarized surgical infection control succinctly: "Antibiotics may be able to convert a third-class surgeon into a second-class—but never into a first-class surgeon."

BIBLIOGRAPHY

1. Dofferhoff AS: Effects of different types and combinations of antimicrobial agents on endotoxin release from gram-negative bacteria: An in-vitro and in-vivo study. Scand J Infect Dis 23:745–759, 1991.
2. Geelhoed GW: New approaches to serious infections in the surgical patient. Clin Ther 12(Suppl B):1–8, 1990.
3. Geelhoed GW: Cultures of the peritoneal cavity. Postgrad Gen Surg 3:167–169, 1992.
4. Jackson JJ, Kropp H: Beta-lactam antibiotic induced release of free endotoxin: In vitro comparison of penicillin binding protein (PBP) 3-specific ceftazidime. J Infect Dis 165:1033, 1992.
5. Onderdonk AB, Kasper DL, Mansheim BF, et al: Experimental animal models for anaerobic infections. Res Infect Dis 1:291–301, 1979.
6. Solomkin JS, Dellinger EP, Christou NV, Busuttil RW: Results of a multicenter trial comparing imipenem/cilastatin to tobramycin/clindamycin for intra-abdominal infections. Ann Surg 212:581–591, 1990.

II. Trauma

15. MULTIPLE TRAUMA

Walter L. Biffl, M.D., and Ernest E. Moore, M.D.

1. Why is trauma an important topic?
Trauma is the leading cause of death in the first four decades of life and is responsible for the loss of more years of productive life than heart disease and cancer combined. Current studies show that one-fourth of trauma deaths can be prevented by an organized approach to care, including appropriate triage, evaluation, resuscitation, definitive treatment, and rehabilitation administered by an experienced, trained trauma team.

2. What is the meaning of trauma center designation?
The American College of Surgeons Committee on Trauma has developed strict criteria to stratify trauma centers as level I, II, III, or IV according to their capability for managing acutely injured patients, providing educational programs, and conducting trauma research. Level I centers are best prepared to treat critically injured patients with multisystem injuries. The goal of regional trauma systems is to triage patients to appropriate trauma centers so that the right patient gets to the right place at the right time.

3. Define triage.
Triage, derived from the French word "trier," means to pick or cull and was used originally to describe how French traders sorted wool into various categories according to quality. In modern trauma systems, triage is used to get the most severely injured patients to the closest trauma center capable of dealing with their injuries. All injured patients should not be directed to a level I center; in general, however, a 25% overtriage rate (sending a less severely injured patient to a regional trauma center) is considered necessary to avoid missing life-threatening injuries.

4. What is the golden hour?
The clock starts ticking at the moment of injury. The golden hour is the first hour after injury, during which the patient must be systematically evaluated and all life-threatening injuries identified. Appropriate triage, rapid transport, and efficient initiation of the airway, breathing, and circulation are essential to maximize survival.

5. Are prehospital care and communication important?
Absolutely. Prehospital providers must relay general information from the scene including age, sex, time and mechanism of injury, level of consciousness, heart rate, blood pressure, respiratory rate, overt and suspected injuries, treatment initiated, and estimated time of arrival. For motor vehicular accidents, additional valuable facts include velocity of and damage to vehicles, use of safety devices (seat belts, air bags, helmets), damage to steering wheel or windshield, ejection, degree of injury to other passengers, and extrication time; whereas for penetrating wounds important aspects include type of weapons(s), depth of penetration, and estimated blood loss at the scene.

6. What is a major mechanism injury?

A major mechanism injury is a big hit. For example, when the victim has bent the steering wheel or another passenger is dead, the patient has a major mechanism injury. No matter how good the patient looks, a high index of suspicion for serious injury is critical.

7. What is an AMPLE medical history?

Allergies, Medications, Past illness and operations, Last meal, and Events preceding the injury.

8. What are the major components of the early phase of trauma management?

Primary survey, resuscitation, secondary survey, definitive management, and tertiary survey.

9. What are the ABCDEs of the primary survey?

Airway, Breathing, Circulation, Disability (neurologic evaluation), and Exposure of the patient. Treatment of all life-threatening conditions (resuscitation) is performed simultaneously.

10. What is the secondary survey?

The secondary survey is a detailed evaluation of the patient's overall condition and identification of potential life-threatening injuries (tubes and fingers in every orifice). The secondary survey includes a head-to-toe physical examination, radiologic screening (after blunt trauma: lateral cervical spine, chest, and pelvis radiographs), laboratory tests (hematocrit, white blood cell count, amylase, blood typing, coagulation profile, toxicology screen, and urinalysis), and special diagnostic tests (peritoneal lavage, ultrasonography, CT scanning, angiography).

11. What lines and tubes are routinely inserted in multiply injured patients?

Supplemental oxygen mask, two large-bore (14- or 16-gauge) peripheral intravenous catheters, and electrocardiographic monitoring leads are routine. Unless contraindicated, nasogastric and urinary bladder catheters are also inserted promptly. A pulse oximeter is important if respiratory compromise is anticipated. Tetanus prophylaxis is mandatory.

12. What is the most common cause of upper airway obstruction in trauma patients?

The tongue, followed by blood, loose teeth or dentures, and vomitus.

13. What initial maneuvers are used to restore an open airway?

The chin lift and jaw thrust physically displace the mandible and tongue anteriorly to open the airway; manual clearance of debris and suctioning of the oropharynx optimize patency. Nasopharyngeal and oropharyngeal airways are useful adjuncts in maintaining an open airway in the obtunded patient. All of these maneuvers can (and must) be accomplished with the patient's head still taped to the backboard (before "clearing" the cervical spine).

14. What does "clearing the C-spine" mean?

Before manipulating the patient's head, injury to the cervical spine (C-spine) must be excluded. Asymptomatic, alert patients without other "significant painful injuries" may be moved without radiographs. Patients with symptoms or a major mechanism injury require a minimum of three views (lateral, anteroposterior, and odontoid) to image the C-spine. Visualization of C7–T1 is mandatory and occasionally requires supine oblique or "swimmer's" views (the patient's arm is placed above the head with the x-ray tube in the axilla). In high-risk patients with continued symptoms, bilateral supine oblique views or focused CT scanning may reveal an abnormality. Upright lateral or delayed flexion/extension films (to rule out ligamentous injury) may be obtained in symptomatic patients with normal five views. In patients with equivocal images or in whom physical examination is not possible, a cervical spine collar should be left in place.

15. Does a Philadelphia collar adequately stabilize the cervical spine?

No. The Philadelphia collar allows approximately 30% of normal flexion and extension, over 40% of rotation, and 66% of lateral motion. Thus, immobilization must also include sandbags taped to a blackboard.

16. What is the preferred method of intubation in spontaneously breathing patients with a known cervical spine injury?
The nasotracheal route, although blind, is safer; it is successful in over 90% of spontaneously breathing patients. The patient must be breathing so that he or she can actually suck the tube into the trachea. If the nasotracheal approach is unsuccessful or the patient is hemodynamically unstable, oral intubation with in-line neck stabilization should be performed immediately.

17. What are the indications and contraindications to cricothyroidotomy?
Extensive maxillofacial trauma, which precludes airway access via the oral or nasal route, is the principal indication for cricothyroidotomy. Furthermore, nasotracheal intubation cannot be performed in apneic patients, and morbid obesity or cervical swelling may limit the feasibility of orotracheal access. Contraindications to cricothyroidotomy include direct laryngeal trauma, tracheal disruption, and age less than 12 years. Tracheostomy or percutaneous transtracheal ventilation are alternatives.

18. What nonairway conditions pose an immediate threat to ventilation?
   Tension pneumothorax, most commonly seen after blunt chest trauma, is treated by tube thoracostomy (36-French tube in the midaxillary line in adult men). An **open pneumothorax** may compromise ventilation if the chest wall defect is greater than two-thirds the diameter of the trachea. The defect should be sealed with petroleum gauze or cellophane wrap taped on three sides to allow the egress of air or, better yet, taped on four sides with concomitant chest tube placement. **Hemothorax** should be drained with a large-bore thoracostomy tube and watched for continued bleeding that may require thoracotomy. Impaired ventilation associated with a **flail chest** is usually due to underlying pulmonary contusion and not to rib fractures.

19. What are the preferred sites for intravenous access?
Peripheral veins (antecubital or cephalic) can be cannulated rapidly and safely with large-bore (14- or 16-gauge) percutaneous catheters. Remember—it is difficult to cannulate empty veins. When vascular collapse precludes percutaneous peripheral access, a saphenous vein cutdown or Seldinger wire access to the femoral vein can be used. Central venous access is primarily indicated to monitor central venous pressure.

20. How is tissue perfusion assessed clinically?
Organ perfusion is not democratic. We preferentially distribute blood flow to coronary and carotid arteries and then (only if cardiac output is adequate) to the liver, kidneys, mesentery, extremities, and big toe. Thus, adequate urine output is evidence of renal perfusion and a warm big toe of hemodynamic stability. Peripheral pulses are useful in predicting blood pressure in adults. A radial pulse indicates BP ≥ 80 mmHg, and a femoral pulse indicates BP ≥ 70 mmHg; a carotid pulse means that the central aortic pressure is ≥ 60 mmHg.

21. What is the most common cause of shock in multiply injured patients? What fluids should be used for initial resuscitation?
Acute blood loss resulting in hypovolemia is the most common cause of postinjury shock. The mainstay of fluid resuscitation is rapid crystalloid infusion. Colloid solutions are costly and have not proved advantageous. Hypertonic saline solutions have shown recent promise but require further study to define appropriate indications. Blood should be administered to optimize oxygen-carrying capacity when crystalloid infusion exceeds 50 ml/kg. Type O-negative blood is acceptable because of its immediate availability—10 minutes before type-specific, non-crossmatched blood and 20 minutes or more before crossmatched blood. In the future, red blood cell substitutes or recombinant hemoglobin my serve as temporizing agents in patients with massive blood loss.

22. What are the most common causes of cardiogenic shock after injury? How are they recognized and treated?
   Tension pneumothorax impairs venous return to the heart. The physical signs are ipsilateral hyperresonance and diminished breath sounds and contralateral tracheal deviation. Empirical

tube thoracostomy is indicated (do not wait for a chest radiograph). Traumatic **pericardial tamponade** is caused by the accumulation of blood (as little as 150 ml) or air in the pericardial sac. The classic Beck's triad (arterial hypotension, central venous hypertension, and distant heart sounds), however, is lacking in most patients (and may have been appreciated only by Beck). Pericardiocentesis frequently stabilizes the patient and confirms the diagnosis for transport to the OR for definitive treatment. **Myocardial contusion** is manifested primarily by dysrhythmias and occasionally by pump failure.

23. What are the indications for thoracotomy in the emergency department?
Thoracotomy should be performed in patients presenting with cardiac arrest or profound hypotension (< 60 mmHg) due to suspected pericardial tamponade, or uncontrolled intrathoracic bleeding that is refractory to initial resuscitative measures. Thoracotomy allows access to decompress the pericardium, to control intrathoracic hemorrhage, to institute open cardiac massage, and to cross-clamp the descending aorta to improve coronary and cerebral perfusion and decrease subdiaphragmatic hemorrhage. Emergency department thoracotomy for blunt trauma has a very low yield, particularly in patients devoid of vital signs (less than 1% survival).

24. When should reevaluation (the tertiary survey) be done?
At 12–24 hours after admission, a complete reevaluation should be done. At this time, patients are usually sober, less distracted by the pain of injuries and interventions, and may have new complaints.

25. What are the most commonly overlooked injuries?
Fractures, most notably cervical spine injuries, underscore the need for the tertiary survey.

26. Following deceleration trauma, occult injuries to what organs should be suspected?
Descending thoracic aorta, pancreas, retroperitoneal duodenum, and renal failure.

CONTROVERSIES

27. Should prehospital fluid resuscitation be withheld in patients with penetrating thoracoabdominal trauma?
Delaying fluid resuscitation until major vascular injuries have been controlled has been proposed in victims of penetrating trauma. It is argued that the increase in perfusion pressure associated with resuscitation dislodges clots and overcomes hemostatic mechanisms, allowing uncontrolled hemorrhage. A recent randomized clinical trial has corroborated animal studies to support this concept, but the study was flawed by excessive times in the emergency department and lack of patient stratification by degree of shock.

28. What is the role of the pneumatic antishock garment?
Also known as MAST (military antishock trousers), the pneumatic antishock garment was once believed to autotransfuse blood from extremities to the central circulation. The MAST garment now appears to increase total peripheral resistance and may be detrimental with major thoracoabdominal injuries. Currently it is used primarily to stabilize and control refractory pelvic venous hemorrhage, but the penalty of soft tissue ischemia is problematic.

29. In a patient in shock with an obvious head injury, grossly positive peritoneal aspirate, and suggestion of a thoracic aortic injury on chest radiograph, what are the priorities after initial resuscitation?
An exploratory laparotomy is indicated based on hemodynamic instability in the face of a grossly positive peritoneal tap. The patient should have a CT scan of the head immediately thereafter, followed by a thoracic aortic arteriogram. Intraoperative intracranial pressure monitoring and intravascular ultrasound may be useful.

BIBLIOGRAPHY

1. American College of Surgeons Committee on Trauma: Advanced Trauma Life Support. Chicago, American College of Surgeons, 1993.
2. Bickell WH, Wall MJ Jr., Pepe PE, et al: Immediate versus delayed fluid resuscitation for hypotensive patients with penetrating torso injuries. N Engl J Med 331:1105–1109, 1994.
3. Eastman AB: Field triage. In Feliciano, Moore, Mattox (eds): Trauma, 3rd ed. Norwalk, CT, Appleton & Lange, 1995.
4. Gould SA, Moore EE, Moore FA, et al: The clinical utility of human polymerized hemoglobin as a blood substitute following trauma and emergent surgery. J Trauma (in press).
5. Mattox KL, Moore EE, Mateer J, et al: Hypertonic saline-dextran solution in the prehospital treatment of post-traumatic hypotension—The USA multicenter trial. Ann Surg 213:482, 1991.
6. Moore EE: Trauma systems, trauma centers, trauma surgeons—Opportunity in managed competition. J Trauma 39:1–11, 1995.
7. Moore FA, Moore EE: Trauma resuscitation. In Wilmore DW, et al (eds): Surgery. New York, Scientific American, 1996.
8. Mulder DS: Airway management. In Feliciano D, Moore E, Mattox K (eds): Trauma, 3rd ed. Norwalk, CT, Appleton & Lange, 1996.
9. Nguyen TT, Zwischenberger JB, Watson WC, et al: Hypertonic acetate dextran achieves high-flow–low-pressure resuscitation of hemorrhagic shock. J Trauma 38:602–608, 1995.
10. Norwood S, Myers MB, Butler TJ: The safety of emergency neuromuscular blockade and orotracheal intubation in the acutely injured trauma patient. J Am Coll Surg 179:646, 1994.
11. Read RA, Moore EE, Moore FA: Early care of multisystem trauma. In Davis JH, et al (eds): Surgery: A Problem-solving Approach, 2nd ed. St. Louis, Mosby, 1995, pp 557–607.
12. Read RA, Moore EE, Moore JB: Emergency department thoracotomy. In Feliciano D, Moore E, Mattox K (eds): Trauma, 3rd ed. Norwalk, CT, Appleton & Lange, 1996.
13. Shackford SR: The evolution of modern trauma care. Surg Clin North Am 75:147–156, 1995.

16. BLUNT THORACOABDOMINAL TRAUMA

Adam Deutchman, M.D., and Jodi A. Chambers, M.D., FACS

1. Should abdominal and thoracic injuries be considered separately?
No. Both make up the torso. The thin diaphragm permits significant transmission of force between the abdomen and chest. Multiple system injury is most likely with a blunt mechanism.

2. What are the major causes of persistent hemodynamic instability in patients with blunt trauma to the torso?
Exsanguination, pericardial tamponade, tension pneumothorax, air embolus, and massive air leak from the tracheobronchial tree.

3. What historical details about the traumatic incident are important?
Much information is obtained from knowing the antecedent mechanism (e.g., auto, auto-pedestrian, fall), the kinetics (e.g., speed of vehicle, height of fall), and details of the scene (e.g., steering wheel and windshield damage, extrication time). The on-scene exam for level of consciousness and vital signs, both initial and en route, are important. It is also important to obtain a standard history when possible (e.g., comorbid conditions, allergies, use of medications, alcohol, and drugs).

4. What are the classic physical findings for tension pneumothorax?
The classic physical findings for tension pneumothorax are distended neck veins, hyperresonance to percussion, absent breath sounds, and hypotension. Although a deviated trachea to the contralateral side is cited in textbooks, it has not been usefully identified by any practicing trauma surgeon since Ambrose Paré performed his first amputation.

5. Is abdominal distention sensitive for hemoperitoneum?
No. Six liters of intraperitoneal bleeding may occur with minimal change in abdominal girth (2 inches or less).

6. Which organs are most commonly injured in blunt abdominal trauma?
The spleen is the correct answer on the in-service exam. With increased use of CT scans for evaluation of blunt trauma, however, the liver appears to be more frequently injured but requires operative intervention less often.

7. What is Kehr's sign?
Pain referred to the left shoulder secondary to diaphragm irritation from hemoperitoneum, usually associated with splenic rupture.

8. Is it necessary to diagnose the source of abdominal bleeding before proceeding to the OR?
No.

9. What is the seat-belt syndrome?
Although appropriate use of seat belts has dramatically reduced injuries, the bowel is occasionally injured in moderate- to high-speed motor vehicle crashes. Crushing or tearing of a hollow viscous occurs between the anterior abdominal wall and the spine during rapid deceleration.

10. Is thoracotomy indicated in blunt trauma patients who are in full arrest on arrival at the emergency department (ED)?
No. The mortality rate under such conditions approaches 100%. Without signs of life at the scene or en route, thoracotomy in the ED is a futile exercise. If vital signs are lost on arrival or shortly before, ED thoracotomy is occasionally life-saving.

11. If the hematocrit is normal, can the patient have significant blood loss?
Yes. It may take up to 6 hours for equilibration and dilution to occur after acute blood loss. Therefore, the initial ED hematocrit may be normal despite significant blood loss.

12. What is the role of diagnostic peritoneal lavage (DPL)?
DPL is a rapid test for determining the presence of hemoperitoneum (intraabdominal bleeding) secondary to blunt injury. Its sensitivity and specificity for the presence of blood are over 95%. DPL is not specific for the source of the bleeding, and its sensitivity for retroperitoneal injury is poor. Therefore, its most significant role is in the rapid evaluation of patients with multiple injuries and hemodynamic instability to determine the immediate need for laparotomy. DPL also may be used to look for hollow viscous injury by evaluating effluent for enteric contents or white blood cell count > 500/ml. Early DPL may miss this injury because of delay in white cell migration and response. Stable patients should be evaluated by either abdominal CT scan or serial physical examinations.

13. What are the criteria for a positive DPL?
Aspiration of 10 ml of gross blood or any enteric contents constitutes a grossly positive lavage. Eighty percent of positive lavages fall into this category. If the initial aspiration is negative, 1 liter of normal saline or Ringer solution (10–15 ml/kg in children) is instilled into the peritoneal cavity and then siphoned and analyzed. Generally accepted criteria for a positive lavage are red blood cell count > 100,000/ml, white blood cell count > 500/ml. Lavage fluid draining from either a chest tube or Foley catheter is obviously another indication for laparotomy. As a general rule of thumb, if one can read newsprint through the lavage effluent, it is probably negative.

14. Are there any contraindications to DPL?
Yes. Patients in shock with an obvious intraabdominal source should go immediately to the operating room. Relative contraindications include advanced pregnancy, cirrhosis, morbid obesity, and previous abdominal surgery.

15. Is CT scan an acceptable alternative to DPL?

Yes—in hemodynamically stable patients. Double-contrast (both intravenous and intragastrointestinal) CT identifies injuries of the liver and spleen and allows visualization of the retroperitoneum, including the duodenum, pancreas, and kidneys. Its weakness, like DPL, is the diagnosis of hollow viscous injuries.

16. If a pelvic fracture is present, can DPL still be performed?

The textbook answer is no, but the practical answer is yes. The incidence of associated intraabdominal injury is 15%. DPL can still be safely performed below the umbilicus in most patients. Lavage above the umbilicus is recommended by some to avoid entering the anterior extension of a large pelvic hematoma.

17. What other modalities are used in evaluation of the patient with blunt abdominal trauma?

1. **Ultrasound.** The use of sonography has gained acceptance for the intraabdominal evaluation of the bluntly injured patient. Ultrasound appears to hold promise as a rapid and sensitive method of detecting hemoperitoneum.

2. **Laparoscopy/thoracoscopy.** Direct visualization of the abdomen or thorax may have a role in the evaluation of the bluntly injured patient. Its value with respect to accuracy, cost, risk, and benefit is questionable, however, compared with other diagnostic tools.

3. **Serial physical examination.** Repeat examinations may be performed in the stable patient without a distracting extremity or head injury.

18. What is the significance of injury to the chest wall?

Blunt injury to the chest most commonly results in rib fracture, either single or multiple. Such injuries are significant, because they often lead to splinting, hypoventilation, atelectasis, and pneumonia. Multiply fractured ribs in two locations are referred to as a flail chest. In patients with flail chest, ventilatory support is frequently needed because of underlying pulmonary contusion and respiratory insufficiency.

19. Thoracic aortic injury is suggested by which radiographic findings?

Classic chest aortogram findings include widened mediastinum, depressed left mainstem bronchus, fractured first or second rib, fractured scapula, loss of contour of the aortic knob, esophageal deviation to the right, pleural cap, and hemothorax. A thoracic aorta injury may exist with none, one, or any combination of the above findings. If an aortic injury is suspected by either mechanism or radiologic findings, an aortogram should be obtained. Transesophageal echo is gaining enthusiastic advocates, but aortography remains the gold standard for diagnosis of a torn aorta.

BIBLIOGRAPHY

1. Feliciano D, Moore E, Mattox K (eds): Trauma, 3rd ed. Norwalk, CT, Appleton & Lange, 1996.
2. Moore JB, Moore EE, Thompson JS: Abdominal injuries associated with penetrating trauma in the lower chest. Am J Surg 140:724, 1980.
3. Root HD, Hauser CW, McKiney CR, et al: Diagnostic peritoneal lavage. Surgery 57:633, 1965.
4. Rozyoki G, Oschsner MG, Haffin JF, et al: Prospective evaluation of surgeons' use of ultrasound in the evaluation of trauma patients. J Trauma 34:516, 1993.
5. Sabiston DC, Spencer FC: Gibbon's Surgery of the Chest, 5th ed. Philadelphia, W.B. Saunders, 1989.
6. Trunkey DD, Lewis FR: Current Therapy of Trauma. St. Louis, Mosby, 1990.
7. Wilmore DW, Brennen MF, Harken AH, et al: American College of Surgeons Care of the Surgical Patient. New York, Scientific American, 1991.
8. Zuidema GD, Rutherford RB, Ballinger WF: The Management of Trauma, 4th ed. Philadelphia, W.B. Saunders, 1985.

17. PENETRATING THORACIC TRAUMA

Adam Deutchman M.D., and Jodi A. Chambers, M.D., FACS

1. What is the most common cause of penetrating chest injury?
In the civilian setting, low-velocity gunshot wounds and stab wounds traditionally have been the most common causes. In a military setting, high-velocity gunshot wounds and shrapnel are more likely agents.

2. Do penetrating thoracic injuries require operative intervention?
No. In 90% of patients placement of a chest tube is the only intervention necessary. Because of the low pressure of the pulmonary vasculature, most injuries tamponade with reexpansion of the lung. Air leaks from pulmonary parenchymal injury also seal and rarely require surgical treatment.

3. What are the operative indications for penetrating thoracic injury?
Generally accepted criteria for thoracotomy are initial drainage of 1000–1500 ml of blood after tube thoracostomy; continued drainage of 200 ml/hour for over 2 hours; evidence of pericardial tamponade; injury to the esophagus, great vessels, and diaphragm; or a missile that traverses the mediastinum.

4. Should a chest radiograph be obtained before placement of a chest tube for penetrating injury?
In hemodynamically unstable patients, no. Death secondary to tension pneumothorax may occur while waiting for a chest film (see the chapter on blunt thoracoabdominal trauma for physical finding of tension pneumothorax). In stable patients with a stab wound, the chest radiograph is valuable because pleural penetration may not have occurred. Observation alone is sufficient. If the patient's stability is questionable, it is always safer to insert a tube.

5. Why should penetrating injury at the base of the neck be included as thoracic trauma?
Many structures at the base of the neck traverse the thorax, including major vessels, trachea, and esophagus; thus, injury to these structures may have consequences in the chest.

6. What is Beck's triad? What is its significance?
Beck's triad consists of elevated central venous pressure (distended neck veins), muffled or distant heart sound, and hypotension. Cardiac tamponade should be considered in this setting. Pericardiocentesis may be both diagnostic and therapeutic.

7. List two other physical signs that may indicate tamponade.
   Pulsus paradoxus. Greater than normal (10 mmHg) decrease in systolic arterial pressure during spontaneous inspiration may be detected by weakening or disappearance of the arterial pulse with inspiration.
   Kussmaul's sign. Failure of venous pressure to decline with inspiration may be reflected by persistently distended neck veins.

8. What structures of the heart are most often injured by a penetrating mechanism?
In order from greatest to least frequency: right ventricle, left ventricle, and right atrium. The most likely (but infrequently) injured vessels of the heart are the left anterior descending and the first diagonal arteries. Such injury patterns reflect the anterior position of the vulnerable structures in the chest.

9. Is placement of a catheter to measure central venous pressure (CVP) sensitive for diagnosing cardiac tamponade in the ED?

No. Although it may be helpful in monitoring the patient over time, the initial readings are frequently falsely elevated by the patient's straining. CVP readings need to be considered along with the clinical status of the patient.

10. What is subcutaneous emphysema?

Subcutaneous emphysema is air within the soft tissue. Palpation of the skin creates a feeling like the crunching of Rice Krispies. Its presence signifies leakage of air either from the lung or airway extrapleurally or from the cervical esophagus into the surrounding soft tissue.

11. Penetrating injury below which intercostal space is associated with intraabdominal injury?

Intraabdominal injury is associated with penetrating injury below the fourth intercostal space anteriorly and the sixth intercostal space laterally. The diaphragm can rise to the level of the nipples at end expiration; therefore, injury to the diaphragm and intraabdominal organs must be kept in mind during evaluation of such injuries.

12. Is ED thoracotomy indicated in trauma patients who arrive in full arrest after a penetrating injury to the chest?

Yes. Unlike blunt trauma, meaningful salvage rates occur in patients with penetrating trauma if hypoxia has not been prolonged. The treatable causes of arrest include tension pneumothorax, tamponade, and hemothorax. Unlike blunt trauma, there is usually a single treatable cause, which accounts for the difference in outcome.

BIBLIOGRAPHY

1. Feliciano D, Moore E, Mattox K (eds): Trauma, 3rd ed. Norwalk, CT, Appleton & Lange, 1996.
2. Moore JB, Moore EE, Thompson JS: Abdominal injuries associated with penetrating trauma in the lower chest. Am J Surg 140:724, 1980.
3. Root HD, Hauser CW, McKiney CR, et al: Diagnostic peritoneal lavage. Surgery 57:633, 1965.
4. Sabiston DC, Spencer FC: Gibbon's Surgery of the Chest, 5th ed. Philadelphia, W.B. Saunders, 1989.
5. Trunkey DD, Lewis FR: Current Therapy of Trauma. St. Louis, Mosby, 1990.
6. Wilmore DW, Brennen MF, Harken AH, et al: American College of Surgeons Care of the Surgical Patient. New York, Scientific American, 1995.
7. Zuidema GD, Rutherford RB, Ballinger WF: The Management of Trauma, 4th ed. Philadelphia, W.B. Saunders, 1985.

18. PENETRATING ABDOMINAL TRAUMA

Walter L. Biffl, M.D., and Ernest E. Moore, M.D.

1. What is the overall management strategy of patients with penetrating abdominal trauma?

Initial management is divided into resuscitation (airway, breathing, circulation), directed physical examination, tailored diagnostic studies, and therapeutic interventions. Hemodynamic stability, the nature of the penetrating object, and the location of wound are key factors in the decision algorithm. Patients with hemodynamic instability, overt peritonitis, massive hemoperitoneum, or other obvious signs of abdominal visceral injury are intubated, volume-loaded, and transported emergently to the OR for exploration. patients who are hemodynamically stable are managed according to the injury mechanism and wound location.

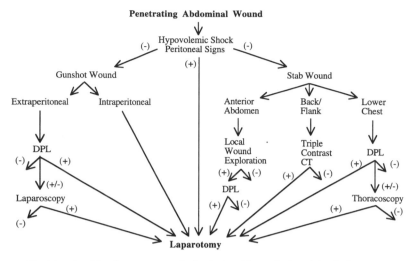

Decision algorithm for management of patients with penetrating abdominal trauma.

2. What is an injury mechanism?

The mechanism is the manner in which the injury was sustained; thus a major mechanism is a big hit.

3. Describe the primary survey and resuscitation phase.

The basics of resuscitation are the same in any severely injured patient: Airway, Breathing, Circulation, Disability, and Exposure. Important historical information includes the time of injury, type of weapon, length or caliber of the weapon, depth of penetration if the weapon was removed, and estimated blood loss at the scene. Each of these descriptors is included in the mechanism of injury. Physical examination must include a comprehensive survey of the neck, chest, axilla, abdomen, flank, back, perineum, rectum, peripheral pulses, and neurologic function. (Remember that in the heat of the battle it is easy to overlook synchronous injuries.) Entrance and exit wounds should be documented carefully. Intravenous access should be secured with two large-bore (14- or 16-gauge) peripheral catheters; central venous catheterization is essential if pericardial tamponade is suspected.

4. When is emergency department (ED) thoracotomy indicated?

Thoracotomy should be performed in the ED when patients present with cardiac arrest or profound hypotension (< 60 mmHg) that is refractory to initial resuscitation. Thoracotomy allows access to decompress the pericardial space (pericardial tamponade), to control intrathoracic hemorrhage, to prevent transpulmonary air embolism, to institute open cardiac massage, and to cross-clamp the descending aorta to improve coronary and cerebral perfusion as well as decrease subdiaphragmatic hemorrhage.

5. What is transpulmonary air embolism?

A laceration of the lung may create a communication between a bronchiole and pulmonary vein. Air entering the pulmonary veins returns to the left atrium and may be pumped out the aorta into the coronary and carotid arteries, with grave consequences. (This occurrence is infrequent, but mention of the possibility is likely to impress the chief resident.)

6. What is the role for presumptive antibiotics?

Antibiotics are given only when the decision has been made to perform a laparotomy. Short courses of high-dose antibiotics are used. The optimal antibiotic has not been established, but coverage of both anaerobic and aerobic flora is desirable. Tetanus prophylaxis should be given to all patients with penetrating injuries.

7. What is the general plan for abdominal exploration?
A midline abdominal incision provides rapid entry and wide exposure and may be extended as a median sternotomy to access the chest or continued inferiorly into the pelvis. The aorta should be palpated to assess blood pressure. Report all findings, including a soft aorta and low blood pressure, to the anesthetist (trauma is both a contact and a team sport). Evacuation of blood with the autotransfusion device (if the patient is hemodynamically stable) is followed by exploration of the wound tract. Actively bleeding areas are packed, and hollow visceral injuries are temporarily isolated with noncrushing clamps. The entire abdomen is systematically explored before undertaking extensive repairs so that injuries can be addressed in the proper sequence.

8. Why is there a different approach to stab and gunshot wounds?
One-third of stab wounds to the anterior abdomen do not penetrate the peritoneum, whereas gunshot wounds violate the peritoneum more than 80% of the time. Furthermore, penetration of the peritoneum by a bullet is associated with visceral or vascular injuries in > 95% of cases, whereas only one-half of stab wounds violating the peritoneal cavity produce significant injury.

STAB WOUNDS

9. What are the indications for immediate laparotomy?
Abdominal distention and hypotension, overt peritonitis, and obvious signs of abdominal visceral injury (hematuria, hematemesis, proctorrhagia, evisceration; palpation of diaphragmatic defect on chest tube insertion; radiologic evidence of injury to GI or GU tracts).

10. What are the appropriate initial studies?
In stable patients, a chest radiograph is mandatory to exclude hemo- or pneumothorax and to determine the position of intravenous catheters and endotracheal, nasogastric, and pleural tubes. In stable patients, biplanar abdominal radiographs are helpful in locating retained foreign bodies and may reveal pneumoperitoneum. Injuries in proximity to the rectum obligate sigmoidoscopy, whereas injuries in proximity to the urinary tract should be evaluated with intravenous pyelography. (See chapter on urinary tract trauma.)

11. How is an anterior abdominal stab wound evaluated?
Physical examination is unreliable, particularly in intoxicated patients. Furthermore, the consequences of false-negative findings are severe; thus, adjunctive tests remain the standard of care. The first step is local exploration of the stab wound to determine peritoneal penetration. If the tract clearly terminates superficially, no further treatment is required. Confirmation of peritoneal penetration is followed by diagnostic peritoneal lavage (DPL) (see below). Double-contrast (oral and IV) CT scanning is not useful because of its relative insensitivity for penetrating hollow visceral injuries. Ultrasonography is useful primarily for detecting blood quickly; thus, most of the tests are helpful only if positive. Laparoscopy in penetrating abdominal trauma has yet to demonstrate distinct advantages over other diagnostic approaches except for the evaluation of suspected diaphragmatic injury. The potential for missed injuries, poor evaluation of the retroperitoneum, and expense (both dollars and time) are major drawbacks.

12. What is a double-contrast CT?
CT scanning is performed after introducing contrast into the GI tract and the circulation. The two markers delineate the position and continuity (leaks) of the GI tract and vasculature.

13. What constitutes a positive DPL after penetrating trauma?
A grossly positive tap (aspiration of > 10 ml of blood or gastrointestinal or biliary contents) mandates immediate exploration. A negative initial aspirate is followed by the instillation of 1000 ml of saline (15 ml/kg in children) into the abdomen through a dialysis catheter, followed by gravity

drainage of the fluid back into the saline bag. The finding of > 100,000 mm³ of red blood cells or the combined elevation of amylase > 20 IU/L and alkaline phosphatase > 3 IU/L is generally considered an indication for exploration. Lower red blood cell counts (5,000–100,000 mm³) may suggest occult injury and should heighten suspicion. Approximately 5% of patients with red blood cell counts < 100,000 ultimately require laparotomy, usually because of perforation of stomach or small bowel. In the case of lower chest stab sounds, a red blood cell count of 1,000–10,000 mm³ mandates further evaluation to rule out diaphragmatic injury.

14. How are flank and back stab wounds evaluated?
The incidence of significant injuries is 10% for stab wounds to the back and 25% for stab wounds to the flank. However, evaluation of such wounds is problematic, because the retroperitoneum is not sampled by DPL and physical examination is even less sensitive. The major concern is a missed colonic perforation. At present, triple-contrast (oral, IV, and rectal) CT and serial physical examination are the two primary modes of assessment.

15. How is the lower chest stab wound evaluated?
The lower chest is defined as the area between the nipple line (fourth intercostal space) anteriorly, the tip of the scapula (seventh intercostal space) posteriorly, and the costal margins inferiorly. Because the diaphragm reaches the fourth intercostal space during expiration (hard to believe, but true), the abdominal organs are at risk after penetrating wounds to this region. Stab wounds to the lower chest are associated with abdominal visceral injury in about 15% of cases, whereas gunshot wounds to the lower chest are associated with abdominal visceral injury in nearly 50%. Thus, wounds to the lower chest should be managed as abdominal wounds for the purposes of evaluating the abdomen.

GUNSHOT WOUNDS

16. What are the indications for immediate laparotomy?
Because of the high incidence of visceral injury, immediate exploration is indicated for all gunshot wounds that violate the peritoneum.

17. What are the appropriate initial studies?
Chest radiographs are mandatory to rule out hemo- or pneumothorax. In stable patients, biplanar abdominal films can be useful in defining the missile trajectory; entrance and exit wounds can be deceiving.

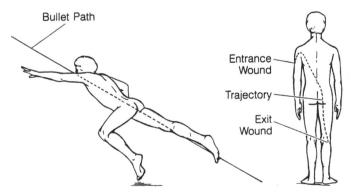

Illustrated is an example of how the path of a bullet through a contorted body can produce confusion when the patient is examined in the emergency room. An entrance wound will be found at the left upper arm and an exit wound at the medial aspect of the right knee. The bullet could have damaged any structure that was in between these two wounds when the patient's body was contorted.

18. What patients with abdominal gunshot wounds are managed nonoperatively?

Stable patients with tangential missile tracts or equivocal peritoneal penetration are candidates for DPL, although many authorities still recommend laparotomy. The cut-off for red blood cell counts is reduced to 10,000/mm³. Patients with a negative DPL are observed for 24 hours. For red blood cell counts of 1,000–10,000/mm³, laparoscopy is used to exclude peritoneal penetration. Newer laparoscopy equipment, which allows examination in the ED under local anesthesia, may broaden its application. Selective management of gunshot wounds to the back and flank are generally based on triple contrast CT. (See algorithm in question 1).

CONTROVERSIES

19. Should prehospital fluid resuscitation be withheld in patients with penetrating abdominal trauma?

Delaying resuscitation until major vascular injuries are under operative control has been proposed to improve outcome in patients after penetrating trauma. it is argued that the increase in perfusion pressure associated with resuscitation dislodges clots and overcomes hemostatic mechanisms, allowing uncontrolled hemorrhage. A recent randomized clinical trial has corroborated animal studies to support this concept, but the study was flawed by excessive times in the ED and lack of patient stratification by degree of shock.

20. What is the role of laparoscopy after penetrating abdominal trauma?

Although an intriguing diagnostic modality with additional therapeutic capabilities, laparoscopy thus far appears to have limited application after trauma. With the exception of the evaluation of suspected diaphragmatic injury, laparoscopy has yet to demonstrate distinct advantages over other diagnostic approaches. The potential for missed injuries, poor evaluation of the retroperitoneum, and expense are major drawbacks. Newer laparoscopy equipment allowing examination in the ED under local anesthesia may broaden its application.

21. What is the role of thoracoscopy after penetrating abdominal trauma?

Like laparoscopy, thoracoscopy has proved a valuable advance in general surgery, but it is unproved in trauma. Its primary indication after penetrating wounds is to search for diaphragmatic injury.

BIBLIOGRAPHY

1. American College of Surgeons Committee on Trauma: Advanced Trauma Life Support. Chicago, American College of Surgeons, 1993.
2. Bickell WH, Wall MJ Jr, Pepe PE, et al: Immediate versus delayed fluid resuscitation for hypotensive patients with penetrating torso injuries. N Engl J Med 331:1105–1109, 1994.
3. Fabian T: Abdominal trauma and indications for celiotomy. In Feliciano DV, Moore EE, Mattox KL (eds): Trauma, 3rd ed. Norwalk, CT, Appleton & Lange, 1995.
4. Moore FA, Moore EE: Trauma resuscitation. In Wilmore DW, et al (eds): Surgery. New York, Scientific American, 1995.
5. Moore JB, Moore EE, Thompson JS: Abdominal injuries associated with penetrating trauma to the lower chest. Am J Surg 140:724–730, 1980.
6. Read RA, Moore EE, Moore JB: Emergency department thoracotomy. In Feliciano DV, Moore EE, Mattox KL (eds): Trauma, 3rd ed. Norwalk, CT, Appleton & Lange, 1995.
7. Read RA, Moore EE, Moore FA: Early care of multisystem trauma. In David JH, et al (eds): Surgery: A Problem-solving Approach, 2nd ed. St. Louis, Mosby, 1995, pp 557–607.

19. SPLENIC TRAUMA

Max B. Mitchell, M.D., and Frederick A. Moore, M.D.

1. What is typical history for splenic trauma?

Any history is consistent with splenic trauma. With blunt abdominal trauma, the spleen is the most commonly injured intraabdominal organ, whereas in penetrating trauma it is injured in fewer than 10% of cases. Localized trauma to the left upper quadrant or left lower chest with associated tenth or eleventh rib fractures or hematuria should arouse suspicion. Delayed hypotension following blunt trauma occasionally occurs when the patient finally decompensates from a persistent, slow, splenic bleed or when a perisplenic hematoma ruptures.

2. How is splenic trauma diagnosed?

History and physical examination are essential. Kehr's sign, pain at the left shoulder often exacerbated by Trendelenburg positioning, is present in fewer than one-half of patients with splenic ruptures. Peritoneal lavage determines significant hemoperitoneum, leading to laparotomy in the majority of cases of splenic trauma; however, it is not organ specific. Overall accuracy is roughly 98%. Ultrasonography can also reliably detect hemoperitoneum. Additionally, ultrasound may delineate specific organ injuries including splenic injuries in the emergency room. CT scanning complements peritoneal lavage and provides organ specificity as well as evaluation of retroperitoneal anatomy. CT grading of the severity of splenic trauma can be helpful in guiding nonoperative management. Alternative organ-specific tests include technetium scanning and selective arteriography. Time, expense, and failure to rule out hollow visceral injuries limit radiographic methods and restrict their use to hemodynamically stable patients.

3. How is splenic trauma classified?

The Organ Injury Scaling Committee of the American Association for the Surgery of Trauma has established five classes of splenic injury:

Classification of Splenic Trauma

Class I:	Nonexpanding subcapsular hematoma < 10% surface area. Nonbleeding capsular laceration with < 1 cm deep parenchymal involvement
Class II:	Nonexpanding capsular hematoma 10–50% surface area. Nonexpanding intraparenchymal hematoma < 2 cm diameter. Bleeding capsular tear of parenchymal laceration 1–3 cm deep without trabecular vessel involvement
Class III:	Expanding subcapsular or intraparenchymal hematoma. Bleeding subcapsular hematoma or subcapsular hematoma > 50% surface area. Intraparenchymal laceration > 3 cm deep or involving a trabecular vessel.
Class IV:	Ruptured intraparenchymal hematoma with active bleeding. Laceration involving segmental or hilar vessels producing major (> 25% splenic volume) devascularization.
Class V:	Completely shattered or avulsed spleen. Hilar laceration devascularizes entire spleen.

4. What is overwhelming postsplenectomy sepsis (OPSS)?

A typical scenario is abrupt onset of fever, chills, nausea, and vomiting following a mild upper respiratory tract infection. This progresses over 12–24 hours to fulminant sepsis associated with shock, disseminated intravascular coagulation (DIC), and adrenal insufficiency. Mortality varies from 40–70%. Fifty percent of cases occur within 1 year of splenectomy, although the syndrome has been reported as late as 37 years postsplenectomy. Encapsulated organisms are most commonly responsible: pneumococcus, 50%; meningococcus, 12%; *E. coli*, 11%; *H. influenzae*, 8%; staphylococcus, 8%; and streptococcus, 7%. Nonencapsulated bacteria, viruses, and protozoa have also been incriminated.

5. In whom does OPSS develop?

In 1952 King and Shumacker made a startling observation. Five children who underwent splenectomy within the first 6 months of life all developed severe sepsis and two died. This stimulated a healthy debate over the spleen's role in infection. Some believed that the increased risk of sepsis was caused by the underlying disease. It was not until 1973, when Singer analyzed 24 series of asplenic patients, that the clear risk of OPSS became apparent. The incidence of severe sepsis was related to the indication for splenectomy. In healthy individuals, and in those with trauma or incidental splenectomy, the risks were 1.5% and 2.1%, respectively. In those with hematologic disorders, the incidence varied from 2.0–7.5%. The incidence is also greater in children under 4 years of age by a factor of 2.5. Everyone agrees that children are at increased risk, but a debate continues about adult trauma. Recent reviews confirm this risk to be in the range of 1–2%.

6. What is the immunologic role of the spleen?

The spleen represents 25% of the reticuloendothelial system, being perfused with 200 ml of blood per minute; 90% of this blood is forced through the cords of Billroth, where fixed macrophages phagocytize particulate matter. Thus the spleen acts as a major immunologic filter. Its second role is that of an immunologic factory, i.e., the site of production of IgM, tuftsin, and properdin. These are critical in opsonization, and thus play a major role in phagocytosis of intravascular antigens. Finally, there is some evidence that the spleen may modulate the ratio of helper T-cells to suppressor T-cells.

7. Can splenic trauma be managed nonoperatively?

Nonoperative management is well established in pediatric trauma patients who are hemodynamically stable with splenic injury documented by an imaging technique and who have no associated serious abdominal injury. Many centers also exclude children with altered levels of consciousness. Nonoperative management involves frequent examination, monitoring, and transfusion therapy. The pediatric spleen has a thicker capsule and more parenchymal smooth muscle compared with the adult spleen. These factors tend to promote hemostasis in the pediatric spleen. Regardless of age, all patients exhibiting hemodynamic instability not correctable with small infusions of crystalloid should undergo prompt celiotomy. Although controversial, nonoperative management is increasingly used in adults. Reported failure rates range widely from 0 to 70%, primarily because of inhomogeneity in patient selection. In patients with class I, II, or III splenic injury secondary to blunt trauma, nonoperative management is appropriate when there is no hemodynamic instability after initial fluid resuscitation, no serious concomitant intraabdominal injury, and no extraabdominal condition that precludes assessment of the abdomen.

8. When should the spleen be salvaged?

In many cases, the spleen can be saved with temporary packing or topical hemostatic agents. If additional techniques are required, it is wise to proceed with splenectomy in the unstable patient with multiple associated abdominal injuries and in patients with extraabdominal trauma such as closed head injuries or a widened mediastinum in whom treatment is uncertain. Obviously some injuries are quite extensive and repair would be unsafe. The risk of repair should not exceed the risk of the asplenic state.

9. How often can the spleen be salvaged and at what risk?

Using the above guidelines, splenic salvage is possible in roughly one-half of acute injuries. The only morbidity appears to be postoperative bleeding, which occurs in less than 3%. This tends to happen in the early postoperative period, when the patient is under close supervision. It is easily detected and therefore easily managed without significant risk of hemorrhagic mortality.

10. What are splenic implants?
They involve autotransplantation of splenic tissue into an omental pouch, which offers a rich blood supply. In both animals and humans these implants survive and are found to increase in size with time.

11. Do splenic implants work?
Numerous animal studies have confirmed the immunologic benefits of splenic implants; however, the extent is variable. Data from studies in humans are limited. Follow-up studies show that IgM, platelet counts, and complement levels normalize. Uniform implant viability is demonstrated by technetium scanning. Target cells and Howell-Jolly bodies disappear. However, more sophisticated studies are needed to confirm whether these implants protect against OPSS.

12. What advice should be given to asplenic patients?
They should be warned of the lifelong risk of OPSS. They should seek medical attention for any lingering infections; early aggressive therapy markedly decreases mortality. Pneumococcal vaccination is recommended but does not give full protection against OPSS. Pneumococcus is the responsible organism in only one-half of cases, and the vaccine does not cover all serotypes. Penicillin prophylaxis may be of benefit in the immunocompromised host.

BIBLIOGRAPHY

1. Cogbill TH, Moore EE, Jurkovich GJ, et al: Nonoperative management of blunt specific trauma: A multicenter experience. J Trauma 29:1312–1317, 1989.
2. Dickermann JD: Traumatic asplenia in adults: A defined hazard. J Trauma 116:361, 1981.
3. Hoffmann R, et al: Blunt abdominal trauma in cases of multiple trauma evaluated by ultrasonography: A prospective analysis of 291 patients. J Trauma 32:452, 1992.
4. King H, Schumacker HB: Splenic studies. Ann Surg 136:239, 1952.
5. McKenney M, et al: Can ultrasound replace diagnostic peritoneal lavage in the assessment of blunt trauma? J Trauma 37:439, 1994.
6. Moore EE, Shackford SR, Pachter HL, et al: Organ injury scaling: Spleen, liver, kidney. J Trauma 29:1664–1666, 1989.
7. Moore FA, et al: Risk of splenic salvage after trauma. Am J Surg 148:800, 1984.
8. Moore FA, Moore EE, Abernathy CM: Injury to the spleen. In Moore EE, Mattox KL, Feliciano DV (eds): Trauma, 2nd ed. Norwalk, CT, Appleton & Lange, 1991.
9. Sherman R: Perspective in management of trauma to the spleen. J Trauma 20:1, 1980.
10. Singer DB: Postsplenectomy sepsis. Perspect Pediatr Pathol 1:285, 1973.
11. Wara DW: Host defense against *Streptococcus pneumoniae*: The role of the spleen. Rev Infect Dis 3:299, 1981.
12. Wessen DE, et al: Ruptured spleen: When to operate? J Pediatr Surg 16:324, 1981.

20. HEPATIC TRAUMA

R. Franciose, M.D., and Ernest E. Moore, M.D.

1. How often is the liver injured in trauma?
Because of its expansive mass and central location, the liver remains the most common site of visceral injury after both blunt and penetrating abdominal trauma. At laparotomy, approximately 35% of patients with either blunt or penetrating trauma have a liver injury.

2. Do the liver and spleen respond similarly to injury?

No. The liver has a unique ability to establish spontaneous hemostasis after superficial laceration. For this reason, the majority of liver injuries in hemodynamically stable patients can be managed nonoperatively. In contrast, splenic fractures continue to hemorrhage; therefore, a greater percentage require operative repair (splenorrhaphy) or splenectomy.

3. What are the major determinants of mortality after acute liver injury?

Mechanism of injury and number of associated abdominal organ injuries are the major determinants of mortality. The mortality rate for stab wounds to the liver is 3%; for gunshot wounds, 10%; and for blunt injuries, 25%. The mortality rate for isolated grade III hepatic injuries is 7%; for grade IV, 30%; and for grade V, 66%. Retrohepatic vena cava injuries carry mortality rates of 80% for penetrating trauma and 95% for blunt trauma. The vena cava (behind the liver) bleeds dramatically and is hard to access surgically.

4. What history and physical signs suggest acute liver injury?

Any patient sustaining blunt abdominal trauma with hypotension must be assumed to have a liver injury until proved otherwise. Specific signs that increase the likelihood of hepatic injury are contusion over the lower right chest, fracture of the right lower ribs (especially posterior fractures of ribs 9–12), and penetrating injuries to the right lower chest (below the fourth intercostal space), flank, and upper abdomen. Physical signs of hemoperitoneum may be absent in as many as one-third of patients with significant hepatic injury.

5. What diagnostic tests are helpful in confirming acute liver injury?

Diagnostic peritoneal lavage (DPL) is the most sensitive test for hemoperitoneum (> 98%). DPL is the diagnostic test of choice for hemodynamically unstable victims of multisystem trauma. Abdominal CT scan is currently used only in hemodynamically stable patients who are candidates for nonoperative management. It is reasonably accurate in defining the grade of liver injury. The major shortcoming of CT is the relatively poor correlation between hepatic CT staging and subsequent risk of hemorrhage. Currently there is much enthusiasm among trauma surgeons for the use of emergency department ultrasonography as an alternative to DPL. Ultrasound is highly sensitive in identifying more than 500 ml of intraperitoneal fluid. It is noninvasive and may be repeated at frequent intervals. It is relatively poor for staging liver injuries. Laparoscopy is an emerging technique, but the equipment is cumbersome and requires general anesthesia.

6. What is the role of hepatic angiography and radionucleotide biliary excretion scans in the diagnosis of liver injury?

Currently, the primary purpose of both procedures is to identify the delayed complications of liver injuries (e.g., arteriovenous fistulas, hepatic artery pseudoaneurysms, hemobilia). Selective hepatic artery embolization is emerging as a therapy for hepatic arterial injuries.

SURGICAL ANATOMY OF THE LIVER

7. How many anatomic lobes are present in the liver? What is their topographic boundary?

The liver is divided into two anatomic lobes, the right and the left. Their boundary lies in an oblique plane extending from the gallbladder fossa anteriorly to the inferior vena cava posteriorly. The three hepatic veins define the division between the lobar segments and the planes of surgical resection. Lobar segments are numbered I–VIII, according to Couinaud's nomenclature.

8. What is the blood supply to the liver and the relative contribution of each structure to hepatic oxygenation?

The hepatic artery supplies approximately 30% of the blood flow to the liver and 50% of its oxygen supply. The portal vein provides 70% of the liver's blood flow and 50% of its oxygen.

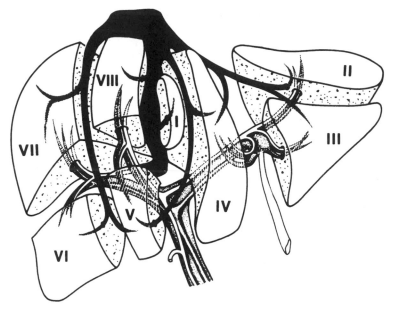

The functional division of the liver and the segments according to Couinaud's nomenclature. (From Bismuth H: Surgical anatomy and anatomical surgery of the liver. World J Surg 6:6, 1982, with permission.)

The relative significance of arterial flow in cirrhotic patients is greater; therefore, hepatic artery ligation in patients with cirrhosis is not recommended.

9. What are the most common variations in hepatic arterial supply to the right and left lobes of the liver?
In most people the common hepatic artery originates from the celiac axis and divides into right and left hepatic arterial branches within the porta hepatis. Approximately 15% of people have a replaced right hepatic artery (sole arterial supply to the right lobe) that originates from the superior mesenteric artery (SMA). A replaced right hepatic artery always supplies a cystic artery, and its ligation should be followed by cholecystectomy. A replaced left hepatic artery (approximately 15% of people) arises from the left gastric artery; it may be the sole blood supply to the left lobe or may contribute to blood supply in conjunction with a normal left hepatic artery. In 5% of people, the hepatic arterial supply does not arise from the celiac axis (either right and left hepatic arteries are replaced, or a single main hepatic trunk derives from the SMA).

10. What is the venous drainage of the liver?
The right, middle, and left hepatic veins are the major venous tributaries and enter the inferior vena cava below the right hemidiaphragm.

OPERATIVE MANAGEMENT OF LIVER INJURY

11. How are acute liver injuries classified?
Liver wounds are generally graded on a scale of I to VI according to the depth of parenchymal laceration and involvement of the hepatic veins or the retrohepatic portion of the inferior vena cava. Optimal methods of obtaining hemostasis vary with the severity of the injury.

12. Do all patients with a traumatic liver injury require surgery?
No. Nonoperative treatment may be considered for victims of blunt trauma who are hemodynamically stable (currently approximately 60% of patients). One-third of such patients require blood

transfusions, but the volume should not exceed 2 units in the first 24 hours. Repeat CT scan should be performed in 5–7 days. Complications, including perihepatic infection, biloma, and hemobilia, have been reported in 10% of nonoperative patients.

13. What are the options for temporary control of significant hemorrhage in victims of hepatic trauma? Why is temporary control important?
Hemorrhage may pose an immediate threat to life. Furthermore, ongoing hemorrhage leads to the vicious cycle of acidosis, hypothermia, and coagulopathy. Temporary control of bleeding allows the anesthesiologist time to restore circulating blood volume. Manual compression, perihepatic packing, and the Pringle maneuver are the most effective temporary techniques until the definitive techniques outlined below can be initiated.

14. What is the Pringle maneuver?
The Pringle maneuver is the manual or vascular clamp occlusion of the hepatoduodenal ligament to interrupt blood flow into the liver. Included in the hepatoduodenal ligament are the hepatic artery, portal vein, and common bile duct. Failure of the Pringle maneuver to control liver hemorrhage suggests either (1) injury to the retrohepatic vena cava or hepatic vein or (2) arterial supply from an aberrant right or left hepatic artery (see question 9).

15. What is the finger fracture technique?
Finger fracture or hepatotomy is the method of exposing bleeding points deep within liver lacerations by blunt dissection. Pushing apart the liver parenchyma enables bleeding points to be identified and ligated. This method is more commonly required for penetrating injuries.

16. What is the role of selective hepatic artery ligation in securing hemostasis in patients with a major liver injury?
Deep lacerations of the right or left hepatic lobes may result in bleeding that cannot be completely controlled by suture ligation of specific bleeding points within the liver parenchyma. In this situation, either the right or left hepatic artery can be ligated for control of the bleeding with little risk of ischemic liver necrosis.

17. Why is retrohepatic vena caval laceration lethal?
The retrohepatic portion of the inferior vena cava is difficult to expose because it is enveloped by the liver. Exposure requires either extensive hepatotomy, extensive mobilization of the right lobe, right lobectomy, or transection of the vena cava. The large caliber and high flow of the inferior vena cava result in prohibitive hemorrhage while surgical exposure is obtained. Most patients (95%) die.

18. What is the physiologic rationale for use of a shunt in attempted repair of retrohepatic vena caval injuries?
Hemorrhage control requires maintenance of venous return to the heart while both antegrade and retrograde bleeding through the laceration is stopped. These requirements are met by shunting blood through a tube spanning the laceration between the right atrium and lower inferior vena cava. New shunts have been devised to allow peripheral insertion through the femoral vein.

19. What is the intrahepatic balloon?
For transhepatic penetrating injuries, a 1-inch Penrose drain is sutured around a red rubber catheter to form a long balloon that is threaded through the bleeding liver injury and inflated with contrast media through a stopcock in the red rubber catheter. The balloon tamponades liver hemorrhage. The catheter is brought out through the abdominal wall, deflated, and removed 24–48 hours later.

20. What are the indications for perihepatic packing?
Liver packing with planned reoperation for definitive treatment of injuries in patients who are hypothermic, acidotic, and coagulopathic is a life-saving maneuver. Laparotomy pads (up to 20)

are packed around the liver to compress and control hemorrhage. The skin of the abdomen is then closed with towel clips (abbreviated laparotomy), and the patient's metabolic abnormalities are corrected with planned reoperation within 24 hours.

21. What is the abdominal compartment syndrome?

A potentially lethal complication of perihepatic packing is the abdominal compartment syndrome, which may occur when intraabdominal pressure exceeds 20 cm H_2O. Intraabdominal pressure increases because of bowel edema secondary to ischemia/reperfusion injury or continued hemorrhage into the abdominal cavity. As pressure increases beyond 20 cm H_2O, venous return, cardiac output, and urine output decrease, whereas ventilatory pressures increase. Patients must return promptly to the operating room for decompression of the abdomen. A manometer attached to the Foley catheter is useful in following intraabdominal pressures.

BIBLIOGRAPHY

1. Bismuth H: Surgical anatomy and anatomical surgery of the liver. World J Surg 6:3–9, 1982.
2. Buechter KJ, Gomez GA, Zeppa R: A new technique for exposure of injuries at the confluence of the retrohepatic veins and the retrohepatic vena cava. J Trauma 30:328, 1990.
3. Burch JM, Ortiz VB, Richardson RJ, et al: Abbreviated laparotomy and planned reoperation for critically injured patients. Ann Surg 215:476, 1992.
4. Burch JM, Moore EE: Hepatic trauma. In Moore EE, Mattox KL, Feliciano DV (eds): Trauma, 3rd ed. Norwalk, CT, Appleton & Lange, 1996.
5. Cogbill TH, Moore EE, Jurkovich GJ, et al: Severe hepatic trauma: A multi-center experience with 1,335 liver injuries. J Trauma 28:1433, 1988.
6. Croce MA, Fabian TC, Kudsk KA, et al: AAST Organ Injury Scale: Correlation of CT-graded liver injuries and operative findings. J Trauma 31:806, 1991.
7. Croce MA, Fabian TC, Menke PG, et al: Nonoperative management of blunt hepatic trauma is the treatment of choice for hemodynamically stable patients. Ann Surg 221:744, 1995.
8. Cue JI, Cryer HG, Miller FB, et al: Packing and planned reexploration for hepatic and retroperitoneal hemorrhage: Critical refinements of a useful technique. Trauma 30:1007, 1990.
9. Fabian TC, Croce MA: Abdominal trauma, including indications for celiotomy. In Moore EE, Mattox KL, Feliciano DV (eds): Trauma, 3rd ed. Norwalk, CT, Appleton & Lange, 1996.
10. Feliciano DV, Mattox KL, Jordan GL, et al: Management of 1000 consecutive cases of hepatic trauma (1979–1984). Ann Surg 204:438, 1986.
11. Feliciano DV, Pachter HL (eds): Hepatic trauma revisited. Curr Probl Surg 26(7), 1989.
12. Hiatt JR, Gabbay J, Busuttil RW: Surgical anatomy of the hepatic arteries in 1000 cases Ann Surg 220:50, 1994.
13. Meldrum DR, Moore FA, Moore EE, et al: Cardiopulmonary hazards of perihepatic packing for major liver injury. Am J Surg 170:537–542, 1995.
14. Meredith JW, Young JS, Bowling J, Roboussin D: Nonoperative management of adult blunt hepatic trauma: The exception or the rule? J Trauma 36:529, 1994.
15. Moore EE, Cogbill TH, Malangoni MA, et al: Organ injury scaling. Surg Clin North Am 75:2, 1995.
16. Morris JA Jr, Eddy VA, Binman TA, et al: The staged celiotomy for trauma. Ann Surg 217:576, 1993.
17. Pachter HL, Hofstetter SR: The current status of nonoperative management of adult blunt hepatic injuries. Am J Surg 169:442, 1995.
18. Poggetti RS, Moore EE, Moore FA, et al: Balloon tamponade for bilobar transfixing hepatic gunshot wounds. J Trauma 33:694, 1992.
19. Rozycki GS, Ochsner MG, Jaffin JH, Champion HR: Prospective evaluation of surgeons' use of ultrasound in the evaluation of trauma patients. J Trauma 34:516, 1993.

21. PANCREATIC AND DUODENAL INJURY

R. *Franciose, M.D., and* Jon M. *Burch, M.D.*

1. How often are the pancreas and duodenum injured in trauma?

Because of the relatively protected deep central retroperitoneal location of the pancreas and duodenum (except for the first portion of the duodenum), traumatic injuries are uncommon. Approximately 7% of patients undergoing laparotomy for trauma have a pancreatic injury. In large trauma centers fewer than 10 severe combined pancreaticoduodenal (PD) injuries are seen each year.

2. What are the determinants of mortality after pancreatic and duodenal injury?

The major determinants of outcome after pancreatic and duodenal injury are mechanism of injury, associated injuries, and combination of pancreatic and duodenal injury. Most early deaths are due to exsanguinating hemorrhage from associated vascular, liver, or spleen injuries. Ninety percent of patients with pancreatic or duodenal injuries have at least one associated injury, with an average of 3–4 associated intraabdominal injuries per patient. The single most important determinant of outcome with pancreatic injury is the presence of a major pancreatic duct injury.

3. What mechanisms and patterns of injury are associated with trauma to the duodenum and pancreas?

Blunt pancreatic and duodenal injuries are caused primarily by deceleration injuries; in fact, at least 60% of blunt pancreatic injuries are due to steering wheel injuries. The three lesions associated with blunt injuries to the pancreas and duodenum are perforation of the duodenum, transection of the neck of the pancreas, and duodenal hematoma. Penetrating injuries to the pancreas and duodenum, most commonly caused by hand guns, result in complex localized tissue disruption with a high incidence of associated vascular injuries.

4. How are pancreatic and duodenal injuries diagnosed?

Because of the predominantly retroperitoneal position of the pancreas and duodenum, such injuries are hard to detect. A high index of suspicion based on mechanism of injury is necessary to prevent a delay in diagnosis. Diagnostic peritoneal lavage may be negative without associated injuries. Double-contrast CT scan and soluble-contrast upper gastrointestinal studies (c-loop study) may be helpful but require expert interpretation. Pancreatic ductal injuries may require endoscopic retrograde cholangiopancreatography (ERCP) or an intraoperative pancreatogram for diagnosis. The most reliable diagnostic maneuver is a thorough exploration of the pancreas and duodenum at laparotomy.

5. What are the four portions of the duodenum and their surgical relationships?

The first portion of the duodenum starts at the pylorus of the stomach (intraperitoneally) and passes backward (retroperitoneally) toward the gallbladder (the remainder of the duodenum is retroperitoneal). The second portion descends 7–8 cm and is anterior to the vena cava. The left border of the duodenum is attached to the head of the pancreas, at the site where the common bile and pancreatic ducts enter; it shares a common blood supply with the head of the pancreas through the pancreaticoduodenal arcades. The third portion of the duodenum turns horizontally to the left, with its cranial surface in contact with the uncinate process of the pancreas, and passes posterior to the superior mesenteric artery and vein. The fourth portion continues to the left, ascending slightly and crossing the spine anterior to the aorta, where it is fixed to the suspensory ligament of Treitz at the duodenojejunal flexure.

6. What is the Kocher maneuver?

The Kocher maneuver is an incision of the lateral parietal peritoneal attachment of the second and third portions of the duodenum; blunt retroperitoneal dissection is carried medially to the level of the vena cava. This approach provides access to the posterior duodenum, distal common bile duct, and head of the pancreas.

7. What are the five parts of the pancreas and their relevant surgical anatomy?

The pancreas is a fixed retroperitoneal organ lying transversely between the duodenal sweep and the spleen. The **head** of the pancreas is firmly fixed to the medial aspect of the second and third portions of the duodenum and lies to the right of the superior mesenteric vessels. The **uncinate process**, an extension of the lower portion of the head, passes behind the portal vein and superior mesenteric vessels and in front of the aorta and vena cava. The **neck** of the pancreas, which overlies the superior mesenteric vessels, is the most common area for blunt traumatic transection. The **body** of the pancreas continues to the left of the superior mesenteric vessels. The body is the portion most readily visible through the lesser sac. The **tail** is relatively mobile and resides in the hilum of the spleen. The splenic artery runs along the upper border of the pancreas, and the splenic vein runs behind the pancreas.

8. How are duodenal perforations treated?

Approximately 80% of duodenal perforations can be treated by primary repair. The remaining 20% are severe injuries that require complex procedures such as pyloric exclusion, Roux-en-y duodenojejunostomy, vascularized jejunal graft, or, in rare cases, pancreaticoduodenectomy (Whipple procedure).

9. What is pyloric exclusion?

A gastrotomy is performed to protect tenuous duodenal repairs, and the pylorus is oversewn with a heavy suture. A gastrojejunostomy is then fashioned to divert the gastric contents away from the repair. The pylorus spontaneously opens within a few weeks in most patients.

10. What is a duodenal hematoma? How is it treated?

Duodenal hematomas are subseromuscular hematomas that cause duodenal obstruction associated with persistent vomiting. Although they may occur in adults after blunt injury, they usually are considered an injury of childhood or child abuse. They are diagnosed with an upper GI contrast study; the "coiled spring" sign is considered pathognomonic. The majority of duodenal hematomas can be treated nonoperatively with continuous nasogastric suction and total parenteral nutrition.

11. How are pancreatic injuries treated?

Minor pancreatic injuries that do not involve the main pancreatic duct can be treated by external drainage or left alone. Injuries involving the neck, body, or tail of the pancreas can be treated with distal pancreatectomy. Extensive injury to the head of the pancreas or proximal main pancreatic duct requires complex reconstruction or, in rare cases, pancreaticoduodenectomy (Whipple procedure).

12. How much pancreas can be resected without subsequent endocrine or exocrine dysfunction?

In most people 80% of the pancreas can be resected without endocrine or exocrine dysfunction. A distal pancreatectomy at the level of the portal vein removes an average of 55% of the pancreas and thus is well tolerated.

13. What complications are specific to pancreatic and duodenal injuries?

Pancreatic injuries are associated with pancreatic fistulas, pancreatitis, and pancreatic pseudocysts. Duodenal injuries are associated with duodenal fistulas. One-third of patients who survive the first 48 hours have a complication related to the pancreatic or duodenal injury. Such complications contribute significantly to the sepsis and multiple organ failure that are responsible for most late deaths.

BIBLIOGRAPHY

1. Asensio JA, Feliciano DV, Britt LD, et al: Management of duodenal injuries. Curr Probl Surg 30:1021–1100, 1993.
2. Berg AA: Duodenal fistula: Its treatment by gastrojejunostomy and pyloric occlusion. Ann Surg 45:721, 1907.
3. Buck J, Sorensen V, Fath J, et al: Severe pancreaticoduodenal injuries: The effectiveness of pyloric exclusion with vagotomy. Am Surg 58:557–560, 1992.
4. Burch JM, Moore EE: Duodenal and pancreatic trauma. In Taylor M, Gollan J, Steer M, Wolfe M (eds): Gastrointestinal Emergencies. Baltimore, Williams & Wilkins, 1996.
5. Cogbill T, Moore E, Feliciano D, et al: Conservative management of duodenal trauma: A multicenter perspective. J Trauma 30:1469–1475, 1990.
6. Cogbill TH, Moore EE, Morris JA, et al: Distal pancreatectomy for trauma: A multicenter experience. J Trauma 31:1600–1606, 1991.
7. Heimansohn D, Canal D, McCarthy M, et al: The role of pancreaticoduodenectomy in the management of traumatic injuries to the pancreas and duodenum. Am J Surg 56:511–514, 1990.
8. Jurkovich GJ: Injury to the duodenum and pancreas. In Feliciano DV, Moore EE, Mattox KL (eds): Trauma, 3rd ed. Norwalk, CT, Appleton & Lange, 1996.
9. Jurkovich G, Carrico C: Management of pancreatic injuries. Surg Clin North Am 70(3):575–593, 1990.
10. Kunin JR, Korobkin M, Ellis JH, et al: Duodenal injuries caused by blunt abdominal trauma. Value of CT in differentiating perforation form hematoma. AJR 160:1221–1223, 1993.
11. Moore E, Cogbill T, Malangoni M, et al: Organ injury scaling. II: Pancreas, duodenum, small bowel, colon, and rectum. J Trauma 30:1427–1429, 1990.
12. Pachter HL, Hofstetter SR, Liange HG, et al: Traumatic injuries to the pancreas: The role of distal pancreatectomy with splenic preservation. J Trauma 29:1342, 1989.
13. Sivit CH, Eichelburger MR, Taylor GA, et al: Blunt pancreatic trauma in children: CT diagnosis. AJR 158:1097–1100, 1992.
14. Stone A, Sugawa C, Lucas C, et al: The role of endoscopic retrograde pancreatography (ERP) in blunt abdominal trauma. Am Surg 56:715–720, 1990.
15. Wisner DH, Wold RL, Frey CR: Diagnosis and treatment of pancreatic injuries. Arch Surg 125:1109–1113, 1990.

22. PENETRATING NECK WOUNDS

Robert A. Read, M.D., and Ernest E. Moore, M.D.

1. Why are penetrating neck injuries unique?

This small area of the body (1% of body surface area) contains numerous vital structures, including the larynx, trachea, thoracic duct, carotid arteries, vertebral and subclavian arteries and veins, external and internal jugular veins, spinal column and cord, cranial nerves, brachial plexus, pharynx, esophagus, thyroid, parathyroid, and salivary glands.

2. What tissue plane of the neck must be penetrated to constitute a penetrating neck wound?

The platysma muscle must be penetrated. This investing fascial layer of the neck is superficial to all vital structures.

3. What are anterior and posterior neck injuries?

The anterior cervical triangle is bounded by the midline, the lower border of the mandible, and the anterior border of the sternocleidomastoid muscle. The posterior cervical triangle is formed by the posterior border of the sternocleidomastoid muscle, the middle one-third of the clavicle, and the anterior border of the trapezius muscle. Wounds in the anterior triangle are more worrisome because of the associated vascular and tracheoesophageal injuries. Wounds in the posterior triangle are associated with fewer life-threatening injuries; however, they may involve major neurologic and vascular structures.

4. What are level I, II, and III injuries?
Level I injuries are inferior to the cricoid cartilage; level II injuries are between the cricoid cartilage and the angle of the mandible; and level III injuries are superior to the angle of the mandible.

HISTORY AND PHYSICAL EXAMINATION

5. What questions in the history are most important?
Dysphagia, dysphonia, hemoptysis, neurologic deficits, and shock or substantial blood loss at the accident scene suggest a serious injury.

6. What physical signs are most important?
Persistent bleeding or shock, dysphonia, hoarseness, stridor, enlarging hematoma, crepitus, and neurologic deficits suggest that a vital structure has been injured.

7. How often do patients with crepitus have an aerodigestive injury?
One-third of patients with crepitus have an injury of the pharynx, larynx, esophagus, or trachea. In two-thirds of such patients, however, the air has been introduced through the wound entrance site and there is no significant underlying injury.

8. Do gunshot wounds and knife wounds cause the same relative injuries?

Injury Patterns for Penetrating Neck Wounds

	GUNSHOT WOUNDS (%)	KNIFE WOUNDS (%)
Artery	18	11
Vein	13	30
Airway	23	7
Esophagus	27	7

9. Which side of the neck is more likely to be injured?
The left side of the neck is more likely to be injured, because most assailants are right-handed.

PATIENT MANAGEMENT

10. Should arteriograms be performed on all patients?
Preoperative arteriograms are generally performed in hemodynamically stable patients with level I or II injuries. Their value in this setting is to identify injuries to major vessels in the thoracic outlet or at the base of the skull that may require a special operative approach.

11. What is the value of other diagnostic studies, such as barium esophageal swallow, esophagoscopy, laryngoscopy, bronchoscopy, and CT scans?
Adjunctive studies are most important in the early diagnosis of occult esophageal injuries, which are associated with a 15–30% mortality risk if not treated promptly. Unfortunately, such studies may be falsely negative in 20–50% of cases.

12. How should deep-neck bleeding be controlled at the accident scene and in the emergency department?
Direct pressure is nearly always successful, even for major arterial lesions. Occasionally, a patient with level I vascular injury (base of the neck) requires an emergency department thoracotomy for adequate control.

13. What are the management priorities in the emergency department?
The ABC (airway, breathing, circulation) principles of trauma resuscitation apply; thus the patient's airway is a top priority. Patients who are neurologically intact (the majority) may be intubated orally. Patients who present with a neurologic deficit require simultaneous protection of the cervical spine and airway; they may require either nasotracheal intubation or cricothyrotomy. Early airway control is particularly critical in patients with an expanding cervical hematoma.

14. What is selective management of penetrating neck wounds?
Most surgeons do not explore all neck wounds. The current literature suggests that up to 50% of penetrating neck wounds are not associated with significant injury. Wounds that result in signs or symptoms of significant injury or that cannot be reliably observed (e.g., in intoxicated patients) are promptly explored in the operating room. Most alert and asymptomatic patients are either evaluated with a combination of diagnostic studies or observed expectantly with frequent serial physical examinations.

15. What are the advantages of selective management?
The morbidity and cost of unnecessary neck surgery are avoided.

16. Should an asymptomatic patient with a penetrating neck wound be sent home from the emergency department?
Life-threatening penetrating neck injuries initially may be clinically silent; therefore, the safest policy is to observe *all* patients in the hospital for at least 24 hours.

BIBLIOGRAPHY

1. Asensio JA, Valenziano CP, Falcone RE, et al: Management of penetrating neck injuries. Surg Clin North Am 71:267–296, 1991.
2. Beitsch P, Weigelt JA, Flynn E, et al: Physical examination and arteriograph in patients with penetrating zone II neck wounds. Arch Surg 129:577–581, 1994.
3. Bishara RA, Pasch AR, Douglas DD, et al: The necessity of mandatory exploration of penetrating zone II neck injuries. Surgery 100:655–660, 1986.
4. Elerding SC, Manart FD, Moore EE. A reappraisal of penetrating injury management. J Trauma 20:695–697, 1980.
5. Feliciano DV, Bitondo CG, Mattox KL, et al: Combined tracheoesophageal injuries. Am J Surg 150:710–715, 1985.
6. Monsour MA, Moore EE, Moore FA, Whitehill TA: Validating the selective management of penetrating neck wounds. Am J Surg 162:517–521, 1991.
7. Ngakane H, Muckar DJ, Luvunno FM: Penetrating visceral injuries of the neck: Result of a conservative management policy. Br J Surg 77:908–910, 1990.
8. Winter RP, Weigelt JA: Cranial esophageal trauma. Arch Surg 125:849–852, 1990.
9. Wood J, Fabian TC, Mongiante EC: Penetrating neck injuries: Recommendations for selective management. J Trauma 29:602–605, 1989.

23. FACIAL LACERATIONS

Lawrence L. Ketch, M.D.

1. What distinguishes facial from other lacerations?
Cosmesis (appearance) is clearly of primary importance. Quality of the final result depends on strict adherence to basic principles of wound management and painstaking technique. Copious irrigation, judicious debridement, gentle tissue handling, meticulous hemostasis, and minimization of sutures combined with early stitch removal are critical to an optimal result. Fine suture and

sharp instruments are to be used, and eversion of the wound margin with layered closure, obliteration of dead space, and lack of tension are mandatory.

2. What factors influence choice of treatment for the wound?

The mechanism of injury, the clinical assessment of contamination, and the time elapsed since wounding dictate treatment. Clean lacerations, heavily contaminated wounds, crush injuries, and bites are all treated differently.

3. How are clean lacerations repaired?

Clean lacerations should be irrigated with normal saline or Ringer's lactate. Only the surrounding skin should be prepared, and no antiseptic should be introduced into the wound. Regional anesthesia is preferred because of the potential for spread of contamination with direct injection of the wound margin. Epinephrine should be avoided, because it devitalizes tissue and potentiates infection. Wounds should be repaired in layers with absorbable suture in the deep tissue. The smallest number of sutures necessary to overcome the natural resting wound tension should be used. Sutures should be removed within 3–5 days and the wound margin supported with Steri-strips subsequently.

4. How are dirty lacerations repaired?

In general, heavily contaminated wounds remain open following irrigation and debridement to undergo delayed closure. However, because of cosmetic considerations, this approach is unacceptable in the face. For this reason, meticulous debridement of devitalized tissue and removal of all foreign bodies are necessary. The wound should be cultured prior to copious irrigation, and a broad-spectrum antibiotic should be instituted prophylactically. The patient must be informed of the potential for a postrepair infection.

5. What factors influence suture selection?

Any method of suturing perpetuates tissue damage, impairs host defense, increases scar proliferation, and invites infection. Presence of a single silk suture in a wound will lower the infective threshold by a factor of 10,000. Therefore, fine, monofilament suture, just strong enough to overcome the resting wound tension, should be used. The amount of suture material placed in the wound should be minimized. Wounds with little or no retraction should be closed with tape, as this is the least injurious approach and produces the best scar.

6. Should eyebrows be shaved when repairing facial lacerations?

No. They provide a landmark for realignment of disrupted tissue edges and do not always grow back.

7. How should crush avulsion injuries with associated skin loss be repaired?

Crush avulsion injuries result in irregular wound edges and devitalized tissue. Nonviable elements must be surgically excised, because they predispose to infection and lead to excessive scarring. If there is doubt concerning viability, the wound should be thoroughly irrigated and left open with continuous moist dressings. A delayed closure can be accomplished when the questionable areas have declared themselves. It is often prudent to close facial tissue as it lies; this technique often produces a less obtrusive scar than straight-line debridement and closure.

8. How should bites be treated?

Both animal and human bite wounds are highly contaminated and prone to infection. Again, because of cosmetic considerations, the wound should be treated as outlined above and closed meticulously. Antibiotic prophylaxis is indicated, and, if the wound becomes infected, the sutures must be removed and the wound allowed to heal. In this circumstance, the patient should be informed that a scar revision will be necessary.

9. Should skin grafts or flaps be used for primary closure of a wound?
Complicated tissue transfer techniques have no place in the acute treatment of the facial wound. Closure should be achieved in the simplest way possible, and complex reconstructive efforts should be deferred until the scar has matured. With tissue loss such that direct closure is impossible, it may be necessary to use a thin split-thickness ski graft to obtain closure.

10. When are antibiotics indicated in the treatment of facial lacerations?
Adherence to previously outlined principles of copious irrigation, debridement, and gentle tissue handling are more pertinent to the prevention of infection than the use of antibiotics in clean and clean-contaminated wounds. Antibiotic coverage is indicated, however, in crush avulsion injuries, bites, and heavily contaminated injuries.

11. What determines the quality of scar?
Location of the wound, age of patient, and type and quality of skin are of great significance in the final outcome. Lesser determinants are the type and quantity of suture material used and the wound care employed. Final appearance depends little on the method of suture. Contusion, infection, retained foreign body, improper orientation of laceration, tension, and beveling of edges predict a poor outcome. Differences among suture materials are negligible. However, the technical factors of suture placement to produce wound eversion and time to removal do affect the final result.

12. When should scars be revised?
A scar usually has its worst appearance at 2 weeks to 2 months after suturing. Scar revision should await complete maturation, which can take 4–24 months. A good rule of thumb is to undertake no revisions for least 6–12 months following initial repair. The maturation of the wound may be assessed by its degree of discomfort, erythema, and induration.

CONTROVERSIES

There is little controversy regarding the care and repair of facial lacerations. Attention to basic principles of wound care usually produces a satisfactory scar. Because of the cosmetic considerations in facial trauma, there are several instances, as elucidated, in which primary repair is undertaken for the sake of appearance despite the risk of infection, which, in other areas of the body, would be deemed unacceptable.

BIBLIOGRAPHY

1. Mason PN: Facial injuries. In McCarthy JG (ed): Plastic Surgery, vol. 2. Philadelphia, W.B. Saunders, 1990, pp 899–916.
2. Davis PKB, Shaheen O: Soft tissue injuries of the face and scalp: Fractures of the larynx. In Rowe NL, Williams JL (eds): Maxillofacial Injuries. New York, Churchill Livingstone, 1985, pp 184–200.
3. Junkiewicz MJ, Krizek TJ, Mathes SJ, Ariyan S: Principles and practice. In Plastic Surgery, St. Louis, Mosby, 1990, pp 244–277.

24. BASIC CARE OF HAND INJURIES

Michael J.V. Gordon, M.D., and Lawrence L. Ketch, M.D.

1. What are the goals of hand repair?
Functional considerations override cosmesis in the treatment of hand trauma. There are no minor hand injuries. Initial diagnosis and management determine the final result; expert secondary repair cannot overcome primary neglect or errors in diagnosis or decision making.

2. What determines the final outcome of a hand injury?
Minimal sacrifice of tissue and primary healing accomplished by early wound closure are essential. Minimization of scar tissue by control of edema, prevention of infection, early wound closure, and vigorous physical therapy produces the optimal functional outcome.

3. What factors influence treatment of hand trauma?
Mechanism, location, and timing of injury and hand dominance, occupation, age, and general health of the patient help to determine treatment plans.

4. How common are occupational hand injuries?
Hand injuries result in more days lost from work than any other type of occupational injury.

5. What are the essentials of examination of the hand?
Inspection of position, color, and temperature often reveals the injury. Location suggests possible injury to underlying structures. Motor, sensory, and Doppler ultrasonic examination are confirmatory. All injuries must be x-rayed, and surgical exploration provides the definitive diagnosis.

6. How and where should hand injuries be explored?
Hand wounds should be explored under tourniquet control with adequate analgesia, using delicate instruments in a well-lighted surgery suite. Visual magnification is usually mandatory.

7. How is emergency hemostasis of the injured hand achieved?
In the acute setting, outside the operating suite, no tourniquet should be applied, and there should be no blind clamping of any structures within the injured part. Hemostasis may be achieved by elevation of the extremity with direct compression of the wound. This approach prevents injury to delicate underlying structures that cannot be identified under such circumstances.

8. How are fingertip injuries treated?
If less than 1 cm of pulp is disrupted, the wound will heal spontaneously with daily cleansing and dressing with nonadherent, moist gauze. Larger defects may require a skin graft, which often can be provided by defatting the amputated piece. Bone exposure necessitates flap coverage if digital length is to be maintained. Digital nerves cannot be repaired distal to the distal interphalangeal joint.

9. What is the classification system for fingertip amputations?

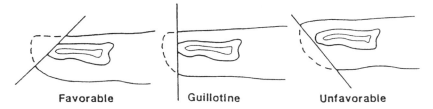

Favorable   Guillotine   Unfavorable

Classification for fingertip amputations based on the amount of remaining sensate volar skin. Although the favorably angulated amputation commonly removes some nail and bone, the volar skin is available for easy coverage. This amputation type is "favorable" for treatment by dressings only, allowing wound repair by contraction and epithelialization. The volarly angulated amputation angle is "unfavorable" for conservative management and usually requires a reconstructive procedure. (From Ditmars DM Jr: Fingertip and nail bed injuries. In Kasdan ML (ed): Occupational Hand and Upper Extremity Injuries and Disease. Philadelphia, Hanley & Belfus, 1991, with permission.)

10. How are nailbed injuries repaired?
Subungual hematoma should be evacuated by a hot-tipped paper clip or battery-powered electric cautery. Repair of the disruption of the sterile or germinal matrix must be meticulously

approximated under magnification and the nailbed splinted, preferably with the avulsed part. The eponychial fold must be maintained for 3 weeks with Xeroform gauze or with the original nail. Often, nailbed disruption cannot be diagnosed without removal of the nail.

11. What is the initial management of flexor tendon laceration?
Flexor tendon laceration is not an emergency, and repair should not be undertaken in the emergency department by an unskilled person. If a hand surgeon is unavailable, the wound should be copiously irrigated and sutured and prophylactic antibiotics instituted. The patient should be referred for definitive repair.

12. What is the proper management of an open fracture?
Open fractures should be cultured and then undergo copious lavage with normal saline or Ringer's lactate. Broad-spectrum antibiotic coverage should be instituted, and the part should be splinted in the position of function with a bulky dressing.

13. What is the proper treatment for hand infection?
The extremity should be immobilized and elevated, and parenteral antibiotics should be given. The patient should be referred immediately for possible surgical drainage.

14. What is the proper management of human bites?
Initial evaluation includes radiographs and cleansing of the wound. The wound should be left open—never closed. Antibiotics are started, and the wound is rechecked at 24 and 48 hours. If evidence of infection is present, parenteral antibiotics should be instituted and referral for possible surgical drainage should be made. The so-called "fight bite" occurs over the metacarpophalangeal (MCP) joint or proximal interphalangeal (PIP) joint when a clenched fist is impaled on the front teeth of the adversary. This injury often inoculates the MCP joint with anaerobic streptococci. When infection is diagnosed, immediate arthrotomy and lavage should be performed.

15. How are injection injuries treated?
Despite their innocuous appearance, injection injuries may cause profound destruction of hand structures. Any such injury requires immediate hospitalization with prompt and extensive decompression and debridement.

16. What is carpal tunnel syndrome (CTS)?
CTS is the most common peripheral compression neuropathy; it is signaled by numbness and tingling of the hand.

17. Is CTS more common in older or younger people? Men or women?
CTS is more common in people over 40 years of age, but an increasing number of young people with CTS have been reported in recent years, usually those whose jobs involve repetitive manual labor. Women are affected approximately twice as often as men.

18. What are the most preventable causes of deformity in hand injuries?
Edema and infection lead to increased scarring and restricted function. Prolonged immobilization in poor position also impairs function, as does delayed skin closure. Failure to obtain a radiograph or a missed diagnosis with delay in recognition of an injury has severe consequences.

19. What is the proper emergency department treatment of all hand injuries?
The patient should be sedated and the wound cultured and irrigated. A thorough examination must be performed and a sterile compression dressing placed. The upper extremity should be splinted, tetanus prophylaxis should be administered, and broad-spectrum antibiotic coverage instituted for crush avulsion or heavily contaminated wounds. A radiograph should be obtained and blood drawn for preoperative laboratory tests.

20. What are the guidelines for replantation of an amputated part?
There are no absolute guidelines. A microsurgeon who is a member of a replantation team should be consulted. If replantation is planned, parts should not be immersed directly in water or put directly on ice or dry ice. The part should be copiously irrigated, wrapped in a moist sponge, and placed in a sterile plastic container; the plastic container should be placed in an ice-water slurry for transport.

BIBLIOGRAPHY

1. American Society for Surgery of the Hand: The Hand: Primary Care of Common Problems. New York, Churchill Livingstone, 1985.
2. Dray GS, Eaton RG: Dislocations and ligament injuries in the digits. In Green DP (ed): Operative Hand Surgery. New York, Churchill Livingstone, 1988.
3. Flatt AE: The Care of Minor Hand Injuries, 2nd ed. St Louis, Mosby, 1963.
4. Flynn JE: Hand Surgery, 3rd ed. Baltimore, Williams & Wilkins, 1982.
5. Green DP: Operative Hand Surgery, 2nd ed. New York, Churchill Livingstone, 1988.
6. Hunter JM, Schneider LH, Mackin EJ, Callahan AD (eds): Rehabilitation of the Hand, 3rd ed. St. Louis, Mosby, 1990.
7. Kasdan ML (ed): Occupational Hand and Upper Extremity Injuries and Diseases. Philadelphia, Hanley & Belfus, 1991.
8. Sinclair TM, Williams HB: Hand infection. In Wilmore DW, Cheung LY, Harken AH, et al (eds): Infection, vol 15. New York, Scientific American, 1995, pp 2–11.

25. FROSTBITE

Ben Eiseman, M.D., and Bruce Paton, M.D.

1. What is frostbite?
Frostbite is local tissue damage due to exposure to a cold environment and freezing of cells.

2. What factors influence the extent of tissue injury after cold exposure?
Factors affecting the extent of damage include the degree of cold (temperature), duration of exposure, windchill factor, protection of the exposed parts, adequacy of circulation, and accelerated heat loss due to contact with water or metal.

3. What is the importance of windchill?
Windchill is a term used to quantify the increased heat loss due to winds of various velocities. Increasing wind velocity does not reduce the temperature but increases the rate of heat loss so that the ambient temperature is equivalent, in terms of heat loss and potential for frostbite or hypothermia, to a much lower temperature.

The effects of windchill can be prevented with suitable protective clothing and protection of exposed parts such as hands, face, and ears. Oil-based protective creams also may alleviate some of the heat loss if applied liberally to nose, lips, cheeks, and ears.

4. Can exposure to temperatures above freezing cause tissue damage?
Prolonged exposure of an extremity to a wet environment at temperatures above freezing may produce damage similar to frostbite (trench foot, immersion foot).

5. What is the cause of tissue damage in frostbite?
Theories include damage due to extracellular ice crystals, red cell sludging, thrombosis, and direct effects of temperatures < 6 C° on cells.Frostbite is a form of ischemic/reperfusion injury similar to tissue damage of the myocardium, kidney, or gut after vascular occlusion and reperfusion.

Frostbite is similarly associated with release of cytotoxic cytokines, such as tumor necrosis factor; various interleukins; adhesive molecules; and cytotoxic substances, such as superoxides and proteases. Neutralizing such cytokines and adhesive molecules before rewarming may attenuate cold injury, but to date this has not proved to be clinically helpful.

6. What are the principles of preventing frostbite?
Avoid exposure of unprotected extremities or exposed parts of the face to cold, wetness, and contact with metal. Keep extremities dry. In military contexts (where frostbite is often of epidemic proportions during a winter campaign) frostbite characteristically occurs in retreating, demoralized troops in whom discipline has broken down.

7. What are diagnostic signs and symptoms?
An exposed extremity initially appears deathly white (ischemic) and then loses both afferent (anesthetic, numb) and efferent (paralytic) innervation.

8. What are the principles of early management of suspected frostbite?
Avoid a freeze-thaw-freeze cycle. Do not rub the part with snow. Once the patient is in a controlled environment and will not be reexposed to cold, immerse the frostbitten extremity in water at 40–45°C (warm to the touch) until it has regained normal body temperature (20–30 minutes). Rewarming often causes pain. Place a sterile or clean nonocclusive dressing over the frostbitten area. Clear blisters may be punctured or unroofed and treated with sterile aloe vera ointment. Keep hemorrhagic blisters that signify deep damage intact.

9. Is any systemic therapy of proven value in the early management of frostbite?
About the only therapy of proven value is rewarming with general support of the patient, avoiding hypothermia, and maintaining circulation. There is no documented benefit of miracle treatments, although many have been suggested, including anticoagulants, sympatholytic drugs, sympathectomy, vasodilators, hyperbaric oxygen, low-molecular-weight dextran, drugs that lower surface tension, and drugs that interfere with platelet activity. It is frustrating, but even the best clinician must stand by and watch. The best that one can do is not to extend tissue injury by ill-advised interference. Give antibiotics only for secondary infection, and tetanus antiserum should be given according to established indications. Daily whirlpool baths provide gentle debridement. Fasciotomy is occasionally necessary if the part is very swollen and circulation is compromised.

10. What is the clinical course of frostbite?
The extent of damage in frostbitten tissue may be slow to declare itself. Blisters develop within 4–8 hours. Clear blisters signify superficial damage, whereas hemorrhagic blisters located proximally on digits indicate deep damage. Blisters shrivel and become escharotic in 7–10 days. Gangrene is obvious in 10–20 days and typically becomes definitive in 30–60 days.

11. What are the long-term residua of frostbite?
1. Hypersensitivity to cold, frequently for life.
2. Hyperhidrosis
3. In children, epiphyseal damage leading to arthritis and faulty digital growth

BIBLIOGRAPHY

1. McCauley RL, Hing D, Robson MC, Heggers JP: Frostbite injuries: A rational approach based on the pathophysiology. Trauma 23:143–147, 1983.
2. Mills WJ, et al: Cold injury. Alaska Med Jan–Mar:5–143, 1993.
3. Paton BC: Pathophysiology of frostbite. In Sutton JR, Houston CS, Coates G (eds): Hypoxia and Cold. New York, Praeger, 1987, pp 329–339.

26. UPPER URINARY TRACT TRAUMA: KIDNEY AND URETER

Norman E. Peterson, M.D.

1. When does one suspect renal trauma?
When hematuria follows trauma (even microhematuria). Certain other injuries often coexist with renal trauma (liver, spleen, colon, spinal transverse process) and may assist diagnosis.

2. How does one investigate renal trauma?
It is traditional for patients with posttraumatic hematuria to undergo cystourethrography and excretory urography (intravenous pyelography [IVP]). Epidemiologic analysis reveals that upper and lower urinary tract injuries rarely coexist in patients who survive. Therefore, diagnostic efforts may be confined to the site of major trauma: IVP or renal CT for abdominal, flank, or thoracic trauma and cystourethrography for lower abdominal and pelvic trauma. Renal integrity is appraised adequately by IVP. In patients undergoing CT scanning (with contrast enhancement) for other injuries, definitive renal examination is incorporated and IVP may be comfortably omitted.

3. What is a single-shot IVP?
A bolus (2 ml/kg Renografin) can be injected intravenously in transit to the operating room. The first film should be obtained at approximately 10 minutes, with additional films at 5–10-minute intervals as necessary for diagnosis. Hypotension or shock contraindicates urography. Intraoperative IVP is recommended when renal injury is suggested (e.g., retroperitoneal hematoma). Intraoperative arteriography also may be accomplished by injecting 5–10 ml of contrast agent directly into the renal artery with immediate film exposure.

4. How is renal trauma classified?
Renal injuries are consistently classified as grade 1 (contusion; 70%); grade 2 (superficial laceration; 15%); grade 3 (deep laceration or collecting system damage; 10%); and grade 4 (stellate parenchymal fragmentation or pedicle interruption; 5%). Grades 1 and 2 injuries are safely amenable to conservative management, whereas grades 3 and 4 require operative intervention for repair or removal. In addition, contrast extravasation is commonly believed to require operative repair. Grade 4 injuries (shattered kidney or pedicle injury) are reflected by ipsilateral urographic nonfunction and the pattern of "big-time" bleed. Therapy predicated exclusively on classification may be delusional, however, because spontaneous resolution is commonplace even with higher grades of injury.

5. Does the magnitude of renal bleeding alone reflect the significance or prognosis of injury?
The pattern of renal hemorrhage is the most reliable prognostic factor. Excluding pedicle interruption, which often is characterized by nominal hemorrhage, the status of renal bleeding within the first few hours after trauma constructively discriminates injuries amenable to spontaneous resolution from injuries requiring operative correction. Gross hematuria that subsides early (often before conclusion of emergency surgery for coexisting injuries) reliably identifies injury that may be exempted from emergency exploration. Conversely, unremitting hemorrhage or hemorrhage that subsides briefly but recurs requires open exploration or arteriography with selective therapeutic embolization.

6. Are there different kinds of renal pedicle trauma?
Yes. The renal pedicle may be interrupted by thrombosis or by complete avulsion; both events are characterized by nonvisualization on IVP and nominal hematuria. Although textbooks commonly

describe absence of hematuria, brief gross hematuria followed by microhematuria is the rule, underscoring the requirement for urinalysis in all circumstances. Left-sided pedicle avulsion produces little retroperitoneal bleeding because of prompt arterial retraction, whereas right-sided injuries often hemorrhage extensively because of avulsion of the vein from the vena cava. No reliable nonoperative method to distinguish pedicle thrombosis from avulsion is available.

7. What is the time limit of renal tolerance of warm ischemia?

Regardless of what transplant surgeons say (they cheat by cooling the kidney), the reversible limit of renal tolerance of warm ischemia is unknown and doubtless subject to several variables. Four hours emerges as a valid standard. It is unlikely that revascularization can be accomplished within this period; therefore, we advocate vascular repair only for selected circumstances (solitary kidney and marginal renal function).

8. Both pedicle trauma and parenchymal shattering are characterized by nonvisualization on IVP. Do they need to be distinguished?

Probably, although the distinction is not clinically obvious, because renal nonfunction is inevitable. As described, pedicle injury commonly produces minimal hematuria. In contrast, shattered kidneys are characterized by extensive and unremitting bleeding in flank, retroperitoneum, and urine; nephrectomy is necessary.

9. What is the significance of delayed gross hematuria?

Traditionally delayed gross hematuria warranted operative intervention and total or partial nephrectomy for unrecognized arteriovenous injury. Our series identified a 50% permanent spontaneous resolution with conservative management. In the remainder, selective therapeutic embolization is often successful. Knife wounds predominate in patients experiencing this complication.

10. What is the recommended response to unexpected intraoperative discovery of retroperitoneal bleeding?

Published discussions of retroperitoneal hematoma consistently refer to expansion and pulsation, both of which are rare. A pulsatile hematoma reflects a major vascular injury, and exploration must be preceded by vascular control and recognition that rapid blood replacement may be needed. Stable hematomas (above the pelvic brim), regardless of size, may remain undisturbed unless the IVP (preoperative or intraoperative) is frightening. When doubt exists, cautious exploration is warranted, with proper respect for the high nephrectomy rate associated with exploration in published series.

11. What is the recommended response to posttraumatic urine extravasation?

When urine extravasation coexists with extensive persistent bleeding into flank and urine, major laceration into the collecting system is likely, and operative correction is advised. Otherwise, urine extravasation commonly resolves promptly.

12. What conditions predispose to traumatic renal injury?

Abnormal renal anatomy tends to increase vulnerability to renal trauma. Preexisting abnormalities are dominated by hydronephrosis (50%) and abnormal position of the kidneys (pelvic, horseshoe). Renal tumors, particularly in children, must always be considered.

13. What is included in conservative management of renal trauma?

When clinical and radiographic appraisal endorses nonoperative management, bed rest is imposed until gross hematuria has subsided. Strenuous activity is avoided until microhematuria has subsided—usually within 3 weeks. Follow-up thereafter is often unnecessary. Patients followed for separated parenchymal fragments should undergo urography at 6 weeks, at which time anatomic restoration is usually complete. Hospitalization is not required during these periods. Conditions responsible for delayed hemorrhage are typically **not** corrected by prolonged bed rest; therefore, early ambulation and limited activity are intended to unmask conditions that may require therapeutic embolization or operative correction.

14. What is the likelihood of subsequent hypertension?
Renal hypertension is a consequence of ischemia rather than infarction, thereby discouraging routine surgical responses to partial or total renal infarction. Authenticated posttraumatic hypertension occurs in under 2% of cases overall. Onset generally occurs within the first several months of injury; blood pressure is often controllable with salt restriction or diuretic therapy.

15. Do blunt and penetrating renal injuries pose different clinical challenges and demand different responses?
No. Injuries to the kidney possess the same prognosis and demand the same responses regardless of the nature of the trauma. Clinical responses should be dictated, as always, by anatomic imaging and status of bleeding.

16. Under what circumstances should ureteral injury be suspected?
Excluding overt operative and endoscopic mishap, guns are the usual mode of ureteral injury. Ninety percent of violent ureteral injuries results from gunshot wounds. Conversely, 2.2–5% of abdominal gunshot wounds involve the ureter. Of all cases of penetrating urologic trauma, the ureter is injured in 17%. Site and tract of injury indicate the possibility of ureteral trauma, particularly when microscopic hematuria is present. Avulsion of the ureter from the renal pelvis may result from blunt forces producing hyperextension of the torso, notably in children. Injury to the distal ureter may occasionally result from fracture of the posterior pelvic ring.

17. How is ureteral injury identified or verified?
Clinical manifestations are characteristically subtle and often obscured by coexisting injury and complaints. Up to 90% of gunshot wounds and 60% of stabbings that injure the ureter also injure bowel, colon, liver, spleen, blood vessels, or pancreas. Hematuria is almost exclusively microscopic (but rarely absent, as many publications promise). IVP within the first 36 hours of injury reveals urinary extravasation in 90% of cases. After 36 hours, the IVP more commonly demonstrates obstruction at the site of injury (no extravasation), with proximal ureterectasis; extravasation is then identified by retrograde ureterography. Bladder and ureteral extravasations are differentiated by comparing cystogram with ureterogram.

18. How is a ureteral injury identified during surgery?
When ureteral injury is suspected during laparotomy without radiographic assistance, retroperitoneal exposure with induced diuresis (Lasix, 20-mg IV bolus) may disclose the site of injury. Indigo carmine (1 vial IV bolus) turns everything blue but may assist in locating the leak.

19. What are the potential consequences of missed ureteral injury?
Complications may include fever, leukocytosis, azotemia, flank pain, ileus, flank mass (urinoma), or urinary fistula. Presentation is often delayed to 2 weeks or more after injury. Fistulous drainage is confirmed as urine by creatinine content exceeding serum levels. In addition, absorption of urinoma or peritoneal extravasation elevates serum blood urea nitrogen (BUN) without corresponding increases in serum creatinine, thereby exaggerating the normal serum BUN/creatinine ratio of 10:1 to levels as high as 30:1.

20. What are the principles of ureteral repair?
The damaged ureter is debrided back to freely bleeding margins. The anastomosis must be a tension-free, spatulated closure with fine absorbable suture and internal ureteral stenting. The rest of the operation requires copious irrigation, adequate drainage, antibiotic coverage, and proper attention to coexisting injuries. Distal injuries are better served by direct tunneled implantation of the ureter into the bladder. Fat, omentum, or peritoneum should be interposed between repair site and adjacent muscle to prevent adhesion and obstruction.

BIBLIOGRAPHY

1. Cass AS, Bubrick M, Luxenburg M, et al: Renal trauma found during laparotomy for intra-abdominal injury. J Trauma 24:651, 1984.
2. Cosgrove MD, Mendez R, Morrow JW: Traumatic renal arteriovenous fistula. J Urol 110:627, 1973.
3. Esho JO, Ireland GW, Cass AS: Renal trauma and pre-existing lesions of the kidney. Urology 1:234, 1973.
4. McAninch JW: Genitourinary trauma. In Moore EE, Mattox KL, Feliciano DV (eds): Trauma, 2nd ed. Norwalk, CT, Appleton & Lange, 1991, p 571.
5. Peterson NE: Blunt renal injuries of intermediate degree. J Trauma 17:425, 1977.
6. Peterson NE: Significance of delayed post-traumatic renal segment. Urology 27:237, 1986.
7. Peterson NE: Fate of the functionless post-traumatic renal segment. Urology 27:237, 1986.
8. Peterson NE: Review article: Traumatic bilateral renal infarction. J Trauma 29:158, 1988.
9. Peterson NE, Norton L: Injuries associated with renal trauma. J Urol 109:766, 1973.
10. Peterson NE, Pitts JC III: Penetrating injuries of the ureter. J Urol 126:587, 1981.
11. Peterson NE, Schulze K: Selective diagnostic uroradiology for trauma. J Urol 137:449, 1987.
12. Whitney RF, Peterson NE: Penetrating renal injuries. Urology 7:7, 1976.

27. LOWER URINARY TRACT INJURY AND PELVIC TRAUMA

Norman E. Peterson, M.D.

1. What clinical circumstances promote suspicion of bladder injury?

Trauma to the lower abdomen or pelvis producing hematuria suggests bladder injury. Other signs may include inability to void or incomplete recovery of catheter irrigation. Associated injuries are sustained in 90% of patients. Trauma need not be excessive: a full bladder (know when to say when) is vulnerable to rupture from modest trauma. Penetrating wounds are also frequently re sponsible.

2. What types of bladder injury may occur?

Laceration or perforation may be either intra- or extraperitoneal. Extraperitoneal injuries constitute up to 85% of all bladder injuries.

3. What is the likelihood of a bladder injury in patients with a fractured pelvis?

Bladder injury coexists in 10% of all patients with pelvic fractures. Conversely, up to 83% of bladder injury results from (or coexists with) pelvic fracture. Intraperitoneal bladder rupture occurs with penetrating trauma or blunt blow-out of a distended bladder; therefore, pelvic fracture is not a requirement. Bladder injuries occur more frequently with parasymphyseal pubic arch fractures and more often with bilateral than unilateral fractures. Isolated ramus fractures produce bladder laceration in 10% of cases.

4. How is bladder injury verified?

Bladder injury should be suspected in patients with hematuria after trauma to lower abdomen or pelvis. Retrograde urethrocystogram provides 95% diagnostic accuracy for bladder rupture. The radiograph should be taken after introduction of 30 ml of a 50% dilution of standard radiocontrast agent by meatal syringe (fortunately trauma is a disease of males). Projections include anteroposterior and oblique films and either projection after voiding or catheter emptying. Extravasation is identified only by postevacuation films in 15% of patients. When renal or distal ureteral injury is suspected, IVP should be obtained before the cystogram. Diagnostic peritoneal lavage is unreliable (33% false-negative results).

5. What are the radiographic patterns of bladder injury?
Lateral contraction of the filled bladder ("teardrop") or elevation out of the pelvis ("pie in the sky") indicates perivesical hemorrhage, but not necessarily a breach of bladder integrity. Extraperitoneal injury allows contrast to escape adjacent to the symphysis, but it is confined to the bladder base by the intact peritoneum. Intraperitoneal extravasation produces a "sunburst" appearance from the bladder dome, which may collect in the paracolic gutters, outline loops of bowel, or pool under liver or spleen. Gross hematuria without extravasation constitutes bladder contusion and may be accompanied by perivesical hematoma.

6. How is bladder rupture managed?
Extraperitoneal lacerations respond to simple indwelling catheter drainage for 7–10 days, at which time cystogram usually confirms resolution of extravasation. Failure to resolve usually reflects a transmural bony spicule necessitating operative correction. Intraperitoneal lacerations are also frequently amenable to nonoperative resolution with catheter drainage. Bladder contusion requires catheter drainage until gross bleeding has subsided.

7. What clinical settings provide a need for appraisal of urethral injury?
Proximal urethral trauma classically accompanies pelvic fractures (crushing or deceleration/impact), with shearing forces focused at the prostatomembranous junction. Straddle injuries produce bulbous urethral damage. Distal urethral trauma is typically an isolated injury, often following assault or self-inflicted mutilation or autoerotic insertions. Urethral injury is heralded by blood at the urethral meatus, digital rectal disclosure of prostatic displacement, perineal ecchymosis, penile and/or scrotal swelling and ecchymosis, and inability to void or to pass a urethral catheter.

8. When a patient presents with a pelvic fracture, is concomitant urethral injury a major concern?
Yes. Urethral trauma occurs in 10% of pelvic fractures. It is more common with anterior disruption of the pelvic ring, including 20% of unilateral and 50% of bilateral parasymphyseal fractures.

9. How is urethral injury best assessed?
Retrograde urethrography must always be performed before inserting a Foley catheter (see question 4). Incomplete urethral transection is reflected by local extravasation accompanied by bladder opacification. Total avulsion produces extensive local extravasation and prevents contrast form entering the bladder. Incomplete transection is more common with anterior (50%) than posterior (10%) urethral injuries.

10. How is urethral injury managed?
For incomplete transection, regardless of site, catheter stenting across the defect is effective definitive therapy. Complete urethral transection should be decompressed initially via a suprapubic cystostomy. The next step is operative restoration of continuity with placement of a bridging urethral catheter. The bridging catheter method prevents complicated scarring, avoids subsequent surgery in many patients, and is easily incorporated into laparotomy for associated injuries.

11. What conditions may complicate urethral rupture or repair?
Complications include stricturing (usually correctable endoscopically), incontinence (uncommon), and impotence (statistically limited to traumatic prostatic displacement). Iatrogenic complications are associated with retropubic dissection or hematoma disturbance. Artificial remedies are available to permanently impotent patients.

12. How is pelvic fracture diagnosed?
Pelvic fracture must be suspected when pain and/or abnormal motion is produced by compression or manipulation of the pelvis and hips. Diagnosis is confirmed by pelvic radiographs or CT scanning.

13. What conclusions may be deduced from the nature of the trauma and type of injury?
Most classifications of pelvic fracture refer to lateral and anteroposterior compression or to vertical shearing. In many systems, acetabular fracture occupies a separate subgroup. Isolated ramus fractures are usually of nominal significance; however, urethral and bladder injury occur in 10%. Malgaigne fractures (any combination of anterior and posterior fractures or dislocations that results in an unstable pelvic ring) result most frequently from vertical shearing forces and may be complicated by vascular injuries.

Anteroposterior compression is often seen with pedestrian accidents and may open the pelvis anteriorly, including symphyseal separation ("open-book" deformity). Lateral compression commonly results from motor vehicle accidents and tends to produce displaced fractures of the anterior pelvic ring. Vertical shearing is characteristically seen with falls from heights and is associated with posterior pelvic (sacroiliac) fractures, notable for their instability.

14. What constitutes pelvic instability?
The pelvic ring must be breached; arbitrary definitions stipulate displacement of 2.5 cm for symphyseal or ramus fractures or 1 cm for sacroiliac joints.

15. What conditions may complicate pelvic fracture?
More extensive comminution and pelvic instability are associated with increasing levels of coexisting injury, blood loss, and morbidity and mortality.

Anorectal injury demands early diagnosis to limit septic complications. Blood on the examining finger warrants endoscopic and radiocontrast inspection; perineal escape of rectal or vesical irrigation is diagnostic. Surgical management includes pelvic irrigation and drainage, colostomy, and antibiotic therapy. Perineal laceration demands digital exploration. Pelvic fracture in women mandates examination for vaginal injury and possible laceration or avulsion of urethra or vesical outlet.

Destabilizing pelvic hemorrhage may persist despite all conservative efforts. Pelvic angiography may then disclose larger vessel involvement that necessitates operative intervention or bleeding from small hypogastric branches that is amenable to therapeutic embolization. Hemorrhage may become extensive when tamponade is prevented by increased pelvic capacity resulting from pelvic ring instability. Blood loss, transfusion requirements, and prognosis correlate with conditions producing expanded pelvic volume. Internal and external pelvic fixation and/or military antishock trousers (MAST) are intended to improve pelvic stability and tamponade of hemorrhage.

BIBLIOGRAPHY

 1. Carroll PR, Lue TF, Schmidt RA, et al: Penile replantation. J Urol 133:281, 1985.
 2. Carroll PR, McAninch JW: Bladder trauma: Mechanisms of injury and a unified method of diagnosis and repair. J Urol 132:254, 1984.
 3. Cryer HM, Miller FC, Evers BM, et al: Pelvic fracture classification: Correlation with hemorrhage. J Trauma 28:973, 1988.
 4. Evers BM, Cryer HM, Miller FB: Pelvic fracture hemorrhage. Arch Surg 124:422, 1989.
 5. Evins SC, Whittle T, Rous SN: Self-emasculation. J Urol 118:775, 1977.
 6. Flint L, Babikian G, Anders M, et al: Definitive control of mortality from pelvic fractures. Ann Surg 211:703, 1990.
 7. Hegmann AD, Bell-Thompson J, Rathod DM, et al: Successful reimplantation of the penis using microvascular techniques. J Urol 118:879, 1977.
 8. Jacob TD, Gruen GS, Udekwu AO, Peitzman AB: Pelvic fracture. Surg Rounds Aug:583, 1993.
 9. Jonassen EA, Fisher RC: Pelvic fractures. In Abernathy CM, Harken AH (eds): Surgical Secrets. Philadelphia, Hanley & Belfus, 1991, p 87.
10. Morehouse DD, Belitsky P, MacKinnon KJ: Rupture of posterior urethra. J Urol 107:255, 1972.
11. Moreno C, Moore EE, Rosenberger A, et al: Hemorrhage associated with major pelvic fracture. J Trauma 26:987, 1986.
12. Peltier L: Joseph Francois Malgaigne and Malgaigne's fracture. Surgery 44:777, 784, 1958.
13. Pennal GF, et al: Pelvic disruption. Clin Orthop Rel Res 151:12–21, 1980.

14. Peterson NE: Traumatic posterior urethral avulsion. Mongr Urol 7:61, 1986.
15. Peterson NE: Current management of urethral injuries. In Rous S (ed): 1988 Urology Annual. New York, Appleton-Century-Crofts, 1988, pp 143–179.
16. Peterson NE: Repair of a traumatically amputated penis with return of erectile function [letter to the editor]. J Urol 147:1628, 1992.
17. Richardson JR, Leadbetter GW: Non-operative treatment of the ruptured bladder. J Urol 114:213, 1975.
18. Spirnak JP: Pelvic fracture and injury to the lower urinary tract. Surg Clin North Am 68:1057, 1988.
19. Turner-Warwick RT: A personal view of the management of traumatic posterior urethral strictures. Urol Clin North Am 4:111, 1977.
20. Wolk DJ, Sander CM, Corriere JN Jr: Extraperitoneal bladder rupture without pelvic fracture. J Urol 134:1199, 1985.

28. BURNS

C. Edward Hartford, M.D.

1. What are the causes of burn injury?
Burns are caused by exposure to excessive heat (flame, scalding liquids, hot surfaces, friction, and electricity). Heat destroys tissues by coagulation of protein. Sunburn and skin cancer are caused by exposure to the same band of ultraviolet light. Exposure to irradiation also may result in destruction of skin. Chemicals injure tissue not by heat but by chemical reactions such as oxidation, reduction, corrosion, salt formation, vesicant activity, and desiccation.

2. What is the incidence of burn injury?
Approximately 0.8% of the population (2,000,000 people) in the United States sustains a burn injury each year. The majority of burns are small and do not require hospital admission for treatment. However, about 55,000 patients are admitted for burn treatment and 5,000 people die from burns each year.

3. How are burns classified?

Classification of Burns

DEPTH OF INJURY	CLINICAL SIGNS AND SYMPTOMS	OUTCOME
First degree (superficial injury limited to epidermis)	Erythema of the skin with mild-to-moderate discomfort.	Wounds heal spontaneously in 5–10 days; the damaged epithelium peels off, leaving no residual effects.
Second degree Superficial (involves entirety of epidermis and superficial portion of dermis)	Wounds are blistered or weeping, erythematous, and painful.	Wounds heal spontaneously within 3 weeks without residual scarring and with good quality skin; pigmentation may be altered.
Deep (involves deeper dermis but viable portions of epidermal appendages remain)	The skin is desiccated, blistered, with eschar often seen. Wounds are occasionally moist and difficult to distinguish from third-degree burns.	Wounds heal spontaneously beyond 3–4 weeks; hypertrophic scarring often occurs and, occasionally, unstable epithelium. For best results, remove eschar by tangential excision and cover with split thickness skin graft.
Third degree (all epidermal appendages destroyed)	Avascular, waxy white, leathery brown or black, insensate eschar.	Unless small in size, wounds require removal of eschar and coverage with skin graft for healing.

4. Under what circumstances should a burn be skin-grafted?

Burns that heal within 3 weeks reestablish good pliability of the skin, usually normal pigmentation, and no hypertrophic scarring (scars that are red, raised, and indurated). The longer the burn wound takes to heal beyond 3 weeks, the greater the incidence of hypertrophic scarring and the poorer the functional and cosmetic results. Therefore, if it appears that the wound will heal within 3–4 weeks, it should be allowed to do so. However, as soon as it can be determined that a wound will not heal within this time frame, the patient should be advised that the burn eschar should be removed surgically and the wound skin-grafted to yield a better cosmetic and functional result.

5. What are the priorities in the initial treatment of burn patients?

As in the treatment of any injured patient, rapid assessment of immediate life-threatening conditions is primary. An airway is established, breathing is ensured, and circulation is evaluated. Children with burns in excess of 10% and adults with burns in excess of 15% of the total body surface area should be given intravenous fluid therapy to prevent or treat hypovolemic shock. A secondary survey, including medical history and complete physical examination, is then done. During the initial phase of treatment, the patient is kept warm, and the burn wounds are covered with a clean dry sheet or wrapped in sterile gauze. Prophylactic antibiotics are not used. Because burns are tetanus-prone wounds, tetanus immunization is updated.

6. How is fluid resuscitation initiated in burn patients?

Because the loss of fluid due to sequestration into the region of a burn wound is rapid, intravenous fluid therapy a large-bore catheter is started. The volume of fluid required for resuscitation can be estimated with the Parkland formula. For the first 24 hours after injury lactated Ringer's solution is given in a volume of 4 ml/kg body weight/% body surface area burn; one-half of the volume is administered during the first 8 hours and the other half during the subsequent 16 hours. However, once fluid resuscitation is initiated, the focus of decision making for fluid management should shift from formula to clinical response. The patient's clinical condition is assessed frequently, with evaluation of vital signs, mental status, cardiorespiratory function, and urine output. Changes in fluid management are based on these functions. The goals are to produce hemodynamic stability and to maintain urine flow in the range of 0.5–1 ml/kg/hr in children and about 50 ml/hr in adults.

7. How does one determine the percentage of body surface area (BSA) affected?

Although other methods to determine the BSA involved by a burn are more precise (e.g., the method of Lund and Browder), the rule of nines is the most easily remembered and practical. The body is divided into areas, each representing approximately 9% or 18% of the BSA. The head and each upper extremity in its entirety are 9% apiece; the anterior aspect of the torso, the back (including the buttocks), and each lower extremity in its entirety are 18% apiece. The area of the palm is equivalent to 1% of the body surface area. Among infants, the relative size of the head is larger (18% for infants vs. 9% for adults), whereas each lower extremity is smaller (14% vs. 18%).

8. Name three important early respiratory complications of flame burn. How are they manifested? How are they treated?

  1. **Upper airway obstruction from edema.** The earliest manifestation of upper airway obstruction is altered phonation. The classic manifestations, such as agitation (a frightening sign of hypoxemia), inspiratory stridor, intercostal retraction, and cyanosis, occur subsequently. Early endotracheal intubation through the third postburn day, until the edema resolves, is often necessary.

  2. **Carbon monoxide poisoning.** Carbon monoxide is a product of combustion of all organic materials and has an affinity for hemoglobin that is about 240 times greater than that of oxygen. This results in reduced arterial oxygen content, which, if uncorrected, may lead to hypoxic encephalopathy and acute tubular necrosis of the kidney. All patients should receive 100% inspired oxygen until the carboxyhemoglobin level is below 5%. The half-life of carbon

monoxide when breathing room air is 250 minutes; with 100% oxygen, it is reduced to 40 minutes.

3. **Smoke inhalation injury syndrome.** Smoke inhalation injury and advanced age are the most dominant predictors of poor outcome in burn patients. Smoke, when inhaled, causes a chemically induced inflammatory response in the airways. Subsequently, the incidence of microbial colonization of the lower airway is high. Pneumonia is the most frequent complication. Smoke inhalation injury is best diagnosed by bronchoscopy. Patients often require ventilatory support.

9. What is an escharotomy?

When skin is destroyed by heat, it loses its elasticity. The resulting rigid eschar is unable to expand to accommodate the edema that is sequestered beneath the burn. As a result, tissue pressure increases, and vascular compromise may occur. Neurovascular damage begins when the level of interstitial tissue pressure reaches 40 mmHg. Because in burn injury the clinical signs of ischemia are unreliable, either Doppler examination of distal pulses or direct measurement of tissue pressure is required to assess the need for escharotomy. An escharotomy through the burn eschar releases the tissues, allowing them to expand and thereby lowering tissue pressure and restoring blood flow. Similarly, circumferential chest burns may drastically increase the work of breathing. Release of the eschar-encased thorax by escharotomy restores thoracic compliance and improves ventilation.

10. How should burn wounds be treated?

Loose, devitalized debris is gently trimmed away. To delay bacterial colonization, a topical antibacterial agent is applied to the wound. Silver sulfadiazine, the most frequently used agent, has broad antimicrobial activity and few side effects. When it is decided that a wound will not heal within 3 weeks, the burn eschar is removed surgically and skin-grafted. Burn eschar is removed either by excision to fascia or by tangential excision, that is, sequential shaving of the wound until viable tissue is encountered. Tangential excision is preferred because it preserves the maximal amount of tissue. Split-thickness skin grafts on fascia tend to have a poorer functional and cosmetic outcome. Among patients with large burns, staged excision of up to 30% of the body surface area is accomplished until all areas of deep burn are removed and skin-grafted. The extent of each operation is limited by intraoperative blood and heat loss.

11. What are the priorities for wound closure?

If the burn injury is not life-threatening, the priorities of wound closure are hands first, face and neck second, and then everything else. Among patients with large, life-threatening burns, the priority is to use the available donor skins to cover as much injured surface as possible.

12. What are the available options for wound coverage?

Autograft skin (the patient's own) is currently the only definitive cover for wounds that will not heal spontaneously. Autograft skin is used as split-thickness skin grafts. Grafts are obtained with a dermatome. Sheet grafts are preferred and are always used to cover the hands, face, and neck. Debrided burns can be temporarily protected by a biologic dressing (cadaver allograft) or synthetic skin substitutes. Eventually, substitute grafts must be replaced by autograft.

13. What is meshing?

When the wound area is large and donor skin is limited, a method of skin expansion is used. The most popular method is meshing. Skin is fed through a device that expands the area by cutting a series of parallel offset slits.

14. What are the metabolic sequelae of burn injury?

Large surface area burn injury causes a hypermetabolic response that typically reaches its zenith 7–10 days after injury. A large burn causes one of the biggest metabolic insults that a patient can sustain. The basal energy expenditure often reaches $2^1/_2$ times the unburned resting state. Contributing factors are an excess of circulating catecholamines, evaporative heat loss through the wound, and inflammatory mediators. Sepsis perpetuates this process. Burn hypermetabolism resolves only after the burns are healed.

15. When should nutritional support be initiated in burn patients?
Nutritional support must be started almost immediately.

16. What is the preferred route of nutritional support?
The preferred route is enteral; however, supplemental central venous alimentation is often required.

17. Why is infection the most common complication in burn patients?
Broad impairment of the immune system is immediate and lasts until after the patient's wounds are healed. The burn eschar is an excellent culture medium for bacteria. Once colonized, the burned skin is incapable of preventing the migration of bacteria through the eschar. Bacteria implanted on a full-thickness, experimental burn wound can be recovered from the regional lymph nodes within 8 hours.

18. How are antibiotics used in the treatment of burn infection?
Antibiotics are used only for specific infection. Prophylactic systemic antimicrobial agents do not prevent sepsis in burn patients. Conversely, prophylactic antibiotics increase the risk of infection by resistant microorganisms. Antibiotics are administered at the first clinical suspicion of infection and modified on the basis of in vitro antimicrobial susceptibility testing of recovered bacteria. The first wave of infection in burned patients is usually caused by gram-positive organisms. Later in the burn course, sepsis is typically from gram-negative aerobic bacilli. In immunocompromised burn patients, prolonged use of broad-spectrum antibiotics often results in candidiasis.

19. Are burned children different?
No. The basic principles of fluid resuscitation, timely skin grafting, nutritional support, and treatment of sepsis also apply to children. Except for infants, the survival prognosis for children and teenagers is exceptionally good.

20. What is the approach to chemical burns?
Experimental evidence suggests that if a chemical can be removed from the skin within 15 seconds of contact, the extent of injury can be minimized. Therefore, immediate lavage of the contaminated area with copious amounts of **water** is the optimal therapy. It is recommended that lavage be continued for 20 minutes. Many chemicals or a moiety of a chemical compound can be absorbed and cause a systemic toxic effect. Therefore, when the chemical burn has been identified, telephone the Poison Control Center for treatment information.

21. What is the difference between a low-voltage and a high-voltage electrical burn? How are they managed?
The extent of tissue necrosis increases directly with the level of electrical energy (amperage) delivered to the tissues. With low-voltage exposure (household current), the risk of cardiac death from ventricular fibrillation is great, but tissue damage is typically small. On the other hand, in high-voltage exposure (industrial levels of electrical energy), the risk of extensive tissue damage is great. The typical injury is a contact wound of electrical entrance, with necrosis extending into the muscle and often even involving bone. When muscle is destroyed, myoglobinemia and myoglobinuria occur, enhancing the risk of acute renal failure. A vigorous diuresis must be provided to clear the myoglobin. In addition, the inevitable metabolic acidosis must be corrected with sodium bicarbonate. As soon as the patient's condition permits, wounds produced by high-voltage electricity should be explored and surgically debrided.

22. What factors determine prognosis in a burn patient?
Age and smoke inhalation dwarf all other outcome variables. The most favorable outcome from burns is among patients between 5 and 34 years of age. Patients over 60 years of age have a substantially increased mortality rate. The larger the area burned and the deeper the burn, the worse the prognosis. Preexisting medical conditions and concomitant injuries that make patients more difficult to treat adversely influence outcome.

CONTROVERSIES

23. Should crystalloid or colloid solutions be used for initial resuscitation of burn patients?
No one knows, but crystalloid is cheaper. Adequate restoration of circulating plasma volume is the primary goal of burn resuscitation and can be achieved with either type of solution or a combination of both. If one uses crystalloid alone, the required volume and the resulting weight gain are much larger.

24. Nutrition for the burn patient: enteral or parenteral?
Total parenteral nutrition (TPN) provides easy intravenous delivery of high-caloric and high-protein nutritional support. However, the expense is great, and the complications associated with a central venous line are significant. Enteral nutritional support is far less expensive and technically simple; it also maintains the integrity of the gastrointestinal tract while theoretically diminishing bacterial translocation. It may be difficult to deliver the large amount of food required for successful treatment of a patient with a large burn by the enteral route alone.

BIBLIOGRAPHY

1. Baxter CR: Emergency treatment of burn injury. Ann Emerg Med 17:1305, 1988.
2. Curreri PW, Luterman A: Burns. In Schwartz SI, Shires GT, Spencer FC (eds): Principles of Surgery, 6th ed. New York, McGraw-Hill, 1994.
3. Deitch EA: The management of burns. N Engl J Med 323:1249–1253, 1990.
4. Demling RH: Burns. In Wilmore DW, et al (eds): American College of Surgeons Care of the Surgical Patients, vol. 3. New York, Scientific American, 1995.

29. HEAD INJURIES

Kerry Brega, M.D., and John Nichols, M.D., Ph.D.

1. Can I skip this chapter?
Absolutely not. Regardless of their field, all clinicians will be called on to evaluate patients with major and minor traumatic brain injuries (TBIs).

2. Is TBI a common problem?
Absolutely. One in 12 deaths in the United States is due to injury. One-third of traumatic deaths are TBI-related. Of deaths resulting from motor vehicle accidents, 60% are due to brain injury. Even more common is minor TBI, which accounts for 70–80% of admissions for head trauma.

3. Why not call a neurosurgeon or neurologist?
Unless one practices in a hospital dedicated to trauma, both can be scarce when they are needed the most. Most deaths due to TBI occur before or in the emergency department. Thus the greatest impact in preventing death is made by emergency physicians, general surgeons, and family practitioners who see patients immediately on arrival.

4. Brain injury is permanent, and the outcome is usually bad. Why waste my time?
True, true, and unrelated. Brain injury occurs in two phases. The primary injury occurs at the moment of impact and is generally irreversible. Secondary injury, however, is treatable, including hypoxia, hypotension, elevated intracranial pressure (ICP), and decreased perfusion to the brain due to ischemia, brain swelling, and expanding mass lesions. Aggressive medical and/or surgical management can be life-saving.

5. How are brain-injured patients managed?
The first step is to recognize the problem by doing a neurologic exam. The neurologic exam in trauma is easy, requiring less than 1 minute to perform, and consists of three important elements: (1) level of consciousness, (2) pupillary exam, and (3) motor exam. Once is not enough! The exam must be repeated every 5–10 minutes. If deterioration is missed and appropriate treatment not quickly initiated, irreversible brain injury may result.

6. Is this exam the same as the Glasgow Coma Scale (GCS)?
No. The GCS is a 15-point scale; 15 is the best score and 3 is the worst. The score is derived from observing the best motor response (1–6 points), best verbal response (1–5 points), and best eye-opening response (1–4 points). The GCS is helpful in communication between physicians, but it leaves out two very important pieces of information: pupillary response and focality. A patient with a perfect score of 15 may have hemiparesis and a life-threatening lesion.

7. Are terms such as semicomatose nonsense?
Yes. Patients are either alert (like most medical students and surgeons), lethargic (arousal is maintained by verbal interaction), obtunded (constant mechanical stimulation is required to maintain arousal), or comatose (neither verbal nor mechanical stimulation elicits arousal). Change in level of consciousness is often the first sign of increasing intracranial pressure; it is also the most poorly documented part of the neurologic exam. Document all findings!

8. What is the significance of anisocoria?
In the context of trauma, anisocoria (unequal pupils) is a true neurologic emergency. Commonly a mass lesion (e.g., subdural or epidural hematoma, contusion, or diffuse swelling of one hemisphere) has led to uncal herniation and stretching of the ipsilateral third nerve. Time is critical in initiating therapy to reduce swelling, making the diagnosis (CT scan), and providing operative intervention if necessary. Get the ball rolling!

9. What if the larger pupil is reactive?
Trick question. If the pupil is reactive, the third nerve is functioning. Think of Horner's syndrome (miosis, ptosis, and anhydrosis) on the other side. This syndrome may be due to injury to the sympathetic nerves traveling with the carotid artery in the neck. Think of carotid dissection.

10. How is motor response tested?
Ascertain the ability to follow commands by asking the patient to hold up fingers and move the legs. Next, if the patient does not follow commands, test response to painful stimulus. The next best response is localization of painful stimulus, followed by withdrawal from pain; flexion posturing (decorticate), which indicates high brainstem dysfunction; extensor posturing (decerebrate), which indicates lower brainstem dysfunction; and last (and least) no response. The patient with no motor response may have a cervical spinal cord injury.

11. Should scalp lacerations be explored in the emergency department?
Yes—but gently. Scalp lacerations should be cleaned and explored to look for underlying fractures. A laceration over a linear nondisplaced fracture can be cleaned and closed. If cerebrospinal fluid (CSF) or brain tissue is evident in the wound or if a significantly depressed fracture is identified, surgical intervention is required to debride the wound and to close any dural tears.

12. What is the significance of periorbital ecchymosis (raccoon eyes) and ecchymosis over the mastoid (Battle's sign)?

In the absence of direct trauma to the eyes or mastoid regions, periorbital ecchymosis and ecchymosis over the mastoid are reliable signs of basilar skull fractures. Between 5–11% of patients with basilar skull fractures have CSF leaks, rhinorrhea, or otorrhea.

13. Which patients need CT scans of the head?

In most centers where CT is readily available, indications include loss of consciousness, amnesia, abnormal neurologic exam, or external craniofacial trauma. The CT scan is used partly as a triage tool with minor brain injuries and can be cost-effective compared with admission to the intensive care unit for observation. Patients with focality on exam (indicating location of brain injury) generally do not proceed to the operating room without a scan. The scan is done first if the patient is hemodynamically stable and if the scan does not significantly delay treatment. Even in these cases operative lesions are uncommon. Making the correct diagnosis is, if possible, preferable.

14. When is intracranial pressure monitoring indicated?

Usually when a patient is unconscious and the threat of elevated ICP exists; in other words, when the neurologic exam becomes insensitive to changes in intracranial pressure.

15. What takes priority in resuscitation of a hypotensive patient with traumatic brain injury?

Hypotension. Never assume that hypotension is due to the brain injury. Hypotension due to brain injury is an extremely terminal event.

16. Describe the treatment of patients with elevated ICP.

First, ensure good perfusion to the brain. The brain, like every other organ, must have adequate blood flow and oxygen delivery. Even in brain injury the ABCs (airways, breathing, circulation) come first. Systolic blood pressures < 90 and partial pressure of oxygen in arterial blood (PaO_2) < 60 are significantly correlated with poor outcomes in patients with TBI.

17. Should all patients with elevated ICP be hyperventilated?

Any patient with depressed level of consciousness and inability to protect the airway should be intubated. Before obtaining a CT scan, patients thought to have a mass lesion by neurologic exam should be hyperventilated. Decreasing the partial pressure of carbon dioxide (pCO_2) is the most rapidly effective treatment for elevated ICP. The goal is usually a pCO_2 of 30 mmHg. Routine prolonged hyperventilation is to be avoided. Extreme hypocapnia may produce brain ischemia.

18. In hemodynamically stable patients, osmotic diuretics are the second medical intervention for controlling ICP. Give examples, with the appropriate dose.

1. Mannitol: 1 gm/kg of body weight IV
2. Urea: 1 gm/kg of body weight IV

Don't forget to insert a Foley catheter in the bladder and limit IV fluids.

19. What is the endpoint of diuresis?

Usually serum sodium levels of 145–150 and serum osmolarities of 290–300 are the upper limits of diuresis. Blood volume should be maintained with colloids to help form an osmotic gradient between the extravascular intraparenchymal space and the intravascular space. Anticipate intravascular hypovolemia, and treat with colloids and blood products.

20. What is the next step?

1. Rule out a surgical lesion.
2. In some cases a ventriculostomy to drain spinal fluid is helpful.
3. Barbiturate coma decreases the metabolic requirements of the brain and decreases blood flow. Beware: the doses necessary to control ICP may induce profound hypotension, which can be treated with colloids and dopamine.

21. Should posttraumatic seizures be treated?
Generally not. Between 10–20% of patients who have seizures within the first 7 days of injury also have late seizures. Because of the adverse effects of antiepileptic medications, routine prophylaxsis is not recommended. Patients with or at risk for increased ICP are treated prophylactically, because seizures increase the metabolic rate of the brain and adversely affect ICP.

22. What is the significance of cerebral perfusion pressure?
Cerebral perfusion pressure (CPP) is the difference between the mean arterial pressure (MAP) and the ICP.

$$CPP = MAP - ICP$$

CPP is an important parameter to follow. The brain can survive CPPs in the 50s but neurologic outcome is superior in patients with CPPs in the 70s. Some patients require treatment with pressors to elevate the CPP.

23. Why should all children with traumatic brain injuries be undressed and thoroughly examined?
Approximately one-half of children presenting with nonaccidental trauma have TBI. A high index of suspicion is warranted.

24. Which coagulopathy is associated with severe brain injury?
Disseminated intravascular coagulation (DIC). The presumed mechanism is massive release of thromboplastin into the circulation from the injured brain. The serum levels of fibrin degradation products roughly correlate with the extent of brain parenchymal injury. All severely brain-injured patients should be evaluated with prothrombin time (PT), partial thromboplastin time (PTT), platelet counts, and fibrinogen levels.

25. Name another medical complication of severe head injury?
Diabetes insipidus (DI) due to the inadequate secretion of antidiuretic hormone is caused by injury to the pituitary or hypothalamic tracts. It results in the inability of the kidney to decrease free water clearance. Usually the urine output is > 200 ml/hr and the urine specific gravity is < 1.003. The serum sodium must be closely monitored as it may rise precipitously if DI is not promptly treated. The treatment of choice in trauma is intravenous infusion of synthetic vasopressin (pitressin), which has a 10–20-minute half-life and can be titrated to produce the appropriate urine output. Because most trauma-induced DI is self-limited, 1-deamino-8-D-arginine vasopressin (DDAVP) (with a 12-hour half-life) is not used acutely.

26. Are gunshot wounds that cross the midline of the brain uniformly fatal injuries?
No. The tract that the bullet takes is important, but in general the kinetic energy (E) of the missile is the most damaging to the brain.

$$E = \frac{1}{2} MV^2$$

Where MV = missile velocity. Weapons with high muzzle velocities may produce relatively minor-appearing bullet tracts and yet result in severe brain injury and vice versa. All gunshot wounds should be examined with CT, because 40% of patients have significant blood clots that may be surgically removed. The CT scan also identifies indriven bone, which may require debridement.

27. In the context of trauma, what else should be considered when the patient has a focal neurologic deficit and a normal CT scan?
An angiogram should be considered to identify a carotid or intracranial vascular lesion.

28. Define concussion.
Concussion is a transient loss of neurologic function without macroscopic brain abnormality.

29. Can patients with minor brain injuries be discharged from the emergency department?
Patients with minor TBIs whose exam (including short-term memory) returns to normal and who have a normal head CT scan can be discharged to home (see question 30).

30. What is the significance of a concussion?
The symptoms of mild TBI are common sequelae of trauma (postconcussive syndrome). In most studies of minor TBI, > 50% of patients have complaints of headache, fatigue, dizziness, irritability, and alterations in cognition and short-term memory. It is important to alert the patient to the likelihood of developing such symptoms. The neurobehavioral problems significantly affect patients' lives. The symptoms usually resolve within 1–6 months after injury.

BIBLIOGRAPHY

1. Barrow DL: Complications and Sequelae of Head Injury. Park Ridge, IL, American Association of Neurological Surgeons, 1992.
2. Chesnut RM, Marshall LF, Klauber MR, et al: The role of secondary brain injury in determining outcome from severe head injury. J Trauma 34:216–222, 1993.
3. Cooper PR: Head Injury. Baltimore, Williams & Wilkins, 1993.
4. Mangaiardi JR: Neurologic injuries. Top Emerg Med 11:1–84, 1990.
5. Rosner MJ, Daughton S: Cerebral perfusion pressure management in head injury. J Trauma 30:933–941, 1990.

30. SPINAL CORD INJURIES

Kerry Brega, M.D., and John Nichols, M.D., Ph.D.

1. What other injuries are commonly associated with cervical spine injury?
Craniofacial injuries. Forces associated with significant head and brain injury may be transmitted through the cervical spine. Approximately 15% of patients with one spine injury have a second injury elsewhere in the spine.

2. What does this association imply?
All victims with evidence of significant craniofacial trauma should be treated initially as if they have a cervical spine injury. Before any movement, the patient should be immobilized with a rigid cervical collar. The thoracic and lumbar spine should be immobilized on a board, and the patient should be log-rolled only.

3. Describe the evaluation of patients with potential spine injuries.
First, be sure that the patient is adequately immobilized. Second, do a neurologic exam, including all four extremities; test strength, sensation (get out a safety pin), and reflexes. Be sure to document the lowest **functional** level. As with brain injury, patients are frequently reevaluated to rule out deterioration. If deterioration occurs, the lowest functional levels change first. All patients should have a rectal exam to evaluate tone. A patulous anus is a good indication of spinal cord or cauda equina injury. Flaccid motor tone and absent reflexes should raise suspicion of spinal cord injury. Such findings are extremely unusual with brain injury. Careful palpation of the spine for areas of tenderness may help to define a level of injury.

4. Are significant spine injuries always tender to direct palpation?
Never say always, but usually yes. Anterior fractures may not be tender to palpation, but the awake and alert patient is likely to complain of pain. All bets are off if the patient is intoxicated.

5. Are cervical spine radiographs necessary if the neurologic exam is normal?
Yes. Patients with fractures, torn ligaments, and even unstable cervical spines may have normal neurologic exams, particularly in the C1 and C2 area, where the spinal canal is comparatively wide.

6. Can a patient have a spinal cord injury and normal plain radiographs?
Yes—with purely ligamentous injuries between vertebrae. Spinal cord injury without radiographic abnormality (SCIWORA) is common in children; 20–30% of children with spinal cord injuries have no radiographic abnormality. SCIWORA is less common in adults. In patients with preexisting bony cervical stenosis, either congenital or degenerative, hyperextension or flexion may result in cord injury without spinal column disruption.

7. What is an adequate radiologic evaluation?
Minimal views include cross-table lateral, anteroposterior, and open-mouth odontoid views. The relationship between C7 and the top of T1 must be visualized. Mild traction on the shoulders with the lateral film or swimmer's views help in patients with large shoulders. If this area cannot be seen on plain films, a lateral tomogram or CT scan may be needed. Oblique views are helpful in viewing the pedicles and facet joints. Patients with evident or possible fractures should have CT scans to define the injury in greater detail.

8. Are MRI scans ever needed in the acute evaluation of cervical spine trauma?
Yes. If plain radiographs and CT scans do not adequately explain the extent of injury noted on the neurologic exam, MRI may be used to evaluate the patient for herniated disks or spinal compressive lesions, such as spinal epidural hematomas. Also, when one vertebral body is subluxed anteriorly on the body below, it is necessary to rule out the presence of a herniated disk before placing the patient in traction. If a herniated disk is present, it may be pulled into the cord when the bodies are realigned in traction. Such herniated disks must be removed.

9. Describe the proper way to read a lateral cervical spine film.
Make a habit of doing a thorough systematic review the same way with every film. First, look at the prevertebral soft-tissue space, which may be the only radiographic abnormality in as many as 30–40% of C1 and C2 fractures. The space anterior to C3 should not exceed one-third of the body. Check the alignment of the anterior, then posterior edges of the vertebral bodies. Be sure that the intervertebral disk spaces are of relatively equal height. Check the spinous processes for alignment and abnormal splaying. Finally, evaluate each vertebra for fracture.

10. What about the anteroposterior (AP) film?
Carefully inspect the alignment of the midline spinous processes. Abrupt angulations suggest unilateral facet dislocation. Fractures of the bodies may be more obvious in the AP view.

11. Fractures of C1 and C2 are best visualized with which view?
The odontoid view. Look for overhang of the lateral mass of C1 off the lateral edges of C2, which should not be greater than 1–2 mm on either side. Abnormal overhang is seen in **Jefferson's fractures** (burst fractures of the C1 ring). The three types of odontoid fractures should be apparent: type I occurs in the body of the odontoid, type II at the junction of the odontoid and the body of C2, and type III through the body of C2 below the odontoid.

12. What is a hangman's fracture?
Bilateral fractures through the pedicles or laminae of C2 are caused by a severe hyperextension injury, usually due to high-speed motor vehicle accidents. Think about the mechanism of injury; the C2–C3 disk space may be disrupted anteriorly. In judicial hangings the fatal injury is the spinal cord stretch caused by the drop and not spinal cord injury caused by the fracture alone. Most patients with hangman's fracture present neurologically intact.

13. Define deficits in complete transverse myelopathy, anterior cord syndrome, central cord syndrome, and Brown-Sequard syndrome.

1. **Complete transverse myelopathy** may result from either transection, stretch, or contusion of the cord. All function below the level of the lesion—motor, sensory, and reflexes—is lost. Complete transverse myelopathy may be accompanied by spinal shock and/or neurogenic shock.

2. **Anterior cord syndrome** results from loss of the anterior two-thirds of the spinal cord (the distribution of the anterior spinal artery), which carries motor, pain, and temperature tracts. The sensation of light touch and proprioception are intact because the posterior columns are preserved.

3. **Central cord syndrome** results from injury to the central area of the spinal cord. Often it is due to injuries in patients with preexisting cervical stenosis due to spondolytic changes. Characteristically, motor deficits are more severe in the upper extremities than in the lower extremities. Motor function is usually affected more than sensory function.

4. **Brown-Sequard syndrome** is characteristically seen in penetrating injuries but also may be seen in blunt injury, especially with unilateral, traumatically herniated disks. The syndrome results from injury to one-half of the spinal cord. Clinically, motor, position, and vibration sense are affected on the side ipsilateral to the injury; these tracts cross in the brainstem. Pain and temperature sensation are abolished contralateral to the lesion; these tracts cross in the cord at or near the level of innervation.

14. What is spinal shock?

Absence of all spinal cord function below the level of the lesion results in flaccid motor tone and areflexia. Neurogenic shock refers to the hypotension that may result from cervical or upper thoracic complete spinal cord lesions. The hypotension is due to the lack of sympathetic vasomotor innervation below the lesion and characterized by bradycardia from unbalanced vagal input to the heart. Fluid resuscitation and pressors with both alpha and beta stimulation work best. Strictly alpha stimulation may result in profound bradycardia or asystole. Usually the spinal shock resolves and vasomotor tone returns over the first few days.

15. What is the role of methylprednisolone in the treatment of acute spinal cord injury?

The results of the Second National Acute Spinal Cord Injury Study suggest that high-dose methylprednisolone results in a statistically significant improvement in outcome. The dose is a 30–40 mg/kg load, followed by 5.4 mg/kg/hr for 23 hours (easy to remember). This regimen should be followed in any patient suspected of having a spinal cord injury. Penetrating trauma was not evaluated in the study.

16. Are patients with spinal cord injuries ever operated upon acutely?

Yes. Patients with deterioration in the neurologic exam may undergo urgent spinal cord decompression. Deterioration may be due to herniated disk material, epidural hemorrhage, or cord swelling in a tight space, which causes cord compression and worsening symptoms.

17. How is the bony injury treated?

The two most important factors in planning treatment of the spine injury are alignment and stability.

1. Bad alignment—traction. If good alignment is obtained, halo with or without operative fixation is recommended. If good alignment is not obtained, open reduction and fixation are required.

2. Good alignment but unstable (significant ligamentous disruption)—halo with or without operative fixation.

3. Good alignment and stable—usually treated in a rigid collar.

18. What is the outcome in patients with spinal cord injury?

With complete lesions (no motor or sensory function below the lesion) the chances of recovery are poor; 2% of patients recover ambulation. Appropriate treatment of bony injuries helps to prevent pain and late neurologic deterioration.

19. What other significant injury may present as a high thoracic cord lesion?
Thoracic aortic dissection may present as a T4 region cord injury. T4 is a watershed zone in the cord between the vertebral arterial distribution and the aortic radicular arteries.

BIBLIOGRAPHY

1. Bracken MB, Shepard MJ, Collins WF, et al: A randomized, controlled trial of methylprednisolone or naloxone in the treatment of acute spinal-cord injury. N Engl J Med 322:1405–1411, 1990.
2. Cooper PR: Head Injury: Epidemiology of Head Injury. Baltimore, Williams & Wilkins, 1993.
3. Harris JH, Edeiken-Monroe B: The Radiology of Acute Cervical Spine Trauma. Baltimore, Williams & Wilkins, 1987.
4. Mangaiardi JR: Neurologic injuries. Top Emerg Med 11:1–84, 1990.
5. Pang D: Disorders of the Preiatric Spine. New York, Raven Press, 1995, pp 509–516.
6. Rea GL, Miller CA: Spinal Trauma: Current Evaluation and Management. American Association of Neurological Surgeons, 1993.
7. Wang AM (ed): Spinal Trauma. Philadelphia, Hanley & Belfus, 1989, pp 189–384.

III. Abdominal Surgery

31. APPENDICITIS

Alden H. Harken, M.D.

1. How do patients with appendicitis typically present?
The classic presentation is periumbilical pain that migrates to the right lower quadrant (RLQ).

2. Where is McBurney's point?
One-third the distance between the anteroposterior iliac spine and the umbilicus.

3. What is McBurney's point?
The typical point of maximal tenderness in appendicitis.

4. Was McBurney a cop from Boston?
Probably. Another McBurney was a surgeon from New York who, in collaboration with a surgeon named Fitz, coined the term "appendicitis" in classic papers published in 1886 and 1889.

5. What are the typical laboratory findings of a patient with appendicitis?
White blood cell count: 12,000–14,000
Negative urinalysis (no white cells)
Negative pregnancy test

6. What layers does the surgeon encounter on exposing the appendix through a Rockey-Davis incision?
Skin, subcutaneous fat, aponeurosis of the external oblique muscle, internal oblique muscle, transversalis fascia and muscle, and peritoneum.

7. Was Rockey-Davis a prizefighter from Philadelphia?
Probably. Another Rockey-Davis was a pair of surgeons—A.E. Rockey and G.G. Davis—who developed RLQ transverse, muscle-splitting incisions that extended into the rectus sheath.

8. What is the blood supply to the appendix and right colon?
The ileocolic and right colic arteries.

9. Does surgery for appendicitis involve a risk of mortality?
No surgical procedure is devoid of risk.

	Mortality
Nonperforated appendix	Less than 0.1%
Perforated appendix	As high as 5%

10. What patient groups are at higher risk of perforated appendicitis?
1. Very young patients (less than 2 years old). This is really veterinary medicine.
2. Elderly patients (over 70 years old), who exhibit dampened abdominal innervation and present late.

3. Diabetic patients, who also present late because of diabetic visceral neuropathy.
4. Patients on steroids. Steroids mask everything.

11. What is the role of ultrasound in the diagnosis of acute appendicitis?
Ultrasound can be both negatively and positively helpful. It is nice to see a perfectly normal right fallopian tube and ovary. It is also reassuring to see an inflamed, edematous appendix.

12. Is laparoscopic appendectomy replacing the traditional open approach?
Surgeons are now facile with laparoscopic cholecystectomy, colectomy, and hiatus herniorrhaphy. The normal appendix can be easily and safely removed via the laparoscope, but the inflamed/perforated appendix is tougher. Laparoscopic appendectomy probably should be reserved for the normal appendix.

13. What is a "white worm"?
A normal appendix.

14. What is the differential diagnosis of right lower quadrant pain?

Meckel's diverticulitis	Tuboovarian abscess
Diverticulitis	Pelvic inflammatory disease
Ectopic pregnancy	Carcinoid tumor
Crohn's disease	Cholecystitis

15. What is a Meckel's diverticulum?
Meckel's diverticulum is a congenital omphalomesenteric remnant that may contain ectopic gastric mucosa. It is found in 2% of the population, 2 feet upward from the ileocecal valve. It becomes inflamed in 2% of patients.

16. Can chronic diverticulitis masquerade as appendicitis?
Yes. Fifty percent of patients aged 50 years have colonic diverticula. The appendix is just a big cecal diverticulum. Thus, it makes sense that appendicitis and diverticulitis should look, act, and smell alike.

17. Can a nun with a negative pregnancy test present with an ectopic pregnancy?
Without intending to sound cynical—yes. Some people believe in miracles; others happen to rely on them. The fallopian tube must be inspected for a walnut-sized lump. Appropriate surgical therapy is a longitudinal incision to "shell out" the fetus with subsequent repair of the tube. This approach (as opposed to salpingectomy) is designed to preserve fertility.

18. Can Crohn's disease initially present as appendicitis
Indeed, this presentation is typical. Crohn's disease is boggy, edematous, granulomatous inflammation of the distal ileum. Traditional surgical dictum suggests that it is appropriate to remove the appendix in patients with Crohn's disease unless the cecum at the appendiceal base is involved.

19. Is it possible to confuse appendicitis with a tuboovarian abscess (TOA)?
Of course. An ovarian abscess buried deep in an inflamed, edematous, matted right adnexa can be treated successfully with intravenous antibiotics alone. Do not drain pus into the free peritoneal cavity—this will only make the patient sicker.

20. How about pelvic inflammatory disease (PID)?
PID can look exactly like appendicitis except for a positive "chandelier" sign. On pelvic examination, manual tug on the cervix moves the inflamed, painful adnexae, and the patient hits the chandelier. PID should be treated with antibiotics (either orally or intravenously, depending on how sick the patient is).

21. How does one deal with an appendiceal carcinoid tumor?

Carcinoid tumors may present anywhere along the GI tract; 60%, however, are in the appendix. An obstructing carcinoid tumor, like a fecalith, can lead to appendicitis—and in 0.3% of appendectomies, carcinoid tumors are the culprit. Most carcinoid tumors are small (< 1.5 cm) and benign; 70% are located in the distal appendix. They are effectively treated with appendectomy alone. A larger carcinoid tumor (> 2.0 cm) at the appendiceal base, especially with invasion of the mesoappendix, must be considered malignant and mandates right hemicolectomy.

22. Can appendicitis be mistaken for acute cholecystitis?

Occasionally, yes. Both entities reflect acute, localized, intraperitoneal inflammation. Laboratory studies may be identical: white blood cell count of 12,000–14,000, negative urinalysis, and negative pregnancy test. Thus, if one is thinking "appendicitis," the major difference may be only right upper versus right lower quadrant pain. Do not attempt to remove an inflamed gallbladder via a right lower quadrant incision. Laparoscopic cholecystectomy is possible for acute cholecystitis, but conversion to an open procedure should be more frequent.

BIBLIOGRAPHY

1. Bailey LE, Finley RK Jr: Acute appendicitis during pregnancy. Am Surg 52:218, 1986.
2. Binderow SR, Shaked AA: Acute appendicitis in patients with AIDS/HIV infection. Am Surg 162:9, 1991.
3. Fitz RH: Perforating inflammation of the vermiform appendix with special reference to its early diagnosis and treatment. Trans Assoc Am Physicians 1:107, 1986.
4. Matsagas MI, Fatouros M, Koulouras B, Giannouras AD: Incidence, complications and management of Meckel's diverticulum. Am Surg 130:143, 1995.
5. Rockey AE: Transverse incisions in abdominal operations. Med Rec 68:779, 1905.

32. GALLBLADDER DISEASE

Rebecca Wiebe, M.D., and Robert McIntyre, M.D.

PATHOGENESIS AND EPIDEMIOLOGY OF GALLSTONES

1. What are the types of gallstones? What is their pathogenesis?

Gallstones are composed of cholesterol, bilirubin, calcium, and mucoproteins. In the United States, 75% of gallstones are cholesterol stones, 20% are black pigment stones, and 5% are brown pigment stones. Black pigment stones are more common in patients with cirrhosis and hemolytic anemia (i.e., thalassemia, sickle-cell anemia). Primary bile duct stones are usually brown pigment stones and are associated with infections.

Cholesterol stones form when the cholesterol concentration in bile exceeds the ability of bile salts to hold it in solution. Normally, cholesterol is held in solution by association with bile salts and phospholipids (i.e., lecithin) in the form of micelles and vesicles. At high concentrations of cholesterol, vesicles fuse to form crystals that aggregate with mucoproteins to form stones. Lithogenic bile may have an increased cholesterol concentration or a decreased bile salt concentration.

2. What is the incidence of gallstones in the United States?

Approximately 11% of the adult population has gallstones. The prevalence varies with age, sex, and ethnic groups.

3. What are the risk factors for cholelithiasis?

The most common factors are female sex, multiparity, age over 40 years, and obesity, otherwise known as the four Fs: female, fertile, forty, and fat. Certain ethnic groups have a high incidence, such as Scandinavians, Hispanics, and Native Americans—particularly the Pima tribe. The incidence is lower in blacks and Asians. Patients who experience rapid weight loss or depend on total parenteral nutrition (TPN) are also more prone to gallstones.

4. Do all gallstones cause symptoms?
Most patients with gallstones have no symptoms. Two percent of patients with gallstones develop symptoms every year, with approximately 20–30% of patients becoming symptomatic during their lifetime.

CLINICAL PRESENTATION

5. What is the most common clinical presentation of patients with symptomatic stones?
Patients most often present with right upper quadrant or epigastric pain. The pain peaks at night and may radiate to the right shoulder. Patients also may report intolerance of fatty foods. Acute complications of gallstones include cholecystitis, jaundice, pancreatitis, and cholangitis.

6. What are the symptoms of acute cholecystitis?
Acute cholecystitis is associated with somatic pain caused by irritation of the peritoneum that overlies the gallbladder. The pain is located in the right upper quadrant, radiates to the back and right shoulder, and usually lasts several hours. It is often associated with nausea, vomiting, and fever.

7. What are the signs of acute cholecystitis?
The signs of acute cholecystitis are fever, tenderness with palpation of the right upper quadrant, and leukocytosis. A tender mass in the right upper quadrant occurs in 20% of patients and is pathognomonic.

8. What is Murphy's sign?
Murphy's sign is pain during deep inspiration when the examiner palpates the right upper quadrant; the pain causes the patient to stop breathing at mid inspiration.

9. Choledocholithiasis (common bile duct stones) is suggested by what symptoms?
Common bile duct obstruction due to stones is suggested by jaundice, dark urine, clay-colored stools, and pruritus.

10. What is Charcot's triad? Reynold's pentad?
Charcot's triad, which suggests infection in the bile duct (cholangitis), consists of right upper quadrant pain, jaundice, and fever. Reynold's pentad adds mental status changes and shock associated with sepsis due to severe cholangitis.

11. What is Courvoisier's law?
In gallstone disease, the gallbladder does not enlarge with obstruction of the common bile duct because of previous inflammation of the gallbladder wall. Obstruction of the bile duct secondary to pancreatic cancer, however, causes distention of the undiseased gallbladder.

DIAGNOSTIC TESTS

12. What are the best laboratory tests for gallbladder disease?
Blood tests cannot detect gallstones but provide evidence of disease. In acute cholecystitis, the white blood cell count, bilirubin, and alkaline phosphatase may be slightly elevated. When the common bile duct is obstructed, liver function tests show an elevation of bilirubin and alkaline phosphatase. In gallstone pancreatitis, amylase levels may be increased.

13. What is the primary method of diagnosing gallstones?

Ultrasound (US) of the right upper quadrant is the gold standard for the diagnosis of all biliary disease. It is 97% sensitive and 95% specific. It is safe and noninvasive. The diagnosis is highly specific if the operator sees a movable echogenic mass that produces a shadow within the gallbladder. US also detects biliary sludge, and thickening of the gallbladder wall suggests inflammation. Dilation of the common bile duct suggests choledocholithiasis.

14. How often are stones seen on plain radiograph?

Ten to 15% of gallstones are sufficiently calcified to be radiopaque.

15. What are the alternatives to US?

Oral cholecystography (OCG) is useful in patients with suspected stones and a negative or equivocal US. An iodinated contrast agent, tyropanoate sodium, is taken the night before the examination. It is absorbed, bound to albumin, taken up by hepatocytes, excreted in the bile, and concentrated in the gallbladder. On OCG, the gallbladder may be seen to contain polyps, stones, or sludge. Alternatively, inability to visualize the gallbladder indicates cystic duct obstruction or cholecystitis.

Nuclear cholescintigraphy permits assessment of gallbladder function in patients with suspected acute cholecystitis. Technetium 99-labeled iminodiacetic acid (HIDA scan) is injected intravenously, excreted in high concentration in the bile, and read by a gamma camera. Nonvisualization of the gallbladder in the setting of right upper quadrant pain with signs of inflammation is 95% specific for acute cholecystitis.

16. What else causes nonvisualization of the gallbladder on HIDA scan?

In addition to acute cholecystitis, nonvisualization of the gallbladder may be due to prolonged fasting and liver disease. Patients may be given a cholecystokinin analog (Kinevac) to stimulate bile flow and improve the accuracy of the test.

17. What does air in the bile ducts on plain radiographs signify?

Air in the bile duct (pneumatobilia) indicates communication with the GI tract. A cholecystoenteric fistula may result from erosion of a gallstone into a loop of adjacent bowel, allowing the stone to pass into the lumen of the bowel. Mechanical obstruction (gallstone ileus) may result, usually at the ileocecal valve. The patient presents with symptoms of small bowel obstruction preceded by symptoms of gallbladder disease. Pneumatobilia also may result from a surgical anastomosis with the common bile duct, such as choledochoduodenostomy.

OTHER DISEASES OF THE GALLBLADDER

18. What is the pathogenesis of acute cholecystitis?

Obstruction of the cystic duct by a gallstone leads to stasis and infection. On the other hand, 10–20% of cases are not associated with gallstones (acalculous cholecystitis). Acalculous cholecystitis occurs in patients hospitalized with other illnesses and may be caused by inspissation of bile by dehydration or bile stasis. It is seen after trauma, severe systemic illness, or major surgery. It may occur more often in patients on TPN.

19. What bacteria are most commonly cultured from bile?

Escherichia coli, Klebsiella sp., enterococci, *Pseudomonas* sp., and *Bacteroides fragilis* are the most common organisms cultured from bile. Second-generation cephalosporins or expanded-spectrum penicillins, such as mezlocillin and piperacillin, are recommended.

20. What is emphysema of the gallbladder?

Clostridia or other gas-forming organisms may infect the gallbladder, causing air to be seen in the wall or the lumen of the gallbladder on plain radiographs.

21. What is empyema of the gallbladder?
A gallbladder filled with pus usually results from delay of treatment. It is often associated with other intraabdominal abscesses and with common duct stones.

22. What is white bile?
Complete cystic duct occlusion leads to collection in the gallbladder of mucus without bile, which has a white or clear appearance.

23. What is biliary dyskinesia?
Biliary dyskinesia is a functional disorder of the bile ducts, sometimes referred to as sphincter of Oddi dysfunction. It is believed to be caused by abnormal and intermittent elevations of pressure within the bile duct and to account for pain that is not relieved by or recurs after cholecystectomy. Diagnosis is difficult, and its existence is questionable.

24. Do patients with AIDS have special issues in regard to the biliary tract?
Patients with AIDS have high rates of biliary infection with cytomegalovirus and *Cryptosporidium* sp. Such infections may result in strictures of the bile duct. The incidence of acalculous cholecystitis, which should be treated with cholecystectomy, seems to be higher.

TREATMENT

25. Who needs treatment for gallstones?
Acute cholecystitis requires cholecystectomy unless the patient's medical condition renders it impossible. Bile duct obstruction and cholangitis from stones in the bile duct also are indications for intervention. Recurrent episodes of upper abdominal pain are the most common indication; however, the pain may subside after several months of observation.

    Prophylactic cholecystectomy for patients with asymptomatic stones is recommended in specific groups, such as children, with a high incidence of developing symptoms or complications. It is recommended for patients with sickle-cell disease and should be done incidentally in patients having surgery for morbid obesity. Prophylactic cholecystectomy is also recommended in patients with high risk for cancer, such as Native Americans (3–5% risk of malignancy) or for "porcelain" gallbladder (calcified gallbladder wall; 50% risk of malignancy). Most authorities do not recommend surgery in diabetic patients with asymptomatic gallstones.

26. How is a cholecystectomy performed?
Open cholecystectomy has been performed with good results throughout this century. The gallbladder is resected from the liver bed with ligation of the cystic duct and artery. Elective cholecystectomy is associated with a morbidity rate of 2% and a mortality rate of 0.2%.

    Laparoscopic cholecystectomy has become the new standard since it was first performed in 1987. The abdomen is insufflated with gas, and four ports are placed through the abdominal wall. A camera is placed through one port and instruments through the others. The gallbladder is resected and removed through one of the ports. Approximately 95% of elective cholecystectomies are performed with laparoscopic techniques.

27. What is the triangle of Calot?
The triangle of Calot is the area between the liver, the cystic duct, and the common hepatic duct. The cystic artery is usually found in this location.

28. What are the ducts of Luschka?
The ducts of Luschka drain directly from the liver into the gallbladder and are sometimes responsible for postoperative bile leaks.

29. What are the benefits of laparoscopic cholecystectomy?

Laparoscopic cholecystectomy avoids an incision in the abdominal wall, which is the primary source of postoperative pain and temporary disability after open cholecystectomy. The patient can leave the hospital the same day and return to work within 1 week.

30. What are the contraindications to laparoscopic cholecystectomy?

A patient who is medically at too high a risk to undergo open cholecystectomy is not a good candidate for laparoscopic cholecystectomy. Several criteria are relative contraindications, including peritonitis, advanced cholecystitis, cirrhosis, cholangitis, pancreatitis, coagulopathy, previous upper abdominal surgery, and pregnancy; experience and selectivity are important factors.

31. What are the most common reasons for conversion from laparoscopic to open cholecystectomy?

Conversion rates as high as 15–30% are reported, depending on selection of patients for laparoscopic cholecystectomy. The most common reasons for conversion are inflammation and adhesions secondary to severe acute and chronic inflammation with the resulting inability to visualize the anatomy. Unfavorable anatomy or complication may necessitate conversion. Preoperative predictors of conversion to an open procedure are acute cholecystitis, increasing age, male sex, and thickened gallbladder wall on ultrasound.

32. What are the complications of cholecystectomy?

The risks of cholecystectomy include bleeding, infection, and bile leak. Rare complications of laparoscopy include injury to bowel or blood vessel by the trocars. The risk of bile duct injury is 0.2–0.4% in large series of laparoscopic cholecystectomy. However, tertiary care centers have reported an increase in bile duct injuries referred for repair. The pneumoperitoneum is usually well tolerated. Insufflation with CO_2 results in predictable cardiovascular changes, such as tachycardia, elevation of central venous pressure, hypertension, and decrease in cardiac output. The respiratory effects include an elevation in PCO_2 and a decrease in pH.

33. What are the indications for intraoperative cholangiograms?

Intraoperative cholangiograms reveal choledocholithiasis in 20–30% of patients with signs of common duct stones: jaundice, hyperamylasemia, multiple small stones, and dilated common bile duct. Some authors suggest that cholangiograms yield anatomic information of significant benefit and should be performed with all laparoscopic procedures.

34. What are the options for treatment of common bile duct stones?

The approach to common bile duct stones in the era of laparoscopic cholecystectomy is evolving and depends on the available resources. There are three potential pathways: (1) laparoscopic cholecystectomy combined with endoscopic retrograde cholangiopancreatography (ERCP), which may be done before or after the operation; (2) laparoscopic cholecystectomy with laparoscopic choledochoscopy via the cystic duct or laparoscopic choledochotomy; and (3) open common bile duct exploration.

BIBLIOGRAPHY

1. Boland GW, Lee MJ, Jeung J, et al: Percutaneous cholecystostomy in critically ill patients: Early response and final outcome in 82 patients. AJR 163:339, 1994.
2. Frazee RC, Nagorney DM, Mucha P Jr, et al: Acute acalculous cholecystitis. Mayo Clin Proc 64:163, 1989.
3. Fried GM, Barkun JS, Sigman HH, et al: Factors determining conversion to laparotomy in patients undergoing laparoscopic cholecystectomy. Am J Surg 167:35, 1994.
4. Hunter JG: Avoidance of bile duct injury during laparoscopic cholecystectomy. Am J Surg 162:71, 1991.
5. Kaplan MM, Johnston DE: Pathogenesis and treatment of gallstones. N Engl J Med 328:412, 1993.
6. NIH Consensus Conference: Gallstones and laparoscopic cholecystectomy. JAMA 266:1018, 1993.
7. Norby S, Herlin P, Holmin T, et al: Early or delayed cholecystectomy in acute cholecystitis? A clinical trial. Br J Surg 70:163, 1983.

8. Ransohoff DF, Gracie WA, Wolfsen LB, Neuhauser D:Prophylactic cholecystectomy or expectant management for silent gallstones: A decision analysis to assess survival. Ann Intern Med 99:199, 1983.
9. Ress AM, Sarr MG, Nagorney DM, et al: Spectrum and management of major complications of laparoscopic cholecystectomy.Am J Surg 165:655, 1993.
10. Shea JA, Berlin JA, Escarce JJ, et al: Revised estimates of diagnostic test sensitivity and specificity in suspected biliary tract disease. Arch Intern Med 154:2573, 1994.
11. Voyles CR, Sanders DK, Hogan R: Common bile duct evaluation in the era of laparoscopic cholecystectomy. 1050 cases later. Ann Surg 219:744, 1994.
12. Woods MS, Traverso LW, Kozarek RA, et al: Characteristics of biliary tract complications during laparoscopic cholecystectomy: A multi-institutional study. Am J Surg 167:27, 1994.

33. PANCREATIC CANCER

Nathan Pearlman, M.D.

1. What are the presenting signs of pancreatic cancer?
   1. Painless jaundice in 30–40% of patients
   2. Pain (epigastric, right upper quadrant, back) and jaundice in 30–40%
   3. Signs of metastatic disease (hepatomegaly, ascites, lung nodules, supraclavicular nodes in 20–30%

2. A patient presents with marked elevation of serum bilirubin and alkaline phosphatase, but only slight abnormalities of other liver functions. There is no history of pain, fever, or similar episodes in the past. What is the next best test to determine the problem?
Ultrasound is 90–95% accurate in detecting dilated extrahepatic bile ducts and stones in the gallbladder or common duct; it is 80% accurate in detecting a mass in the head of the pancreas. CT scan and/or endoscopic retrograde cholangiopancreatography (ERCP) provide much of the same information but are far more expensive and probably not warranted as initial tests.

3. Ultrasound shows a dilated common duct, stones in the gallbladder but not the common duct, and an ill-defined mass in the head of the pancreas. Why not proceed to the operating room?
Not all such patients have cancer of the pancreas. Some have stones impacted in the distal common bile duct (despite what ultrasound shows), some have pancreatitis, and some may have cancer of the distal bile duct instead of the pancreas. In patients with pancreatic cancer, it is useful to know whether the cancer has spread to other sites if surgery is contemplated.

4. If surgery is not the next step, what is?
ERCP or transhepatic cholangiogram is the next step, followed by CT scan. ERCP and transhepatic cholangiogram define the level of obstruction (high or low in the common duct) and its likely cause (stone, tumor, stricture). The biliary tract also can be decompressed at this time, allowing liver function to improve before any planned therapy is initiated. CT scan helps to define the extent of any tumor present and the likelihood of successful resection.

5. ERCP and CT scan merely confirm what ultrasound showed: extrahepatic biliary obstruction and a mass in the head of the pancreas. Why not try to get a diagnosis by percutaneous fine-needle aspiration (FNA)?
The information will not change what is done if the patient is an average or better operative risk. If the FNA shows cancer, surgery is in order to remove it, if possible, or to bypass it, if not resectable. If the FNA shows only benign pancreatic tissue or is indeterminate, surgery is still indicated, because the needle may have missed the lesion. In addition, FNA not infrequently causes

hemorrhage in the pancreas, adding to the difficulty of pancreaticoduodenectomy. A transabdominal FNA may be of benefit, however, if the patient is a poor operative risk. In such cases, resection is unlikely, and one can use endoluminal stents—placed at ERCP or by the radiologist—to achieve biliary decompression and thereby avoid surgery.

6. The surgical team proceeds to the operating room without an FNA and opens the abdomen. They find a 3-cm mass in the head of the pancreas, no ascites, and no liver metastases. What next?
Take down the gastrohepatic ligament and evaluate the rest of the pancreas. If the mass is rock-hard but the body and tail look and feel relatively normal, the patient has cancer. If the rest of the pancreas is diffusely indurated and almost as hard as the mass, the problem is more likely to be chronic pancreatitis. Many surgeons try to get a definitive tissue diagnosis at this point with a transduodenal or direct needle biopsy and frozen section.

While the pathologist is trying to decide between cancer and pancreatitis (the distinction can be difficult), try to determine whether the tumor is resectable for cure, if a diagnosis of cancer is reported. Grab the mass and try to move it up and down to see if it is free of retroperitoneal structures. Check for suspicious nodes and/or suspicious induration around the celiac axis, at the root of the mesentery, and in the hilum of the liver. If nodes are present, do not automatically assume that they are cancerous; biopsy and send for frozen section.

7. Biopsy of nodes at the celiac axis, root of the mesentery, or hilum of the liver shows cancer on frozen section. Is the tumor resectable for cure? If not for cure, for palliation?
No and no.

8. Biopsy of the nodes shows no cancer, and the pathologist reports finding only pancreatitis in the needle biopsy. Is it justified to proceed with resection or bypass on the basis of clinical judgment alone?
For many experienced pancreatic surgeons, the answer is yes. Most pancreatic cancers are surrounded by a rim of pancreatitis, which often feels like tumor and is easy to biopsy instead of the tumor. In addition, clinical judgment in this situation is about 90% accurate (i.e., in 10% of cases, resection is carried out and no tumor is found). Others, however, say no; operative mortality is too high to warrant resection unless cancer is definitely present. In the past, this argument had some merit, because pancreatic resection in the 1960s and 1970s had a mortality rate of 10–20%. In the last 10–15 years, however, resection has become safer, and many centers now report an operative mortality rate of less than 3%.

9. The pathologist asks whether the surgeon is going to carry out a Whipple procedure. If so, he wants to call in blood donors (he remembers the surgeon's last attempt).
Once again, the argument that a Whipple procedure (i.e., pancreatic resection) was a bloody and dangerous undertaking had some merit in the past. Once again, this has changed in recent times; fully one-half of such resections no long require transfusions.

10. What is a Whipple procedure? What is a total pancreatectomy?
The Whipple procedure is en bloc removal of the gallbladder, distal common bile duct, duodenum, and head of the pancreas. A total pancreatectomy removes these structures plus the body and tail of the pancreas and the spleen. In many instances, removal of the antrum of the stomach, with or without a vagotomy, is added to either procedure.

11. What are the advantages and disadvantages of each procedure?
Theoretically, 20% of patients have multifocal disease involving the body and tail of the pancreas, which are left behind with a Whipple procedure. In addition, a major source of operative morbidity after this procedure has been leakage from the anastomosis of pancreatic remnant to small bowel. Both problems are avoided if a total pancreatectomy is performed.

Total pancreatectomy, on the other hand, produces insulin-dependent diabetes, which may be difficult to manage when accompanied by other problems, such as postgastrectomy dumping, diarrhea, and pancreatic insufficiency. In addition, despite its theoretic advantages, to date total pancreatectomy has led to no better survival rates than the Whipple procedure. Finally, leaks from the pancreaticojejunostomy are no longer much of a problem. For these reasons, the author believes that the morbidity of total pancreatectomy outweighs its potential benefits and performs a Whipple procedure whenever possible.

12. Why take out the gallbladder, duodenum, and stomach if the tumor is in the pancreas?
Once the ampulla of Vater is removed, the gallbladder does not function well and forms stones. The second and third portions of the duodenum share a blood supply with the pancreatic head and are usually devascularized when the pancreatic head is removed. Historically, the gastric antrum was removed to achieve a better margin around the tumor. Vagotomy was added to reduce the incidence of marginal ulceration at the site where the gastric remnant is sewn to the bowel. Marginal ulceration, however, primarily reflects the site where bile and pancreatic ducts join the gut (upstream from the gastroenterostomy, so that alkaline secretions neutralize the gastric acid washing the suture line, or downstream, where no neutralization occurs). In addition, preserving the antrum does not compromise resection margins. Thus, many surgeons now perform pylorus-preserving Whipple procedures, in which the antrum and first portion of the duodenum are saved and vagotomy is omitted. Survival with this approach is the same as with the more radical procedure, and long-term function is somewhat better.

13. The tumor is mobile and node biopsies are negative. Does the surgeon need to know anything else at this point?
The surgeon needs to know whether the superior mesenteric vein and portal vein are free of invasion at the site where they pass behind the neck of the pancreas.

14. The portal vein seems stuck to the tumor. Is the tumor unresectable?
A few surgeons would consider removing the affected portion of the portal vein en bloc with the tumor, if it were the only sign of unresectability. The vein is then repaired by sewing the two ends together or using a graft. Such an undertaking generally requires special circumstances (a young, otherwise healthy patient with clean dissection planes), however, for resection of the portal vein has yet to be shown to improve survival rates. Thus, in most patients tumor attachment to the portal vein connotes incurability.

15. During mobilization of the mass the surgeon finds adherence to the portal vein and decides that the tumor is unresectable. Should anything else be done?
At a minimum, a biliary-enteric bypass (cholecystojejunostomy or choledochoenterostomy) should be done. It is preferable not to use the duodenum for the bypass, because tumor tends to grow upward toward the anastomosis and obstruct it. However, the duodenum may be the best choice when the root of the mesentery is invaded and small bowel mobility is limited.

Some authors also recommend a routine gastric bypass (gastroenterostomy), because 30% of patients develop gastric outlet obstruction secondary to tumor growth at a later date. The author prefers to treat this problem when it occurs, however, because gastroenterostomy in the asymptomatic patient may create as many problems as it solves.

Finally, if the patient had pain before surgery, alcohol injection of the celiac ganglion may provide some benefit. Unfortunately, sensory denervation often works better in theory than in practice.

16. The patient recovers nicely from the bypass procedure(s) and wants to know whether anything else can be done. What is available for locally unresectable pancreatic cancer?
Both radiotherapy and chemotherapy (5-fluorouracil or a combination of 5-fluorouracil, Adriamycin, and mitomycin-C) prolong survival by 3–4 months but offer little, if any, hope of cure.

17. What would the outlook be if resection had been possible?
The survival rate at 1 year is 70–80%; at 2 years, 40–60%; and at 5 years, 20–50%. The lower numbers are for carcinoma of the pancreas itself; the higher numbers are for carcinoma of the ampulla of Vater or distal common bile duct.

18. The survival rates are not great, particularly for cancer of the pancreas. Why are surgeons so eager to "do a Whipple"?
First, it is not always clear that the patient has a pancreatic tumor (with a relatively bad prognosis) rather than a distal bile duct cancer (with a relatively good prognosis), because the two sites are in close proximity. Second, median survival when the tumor cannot be removed is only 8–12 months, with or without chemotherapy and/or radiation. Thus, as bad as the figures are, they are better than with any other form of treatment.

BIBLIOGRAPHY

1. Brennan MF, Pisters PW, Posner M, et al: A prospective randomized trial of total parenteral nutrition after major pancreatic resection for malignancy. Ann Surg 220:436–444, 1994.
2. Cameron JL, Pitt HA, Yeo CJ, et al: One hundred and forty-five consecutive pancreaticoduodenectomies without mortality. Ann Surg 217:430–438, 1993.
3. Crist DW, Stizmann JV, Cameron JL: Improved hospital morbidity, mortality, and survival after the Whipple procedure. Ann Surg 206:358–365, 1987.
4. Cubilla AL, Fitzgerald PH: Cancer of the exocrine pancreas: The pathologic aspects. Cancer 35:2–18, 1985.
5. Evans DB, Termuhlen PM, Byrd RD, et al: Intraoperative radiation therapy following pancreaticoduodenectomy. Ann Surg 218:54–60, 1993.
6. Fortner JG: Regional, total and subtotal pancreatectomy. Cancer 47:1712–1718, 1986.
7. Hansson JA, Hoevels J, et al: Clinical aspects of nonsurgical percutaneous transhepatic bile drainage in obstructive lesions of the extrahepatic bile ducts. Ann Surg 189:58–61, 1979.
8. Haslam JB, Cavanaugh PH, Strapp SL: Radiation therapy in the treatment of unresectable adenocarcinoma of the pancreas. Cancer 32:1341–1345, 1973.
9. Neuberger TJ, Wade TP, Swope TJ, et al: Palliative operations for pancreatic cancer in the hospitals of the U.S. Department of Veterans Affairs from 1987 to 1991. Am J Surg 166:632–637, 1993.
10. Peters JH, Carey LC: Historical review of pancreaticoduodenectomy. Am J Surg 161:219–225, 1991.
11. Proctor HJ, Mauro M: Biliary diversion for pancreatic carcinoma: Matching the methods and the patient. Am J Surg 159:67–71, 1990.
12. Traverso LW, Longmire WP: Preservation of the pylorus in pancreaticoduodenectomy. A follow-up evaluation. Ann Surg 192:306–309, 1980.

34. ACUTE PANCREATITIS

Jon M. Burch, M.D., and Lawrence W. Norton, M.D.

1. What are the common causes of acute pancreatitis?
   1. Gallstones (50%)
   2. Alcohol (35%)

2. What are the uncommon causes of pancreatitis?
Hyperlipemia (types I and V), hyperparathyroidism, familial susceptibility, drugs (diuretics, sulfonamide, azathioprine, tetracycline, estrogens), and surgery. About 10% of cases are considered idiopathic.

3. What are the characteristic symptoms of acute pancreatitis?
Moderate-to-severe epigastric or right upper quadrant pain, which is boring in nature and may radiate through or around to the back, is almost always associated with nausea and vomiting.

4. Does hyperamylasemia in a patient with abdominal pain confirm pancreatitis?

No. Amylase levels can be elevated as a result of perforated peptic ulcer, bowel obstruction, salpingitis, and parotid inflammation. An amylase greater than 500, however, points to pancreatitis.

5. Do all patients with acute pancreatitis have hyperamylasemia?

No. Normal amylase levels occur in 5–30% of patients and are found most frequently in alcoholics with chronic pancreatitis (a "burned-out" pancreas cannot elaborate amylase) and in patients with lipemic serum.

6. How is hyperamylasemia due to pancreatitis identified?

Hyperamylasemia due to pancreatitis is identified by measurement of the pancreas-specific isoenzyme. Formerly this assay was complex and not widely available. Current methods use monoclonal antibodies to suppress the activity of the salivary fraction. The specimen can then be run on any standard autoanalyzer.

7. What are the frequency and mortality rate of severe (necrotizing) pancreatitis?

Frequency, < 10%; mortality rate, 10–15%.

8. What are the indications for operation in patients with acute pancreatitis?

The major indications for operation are uncertainty about diagnosis, local complications, and infected pancreatic necrosis. Cholecystectomy is performed in patients with gallstone pancreatitis after resolution of the acute attack.

9. By what means can severe pancreatitis be predicted?

Virtually all cases of severe or life-threatening pancreatitis are caused by pancreatic necrosis. At present the best method for identifying this entity is intravenous bolus, contrast-enhanced computed tomography, also known as dynamic pancreatography. The contrast highlights perfused areas of viable pancreas. Blotchy zones of necrotic pancreas portend trouble. Ranson's criteria, the APACHE II score, and other multiple parameter prognostic systems are similarly predictive but not diagnostic. They are also predictive of necrotizing pancreatitis.

10. What are Ranson's indices?

Ranson's indices are 11 physiologic measurements or blood chemistries that are useful in predicting the occurrence of severe pancreatitis:

On admission	After initial 48 hours
Age > 55 yr	Blood urea nitrogen > 5 mg/dl
White blood cell count > 16,000/mm^3	Hematocrit fall > 10%
Glucose > 350 IU/L	Serum calcium < 8 mg/dl
Lactate dehdyrogenase > 350 IU/L	Arterial partial pressure of oxygen < 60 mmHg
Serum glutamate oxaloacetate	Base deficit > 4 mEq/L
transaminase > 250 Frankel U/dl	Fluid sequestration > 6,000 ml

11. What is the best drug to relieve pain in mild pancreatitis?

Meperidine (Demerol) may have some theoretical advantage over morphine, because it causes less constriction of the sphincter of Oddi. The difference in effectiveness of the two analgesics is not clinically significant.

12. Should antibiotics be given to patients with mild pancreatitis?

No. Antibiotics neither improve the early course of disease nor prevent later septic complications.

13. Is nasogastric suction effective treatment of mild pancreatitis?

No. Controlled prospective studies show no advantage of nasogastric suction in patients with mild disease, although it may relieve nausea and vomiting.

14. What are possible complications of necrotizing pancreatitis?
Hemorrhage from adjacent vessels
Colonic perforation, fistula, or obstruction abscess
Pancreatic fistula or pseudocyst
Infected pancreatic necrosis

15. What is the significance of hypoxemia early in the course of pancreatitis?
Both necrotizing pancreatitis and infected pancreatic necrosis are capable of inducing either respiratory failure alone or the entire spectrum of multiple organ failure. Hypoxemia is an ominous sign.

16. What is the cause of hypocalcemia in severe disease?
No single explanation of hypocalcemia is accepted. Possible causative factors include (1) saponification "soap" formation in the lesser sac, (2) calcium release stimulated by glucagon, (3) hypomagnesemia, (4) hypoalbuminemia, (5) decreased levels of parathormone, and (6) hypovolemia.

17. Why does shock occur in severe pancreatitis?
The answer is multifactorial: (1) fluid sequestration in the abdominal cavity causes hypovolemia; (2) myocardial function is impaired; and (3) peripheral vascular resistance is often decreased.

18. What is the natural history of gallstone pancreatitis?
Attacks recur. Removal of the gallbladder cures the disease.

19. What is the natural history of alcoholic pancreatitis?
Attacks recur if the patient continues drinking. Many patients develop chronic pancreatitis.

20. What is the optimal method for diagnosing infected pancreatic necrosis?
The optimal method of diagnosis is CT-directed needle aspiration of suspicious areas for Gram stain and culture. This technique may be repeated as indicated during the course of the disease.

CONTROVERSIES

21. Terminology.
The greatest hindrance to advancement in the treatment of acute pancreatitis has been the lack of consistent terminology. To eliminate this confusion, new definitions have been proposed:
    Acute interstitial pancreatitis: acute inflammation and edema of the pancreas with or without fat necrosis.
    Necrotizing pancreatitis (or pancreatic necrosis): inflammation with devitalized pancreatic and/or peripancreatic tissue.
    Infected pancreatic necrosis: necrotizing pancreatitis plus diffuse bacterial infection.
    Pancreatic abscess: purulent material in the region of the pancreas enclosed by an inflammatory wall.
    Acute pseudocyst: effusion of pancreatic juice enclosed by an inflammatory wall.
    Fat sequestration: necrotic fat enclosed by an inflammatory wall.
    The original and recently revised versions of the Marseilles classification are not clinically relevant and should be abandoned.

22. Timing of cholecystectomy for patients with gallstone pancreatitis.
A prospective randomized study by Kelly demonstrated that cholecystectomy should be performed during the same admission after the acute illness has resolved. For most patients this requires 2 or 3 days; for patients with necrotizing pancreatitis, several days or even weeks may be necessary.

23. Somatostatin.
Somatostatin suppresses elaboration of essentially all GI hormones. Although early administration of somatostatin in patients with acute pancreatitis may decrease the incidence of local complications, it does not improve survival rates.

24. Peritoneal lavage.
Dilution of vasoactive peptides and enzymes elaborated by the severely inflamed pancreas is the rationale for therapeutic peritoneal lavage. Results in patients with severe pancreatitis were encouraging initially. However, recent reports demonstrate no improvement in survival rates.

25. Pancreatic resection.
Most patients with necrotizing pancreatitis (pancreatic necrosis) can be successfully managed with operative intervention. An occasional patient with refractory single or multiple organ failure may benefit from debridement of necrotic (even noninfected) pancreatic and peripancreatic tissue. There is universal agreement that infected pancreatic necrosis must be surgically debrided. Excellent results are currently obtained with debridement with drainage alone, open packing, or postoperative irrigation.

BIBLIOGRAPHY

1. Acosta JM, Rossi R, Galli OMR, et al: Early surgery for gallstone pancreatitis: Evaluation of a systematic approach. Surgery 83:367–370, 1978.
2. Beger HG: Surgical management of necrotizing pancreatitis. Surg Clin North Am 69:529–549, 1989.
3. Bradley EL, Murphy F, Ferguson C: Prediction of pancreatic necrosis by dynamic pancreatography. Arch Surg 210:495–504, 1989.
4. Choi TK, Mok F, Zhan WH, et al: Somatostatin in the treatment of acute pancreatitis: A prospective randomized controlled trial. Gut 30:223–227, 1989.
5. Demmy TL, Burch JM, Feliciano DV, et al: Comparisons of multiple-parameter prognostic systems in acute pancreatitis. Am J Surg 156:492–496, 1988.
6. Howard JM: Delayed debridement and external drainage of massive pancreatic or peripancreatic necrosis. Surg Gynecol Obstet 168:25–29, 1989.
7. Howes R, Zuidema GD, Cameron JL: Evaluation of prophylactic antibiotics in acute pancreatitis. J Surg Res 18(2):197–200, 1975.
8. Kelly TR, Wagner DS: Gallstone pancreatitis: A prospective randomized trial of the timing of surgery. Surgery 104:600–605, 1988.
9. Luiten EJ, Hop WCJ, Lange JF, Bruining HA: Controlled clinical trials of selective decontamination for the treatment of severe acute pancreatitis. Ann Surg 222:57–65, 1995.
10. Normal JG, Franz MG, Fink GS, et al: Decreased mortality of severe acute pancreatitis after proximal cytokine blockade. Ann Surg 221:625–634, 1995.
11. Stanten R, Frey CF: Comprehensive management of acute necrotizing pancreatitis and pancreatic abscess. Arch Surg 125:1269–1275, 1990.

35. CHRONIC PANCREATITIS

Jon M. Burch, M.D., and Lawrence W. Norton, M.D.

1. What is chronic pancreatitis?
The classic syndrome consists of abdominal pain, diabetes, steatorrhea, and pancreatic calcification. Frequently, one or more of the latter three symptoms are absent. Diabetes occurs with extensive damage (90%) of the pancreas and is found in about one-third of patients. Calcification may be due to a decrease in pancreatic stone protein, which normally prevents formation of insoluble calcium salts.

2. Is chronic pancreatitis the result of acute pancreatitis?

Many patients have not had acute pancreatitis, although alcoholism is common to both. The average age for chronic pancreatitis is 13 years less than for acute pancreatitis.

3. What are the signs and symptoms of steatorrhea?

Steatorrhea is frequently but not invariably associated with pancreatic insufficiency. Stools typically are soft, greasy, and foul-smelling. An oily ring is left in the toilet bowl.

4. What test confirms steatorrhea?

Increased neutral fat (triglyceride) in the stool can be detected microscopically or biochemically. A fecal fat concentration in excess of 10% is characteristic of pancreatogenous steatorrhea.

5. What tests help to differentiate various causes of steatorrhea?

The D-xylose test is positive in the presence of small bowel disease and usually is normal in patients with pancreatic exocrine insufficiency. The Schilling test for vitamin B12 absorption shows decreased urinary secretion of labeled cyanocobalamin in 40% of patients with chronic pancreatitis but also may be positive in the presence of anemia, bacterial overgrowth, or ileal disease.

6. In patients with abdominal pain due to chronic pancreatitis but no steatorrhea , is there any means of detecting pancreatic insufficiency?

The secretin stimulation test becomes abnormal when more than 75% of pancreatic function is lost. Normally, the peak concentration of bicarbonate in pancreatic juice is greater than 80 mEq/L. Patients who have abdominal pain secondary to chronic pancreatitis but no steatorrhea have bicarbonate concentrations in the range of 60–80 mEq/L. Such patients have normal levels of pancreatic polypeptide.

7. Is serum amylase elevated in chronic pancreatitis?

No. Serum pancreatic isoamylase is usually normal or decreased ("burned-out" pancreatitis).

8. What is the treatment of steatorrhea?

Most patients respond to replacement of pancreatic enzymes. If this approach fails to reduce fecal fat excretion to less than 15–20 gm/day, fat content in the diet is decreased. If steatorrhea persists, aluminum-containing antacids and, finally, cimetidine are introduced.

9. How is pain relieved?

Pancreatic enzymes, acting in a feedback loop, may relieve pain. Because the narcotic bowel syndrome may contribute to pain, alcohol and narcotics should be withdrawn (under cover of clonidine). Medically intractable pain suggests the need for operation.

10. What local complications may result from chronic pancreatitis?

Pancreatic pseudocyst or fistula (pancreatic ascites) may occur. Fibrosis may constrict the distal common bile duct as it passes through the gland, causing obstructive jaundice. Splenic vein thrombosis and duodenal obstruction occur rarely.

11. What information is essential before operating on a patient with chronic pancreatitis?

A radiographic contrast study of the pancreatic duct should be obtained. The best approach is by endoscopic retrograde cholangiopancreatography (ERCP). During operation, the duct can be visualized by (1) direct needle injection of contrast material into the enlarged duct, (2) duct cannulation via duodenotomy, or (3) cannulation of the distal duct after amputation of the tail of the gland.

12. Which procedure is indicated for multiple duct obstructions that result in the "chain-of-lakes" appearance?
The Peustow operation opens the obstructed duct system longitudinally and provides drainage from the head to the tail via a Roux-en-Y pancreaticojejunostomy.

13. Which procedures may be useful for patients with a normal pancreatic duct?
Pancreatic resections of varying extent have relieved pain to a similar extent as decompressive procedures. Total pancreatectomy should be avoided, because results are no better than with more limited resections and the resultant diabetes tends to be very brittle.

14. What is the usual result of such operations?
Pain relief in 70% of patients at the end of 1 year and in 50% at the end of 5 years.

CONTROVERSIES

15. Visceral ganglionectomy.
Neurectomy of sympathetic fibers supplying the pancreas is sometimes performed at the level of the celiac axis for pain relief in patients failing resection or as an alternative to pancreatic operations. Pain relief is variable (50–90%).

16. Ligation of pancreatic duct.
Ligating the ducts of Wirsung and Santorini as they penetrate the wall of the duodenum causes atrophy of acini and ducts (exocrine function) but preserves islet cell (endocrine) function. Results of this procedure for pain relief are not encouraging.

17. Autotransplantation.
Segmental pancreatic autotransplantation after duct occlusion may prevent diabetes after partial pancreatectomy. Limited experience with the technique is encouraging. An alternative means to preserve islet cell function is autotransplantation of islet cells alone. This technique is accomplished by injecting islet cell preparations either into the portal vein (hopefully they seed the liver) or under the highly vascular renal capsule.

BIBLIOGRAPHY

1. Ammann RW, Akovbiantz A, Lariader F, et al: Course and outcome of chronic pancreatitis. Gastroenterology 86:820–828, 1984.
2. Arnaud J-P, Bergamaschi R, Serra-Maudet V, Casa C: Pancreaticoduodenectomy for hemosuccus pancreaticus in silent chronic pancreatitis. Arch Surg 129:333–334, 1994.
3. Bradley EL III: Long-term results of pancreaticojejunostomy in patients with chronic pancreatitis. Am J Surg 153:207–213, 1987.
4. Cooperman A: Chronic pancreatitis. Surg Clin North Am 61:71, 1981.
5. Fernandez-del Castillo C, Rattner DW, Warshaw AL: Standards for pancreatic resection in the 1990s. Arch Surg 130:295–300, 1995.
6. Niederau C, Grendell JM: Diagnosis of chronic pancreatitis. Gastroenterology 88:1973–1995, 1985.
7. Rossi RL, Meiss FW, Braasch JW: Surgical management of chronic pancreatitis. Surg Clin North Am 65:79, 1985.
8. Sarles H: Etiopathogenesis and definition of chronic pancreatitis. Dig Dis Sci 31(Suppl): 91, 1986.
9. Stone WM, Sarr MG, Nagorney DM, et al: Chronic pancreatitis: Results of Whipple's resection and total pancreatectomy. Arch Surg 123:815–819, 1988.
10. Warshaw RL: Pancreatic surgery: A paradigm for progress in the age of the bottom line. Arch Surg 130:240–246, 1995.
11. Warshaw AL, Popp JW, Schapiro RH: Long-term patency, pancreatic function and pain relief after lateral pancreaticojejunostomy for chronic pancreatitis. Gastroenterology 79:289–293, 1980.

36. PORTAL HYPERTENSION AND ESOPHAGEAL VARICES

James B. Downey, M.D., and Greg Van Stiegmann, M.D.

1. What is the blood supply to the liver?
Total hepatic blood flow is roughly one-fourth of cardiac output at 1500 ml/min. The hepatic artery supplies approximately 30% of blood flow but delivers 70% of oxygen to the liver, whereas the portal vein supplies 70% of blood flow and delivers 30% of oxygen.

2. What is portal hypertension?
Normal portal venous pressures range from 7–10 mmHg. In portal hypertension, pressures average 20 mmHg. This elevation of pressure may result in retrograde blood flow in the collateral vessels supplying the portal vein.

3. Describe the collateral flow between the portal and systemic venous systems and its clinical significance.
Four collateral venous systems connect the portal and systemic circulations:

1. Portal → coronary (left gastric) → esophageal → azygous and hemiazygous veins (leads to esophageal varices).

2. Portal → inferior mesenteric → superior hemorrhoidal → submucosal hemorrhoidal plexus → middle and inferior hemorrhoidals → hypogastric vein (leads to hemorrhoids).

3. Portal → umbilical → superficial veins of abdominal wall → superior and inferior epigastrics (leads to periumbilical caput medusa).

4. Portal → mesenteric → veins of Retzius → peritoneal → inferior vena cava.

Esophageal and gastric varices form when portal pressures exceed 12 mmHg. Hemorrhoids and periumbilical caput medusa are common in portal hypertension.

4. What are the causes of portal hypertension?
Elevated portal venous pressures may arise from increased portal blood flow, increased resistance to flow, or both. Increased flow is seen with arteriovenous fistulas (congenital or traumatic) or increased splenic blood flow. Increased resistance to flow is divided into three categories:

1. **Prehepatic:** portal vein thrombosis, extrinsic compression of the portal vein by tumor or pseudocysts

2. **Hepatic:** cirrhosis, schistosomiasis, hepatic fibrosis

3. **Posthepatic:** hepatic vein thrombosis (Budd-Chiari syndrome), constrictive pericarditis, right-heart failure

5. What is the most common cause of portal hypertension in the United States in adults? In children? In the world?
Laennec's (alcoholic) cirrhosis is the most common cause of portal hypertension in Western countries, accounting for 85% of cases in the U.S. Chronic alcoholism results in obstruction of postsinusoidal hepatic blood flow. Extrahepatic portal venous occlusion, usually due to cavernous malformation of the portal vein, is the most common cause in children. Worldwide, schistosomiasis is the most common cause of portal hypertension.

6. What are the complications of portal venous hypertension?
Hemorrhage from esophageal varices is the most catastrophic complication. Other complications include ascites, hypersplenism, hemorrhoids, gastritis, and portosystemic encephalopathy.

7. How common are esophageal varices? How often are they symptomatic?
Sixty percent of cirrhotic patients have varices. Hemorrhage from varices occurs in 30% of patients within 1 year of diagnosis; without treatment 40–60% will subsequently rebleed. Despite recent advances, each bleed from esophageal varices carries a 30–40% mortality rate.

8. Is upper gastrointestinal bleeding in cirrhotic patients always due to varices?
No. Twenty-five percent of cirrhotic patients bleed from another source. Endoscopy is crucial in diagnosing the etiology of the bleed. Ninety-five percent of esophageal varices are within 3 cm of the gastroesophageal (GE) junction.

9. What is the initial treatment of patients with suspected esophageal variceal hemorrhage?
The initial treatment is aggressive resuscitation, which consists of large-bore or central venous access, invasive monitoring, Foley catheterization, and judicious replacement of blood volume and blood products. Gastric lavage should be performed with a large-bore nasogastric (Ewald) tube. Endoscopy should be performed as soon as the patient is hemodynamically stable. If variceal hemorrhage is diagnosed, mechanical, pharmacologic, endoscopic, radiologic, and surgical treatment options are available.

10. What is a Sengstaken-Blakemore tube?
The Sengstaken-Blakemore (SB) tube is used for mechanical tamponade of variceal hemorrhage. It consists of two balloons and is placed nasally into the stomach. When its position in the stomach has been confirmed radiographically, the distal gastric balloon is inflated with 250 ml of air, drawn tight against the GE junction, and placed on traction. If the gastric balloon alone does not control the hemorrhage, the proximal esophageal balloon is inflated to a pressure of 20 mmHg. Balloon tamponade is a temporary measure to control bleeding and can be applied for 12–24 hours. Fifty percent of patients rebleed after balloon deflation. Risks include esophageal perforation and necrosis of esophageal mucosa from overinflation of the balloon.

11. What pharmacologic agents are used in the treatment of variceal bleeding?
Medical therapy alone is successful in controlling roughly 50% of acute bleeds. However, 30–50% of patients rebleed within 7–10 days. Commonly used agents include the following:
Vasopressin (0.4–0.8 U/min IV) is a potent vasoconstrictor that decreases splanchnic blood flow. However, it has severe systemic side effects, such as peripheral vasoconstriction, decreased coronary blood flow, decreased cardiac output, hypotension, and intestinal cramping. Nitroglycerin, a vasodilator, further reduces portal pressures and ameliorates the side effects of vasopressin.
Glypressin (2 mg IV every 4 hours) is a synthetic analog of vasopressin with a longer half-life, simpler administration, and fewer systemic side effects. Nitroglycerin is also used in conjunction.
Somatostatin (250 µg IV bolus, then 250 µg/hour IV) decreases portal blood flow by selective splanchnic vasoconstriction and is free from systemic side effects.
Octreotide is a new synthetic analog of somatostatin under clinical investigation.

12. What endoscopic treatments are available?
The available endoscopic treatments are sclerotherapy and endoscopic band ligation (EBL). Intravariceal injection of a sclerosant (5% ethanolamine oleate, sodium morrhuate, or tetradecyl sodium) promotes thrombosis. Strangulating varices with rubber bands is an extension of the well-recognized method of ligating anal hemorrhoids. The goal of both treatments is to replace varices with fibrous scar tissue.

13. What are the results of endoscopic therapy?
Acute variceal hemorrhage is controlled with a single endoscopic treatment in 75–95% of cases. Four to eight subsequent sessions of endoscopic therapy at weekly or monthly intervals may

obliterate varices. Fifty percent of patients rebleed, but the bleeding tends to be less severe and less frequent than in untreated patients.

14. Is one form of endoscopic therapy superior?

Yes. EBL is safer, faster, and cheaper. It also offers better control of variceal hemorrhage, and the resultant scar tissue is confined to the mucosa and submucosa. As a result, complications seen with sclerotherapy, such as esophageal strictures and dysmotility, have not been reported with EBL. Banding takes less time to learn and to perform. EBL requires fewer treatment sessions than sclerotherapy to eradicate varices, and the period between sessions is shorter. Such features make EBL less expensive than sclerotherapy. Finally, most authors report not only improved control of acute variceal hemorrhage but also improved survival rates with fewer recurrent bleeds after EBL.

15. What is the role of radiologic and surgical procedures in the treatment of esophageal varices?

Endoscopic therapy is the first-line treatment of choice in most centers. Radiologic procedures and surgical shunts are usually reserved for patients who fail endoscopic therapy or live in remote areas.

16. What is TIPS?

Transjugular intrahepatic portosystemic shunt (TIPS) is a minimally invasive technique for the treatment of portal hypertension. An 8–10-mm stent is placed flouroscopically from the hepatic venous system, through the hepatic parenchyma, and into the portal venous system. The goal of TIPS is relief of ascites and variceal bleeding by decompressing the portal pressure to less than 15 mmHg. Rebleeding, usually due to shunt thrombosis, occurs in 25% of cases. Stents with increased diameter result in higher flow and greater decompression of the portal venous system with a lower incidence of thrombosis but a higher incidence of hepatic encephalopathy.

17. What is the Child's classification?

The Child's classification assesses the severity of liver failure and the associated operative risk by using several parameters of hepatic function and nutrition:

Child's Classification

	A	B	C
Serum bilirubin (md/dl)	Below 2.0	2.0–3.0	Over 3.0
Serum albumin (mg/dl)	Over 3.5	3.0–3.5	Under 3.0
Ascites	None	Easily controlled	Poorly controlled
Encephalopathy	None	Minimal	Advanced
Nutrition	Excellent	Good	Poor

Patients in Child's class A are good risks and have low operative mortality rates, whereas patients in class C have significantly higher mortality rates.

18. What surgical shunt operations are available to treat portal hypertension? What is the difference between selective and central (nonselective) shunts?

Portacaval and mesocaval central shunts nonselectively decompress the portal venous system. However, they often result in stagnation or reversal of portal blood flow, thus worsening hepatic failure and encephalopathy. The selective splenorenal (Warren) shunt decompresses esophageal varices while allowing prograde portal blood flow to the liver. The procedure involves anastomosis of the distal (splenic side) splenic vein to the left renal vein with ligation of the coronary (left gastric) veins. This technique allows decompression of the esophageal varices via the short gastric veins into the spleen and hence from the newly anastomosed splenic vein into the renal vein and systemic circulation. High pressures are maintained in the portal vein, which continues to perfuse the liver.

19. What is the operative mortality rate for elective portosystemic shunts? What percent rebleed? What is the cause of rebleeding?
The operative mortality rate for in elective portosystemic shunts is 5% for Child's A patients, 10% for Child's B patients, and 20–40% for Child's C patients. Rebleeding occurs in approximately 5% of patients and, as in TIPS, is usually due to thrombosis of the shunt.

20. What operations are used for emergency treatment of variceal bleeding?
The goal in emergency operations is control of bleeding and prevention of exsanguination; less concern is given to the possible postoperative sequelae (e.g., encephalopathy). A nonselective (central) portosystemic shunt is used. The most expeditious and popular shunt is performed by placing a prosthetic graft between the proximal superior mesenteric vein and the inferior vena cava (mesocaval shunt). Other emergent procedures include direct varix ligation, splenectomy, or esophageal transection with a surgical stapler, but these techniques are used infrequently and only in desperation.

21. What is the operative mortality rate in emergency shunt procedures for acute hemorrhage?
Emergency shunt procedures have a mortality rate of 50%. Hepatic failure is the cause of death in two-thirds of cases.

22. What is the role of liver transplantation in the treatment of portal hypertension?
Liver transplantation is the only therapy that cures both portal hypertension and underlying liver disease. All Child's B and C patients should be assessed as potential transplant recipients. However, organ supply is limited, and less than 10% of patients who would benefit receive liver transplants. Prior TIPS or portosystemic shunts do not preclude transplantation but make the procedure technically challenging.

23. Devise an algorithm for the treatment options in patients with portal hypertension and bleeding esophageal varices.
Child's A patients who fail endoscopic therapy are best treated with elective portosystemic shunting. In patients with favorable anatomy (patent splenic vein, normal renal vein), a selective splenorenal shunt is preferred because of the lower incidence of encephalopathy. In Child's C patients, elective shunt operations carry a high operative mortality rate, have not been shown to improve survival, and thus are not warranted. Patients with Child's B and C liver disease who are good operative candidates are best treated with liver transplantation. TIPS can be used as a bridge to transplantation or as primary treatment in patients deemed to be poor operative candidates.

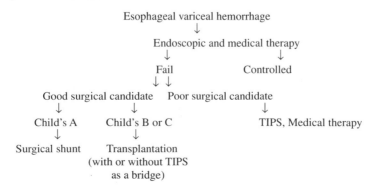

BIBLIOGRAPHY

1. Arroyo V, Bosach J, Rodes J: Treatments in Hepatology. Masson, 1995.
2. Chojkier M, Conn HO: Esophageal tamponade in the treatment of bleeding varices: A decadal progress report. Dig Dis Sci 25:267, 1980.
3. Knechtle S, et al: Portal hypertension: Surgical management in the 1990's. Surgery 116:687, 1994.
4. Schwartz SI: Principles of Surgery, 6th ed. New York, McGraw-Hill, 1994.
5. Stiegmann GV, et al: Endoscopic sclerotherapy as compared with endoscopic ligation for bleeding esophageal varices. N Engl J Med 326:1527, 1992.
6. Stiegmann GV: Endoscopic management of esophageal varices. Adv Surg 27:209, 1994.
7. Terblanche J: The surgeon's role in the management of portal hypertension. Ann Surg 209:381, 1989.
8. Warren WD, et al: Distal splenorenal shunt vs. endoscopic sclerotherapy for long term management of variceal bleeding. Ann Surg 203:454, 1986.

37. GASTROESOPHAGEAL REFLUX DISEASE

Lawrence W. Norton, M.D.

1. What symptoms suggest gastroesophageal reflux (GERD)?

Substernal burning discomfort after meals or at night, associated occasionally with regurgitation of gastric juice, is a frequent symptom of GERD. Discomfort is relieved by standing or sitting. Dysphagia, a late complication of GERD, is caused by mucosal edema or stricture of the distal esophagus.

2. What is the difference between heartburn and GERD?

Heartburn is a lay term for mild, intermittent reflux of gastric content into the esophagus without tissue injury. It is relatively common among adults. GERD implies esophagitis with varying degrees of erythema, edema, and friability of the distal esophageal mucosa. It occurs in 5–10% of the population.

3. What causes GERD?

The underlying abnormality of GERD is functional incompetence of the lower esophageal sphincter (LES), which allows gastric acid, bile, and digestive enzymes to damage the unprotected esophageal mucosa. Achalasia, scleroderma, and other motility disorders of the esophagus are sometimes associated with gastroesophageal reflux disease.

4. Is hiatal hernia an essential defect in GERD?

No. Hiatal hernia is present in only about 50% of patients with GERD.

5. What studies are useful to diagnose GERD?

Endoscopy with biopsy is the essential element in diagnosing GERD. Barium swallow with or without fluoroscopy can diagnose reflux but cannot identify gastritis. Twenty-four hour esophageal pH testing associates reflux with symptoms and is useful in some but not all patients. Manometry of the esophagus and LES is required whenever an esophageal motility disorder is suspected. Gastric secretory or gastric emptying tests are occasionally helpful.

6. What is the initial management of a patient suspected to have GERD?

  • Change diet to avoid foods known to induce reflux (e.g., chocolate, coffee)
  • Avoid large meals before bedtime.
  • Stop smoking.
  • Do not wear tight, binding clothes.

• Elevate the head of the bed 4–5 inches.
• Take antacids when symptomatic.

7. If initial treatment fails, what should be recommended?
About 50% of patients show significant healing with H_2-blockers. Only a small number of these patients (10%) remain healed over the course of 1 year. Metoclopramide or cisapride may be prescribed to stimulate gastric emptying. Neither agent relieves symptoms consistently in the absence of acid reduction.

8. What is the role of omeprazole in GERD?
Omeprazole, which irreversibly inhibits the parietal cell hydrogen ion pump, is over 80% successful in healing severe erosive esophagitis. Two-thirds of patients who continue the mediation remain healed. A concern in prolonged omeprazole therapy is hypergastrinemia secondary to alkalinization of the antrum. The fact that gastrin is trophic to gastrointestinal mucosa raises the fear of later neoplasia.

9. When should operation for GERD be recommended?
Failure of nonoperative therapy is the primary indication for operation. Noncompliance with prescribed treatment is a frequent cause of failure. Stricture unresponsive to dilation is another indication for operation.

10. What is the goal of surgical treatment?
Operations for GERD attempt to prevent reflux by mechanically increasing LES pressure and, in most procedures, to restore a sufficient length of distal esophagus to the high-pressure zone of the abdomen. Hiatal hernia, when present, is reduced simultaneously. The crura of the diaphragm sometimes can be approximated to act as a pinchcock on the LES.

11. What procedures can accomplish this goal? How do they do it?
    1. In the **Nissen fundoplication**, which is used in over 95% of patients, the fundus of the stomach is mobilized, wrapped around the distal esophagus posteriorly, and secured to itself anteriorly. The procedure alters the angle of the gastroesophageal junction and maintains the distal esophagus within the abdomen to prevent reflux. The operation is done transabdominally by either laparotomy or laparoscopy.

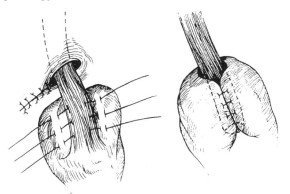

Nissen fundoplication. (This figure and the figures illustrating the Belsey Mark IV operation and the Hill gastropexy were redrawn from Nardi GL, Zuidema GD (eds): Surgery: Essentials of Clinical Practice. Boston, Little, Brown, 1982, pp 404–405.)

    2. The **Belsey Mark IV operation** accomplishes the same anatomic changes but is done via a thoracotomy.

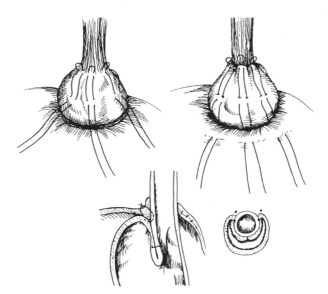

Belsey Mark IV operation.

3. The **Hill gastropexy** restores the esophagus to the abdominal cavity by securing the gastric cardia to the preaortic fascia.

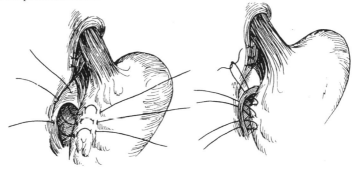

Hill gastropexy.

4. The **Angelchik prosthesis** is a silicone-filled collar placed around the distal esophagus within the abdominal cavity.

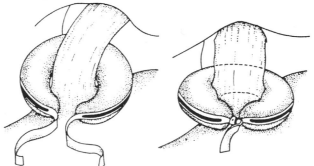

Angelchik prosthesis. (From Angelchik JP, Cohen RC: Surg Gynecol Obstet 148:246–248, 1979, with permission.)

12. What are the success rates for such procedures?
All of the procedures described in question 11 eliminate GERD in about 90% of patients who are
followed for 10 years. The Nissen fundoplication is considered to be the most effective in comparison studies.

13. What are the long-term complications of such procedures?
The repair may fail, with recurrence of reflux, after each operation. Incorrect placement or slippage of the stomach wrap can complicate Nissen fundoplication and the Belsey Mark IV procedure. Dysphagia and the inability to belch (gas-bloat syndrome) result from too tight a wrap. The
Angelchik prosthesis may erode into a viscus or become displaced.

14. How can stricture from GERD be managed?
Pliable (unfixed) strictures can be dilated. Fixed strictures require surgical repair. One such operation is to patch the narrowed esophagus with stomach wall (Thal).

CONTROVERSIES

**15. Is GERD better treated in the long term by omeprazole therapy or Nissen fundoplica-
tion?**
The effectiveness of omeprazole in resolving esophagitis and eliminating symptoms of GERD is
excellent, but the side effects of the medication taken over years are not fully known.
Fundoplication frees the patient from the need for daily medication but causes morbidity in about
5–10%.

16. Is Nissen fundoplication better done by laparoscopy or laparotomy?
Exactly the same procedure can be accomplished by either approach. The incidence of postoperative morbidity and mortality is comparable. The distinct advantages of laparoscopy are less
postoperative pain, shorter hospitalization, and earlier return to work.

BIBLIOGRAPHY

1. Bremner RM, DeMeester TR, Crookes F, et al: The effect of symptoms and nonspecific motility abnormalities on outcomes of surgical therapy for gastroesophageal reflux. J Thorac Cardiovasc Surg
107:1244, 1994.
2. Collard JM, Verstraete L, Otte JB, et al: Clinical, radiological and functional results of remedial antireflux
operations. Int Surg 78:298, 1993.
3. Hetzel DJ, Dent J, Reed WED, et al: Healing and relapse of severe peptic esophagitis after treatment with
omeprazole. Gastroenterology 95:903, 1988.
4. Hinder RA, Filipi CJ, Wetscher G, et al: Laparoscopic Nissen fundoplication is an effective treatment for
gastroesophageal reflux disease. Ann Surg 220:472, 1994.
5. Liegermann DA: Medical therapy for chronic reflux esophagitis: Long-term follow-up. Arch Intern Med
147:1717, 1987.
6. Spechler SJ: Comparison of medical and surgical therapy for complicated gastroesophageal reflux disease
in veterans. N Engl J Med 326:786, 1992.
7. Urschel JD: Complications of antireflux surgery. Am J Surg 166:68, 1993.

38. ESOPHAGEAL CANCER

James R. Denton, M.D.

1. Describe the epidemiology of esophageal cancer.
Esophageal cancer accounts for 1% of all cancers and 2% of all cancer-related deaths. Approximately 10,000 new cases and 9,500 deaths are reported each year. In the United States there is definite race and sex predisposition: four times more common in men, three times more common in blacks. Iran, North China, and the Cape Province of South Africa all have an unusually high incidence.

2. Esophageal cancer has one of the poorest cure rates and shortest survivals of all malignancies. Why?
Esophageal cancer is an aggressive malignancy that typically presents at advanced or unresectable stages. The physiologic status of the typical patient with esophageal cancer is poor. Patients frequently have significant cardiopulmonary disease as well as a debilitated nutritional status.

3. What disorders of the esophagus are considered premalignant?

Barrett's esophagus	Caustic injuries
Leukoplakia	Scleroderma
Achalasia	Strictures
Plummer-Vinson syndrome	Tylosis

4. What is Barrett's esophagus? What type of carcinoma arises from Barrett's esophagus?
Barrett's esophagus is a form of glandular metaplasia of the esophageal mucosa resulting from chronic gastroesophageal reflux and esophagitis. There is a 40-fold increase in the incidence of carcinoma in patients with a columnar-lined distal esophagus. Adenocarcinoma arises from the glandular metaplasia; unlike squamous carcinoma, the incidence of adenocarcinoma of the esophagus is increasing

5. What other factors have been incriminated in the etiology of esophageal cancer?
Alcohol consumption increases risk by 10 times and tobacco by 10 times. Vitamin and trace element deficiencies as well as chemical toxins also have been associated with esophageal malignancy.

6. What is the anatomic distribution of esophageal cancer?
For anatomic purposes, the esophagus is divided into upper, middle, and lower thirds. Fifteen percent of cancers arise in the upper third, 50% in the middle third, and 35% in the lower third.

7. Describe the histopathology of esophageal cancer.
Seventy-five percent of esophageal cancer is of the squamous cell variety. If one limits the survey to the distal third of the esophagus and includes the gastroesophageal junction and cardia, far more than 50% of cases are adenocarcinoma. Unusual types of esophageal cancer include mucoepidermoid, carcinoid, leiomyosarcoma, melanoma, rhabdomyosarcoma, lymphoma, and anaplastic carcinoma, but these are rare.

8. What are the most common presenting symptoms of esophageal cancer?

Dysphagia—85%	Regurgitation—25%
Weight loss—60%	Hoarseness—5%
Pain—25%	Cough—3%

9. How does the presenting symptom correlate with potential resection for cure?
Dysphagia for both solids and liquids or evidence of near total obstruction by either GI series or endoscopy often signifies a circumferential lesion with local invasion. Similarly, pain may be an indication of spread beyond the confines of the esophagus. Hoarseness represents recurrent laryngeal nerve invasion and bodes poorly for resection for cure. Cough may represent either aspiration from obstruction or a tracheoesophageal fistula—both ominous prognostic signs.

10. What is the natural history of esophageal cancer?
Natural history data are obtained by following untreated patients with documented esophageal cancer. In a collected series of almost 1,000 patients, the 1- and 2-year survival rates were 6% and 0.3%, respectively. Untreated patients typically succumb to progressive malnutrition complicated by aspiration pneumonia, sepsis, and death. Formation of a fistula between the aorta or pulmonary artery and the esophagus or pulmonary tree is a somewhat more dramatic and perhaps merciful mode of exit.

11. After traditional esophagogastrectomy, what is the survival rate by stage?

Survival Rates after Surgery by Stage

	2 YEARS (%)	5 YEARS (%)
Stage I	29	12
Stage II	20	6
Stage III	6	0

12. Since the potential for cure is poor, what is the primary goal of therapy?
Durable palliation should be foremost in the physician's mind when planning therapy for the majority of patients with esophageal cancer. The ability to swallow secretions and to maintain adequate oral nutrition is of paramount importance.

13. What are the various treatment options?
Treatments include resection, radiation, chemotherapy, laser recanalization, esophageal stents, and dilation. The latter three are clearly directed at palliation alone. Surgery, chemotherapy, radiation, and combinations thereof provide an opportunity for durable palliation in most patients and a chance for cure in a fortunate few. The advent of transhiatal esophagectomy has expanded the group of patients suitable for surgery. By avoiding thoracotomy, the morbidity and mortality of resection for either palliation or cure have been significantly decreased. Long-term survival is similar to patients undergoing the more traditional esophagogastrectomy via thoracotomy. Radiation and chemotherapy may provide some palliation in patients unable to undergo surgical resection.

14. Which sites are most commonly involved in distant metastatic spread of esophageal cancer?
Lung, liver, and bone.

15. How does the surgeon access the esophagus?
The esophagus passes behind the aortic arch as it curves and descends into the posterior mediastinum. The aortic arch and its branches effectively shield the upper two-thirds of the esophagus from left thoracotomy access. Right-sided access is limited only by the azygous vein, which can be ligated without sequelae.

16. Define multimodality therapy. What are its results?
Multimodality therapy combines neoadjuvant chemotherapy and radiation followed by resection. Initial results in selected patients are encouraging. The 3-year survival rate approaches 45% compared with 20% in a similar group treated with esophagectomy alone.

17. What evidence suggests that chemotherapy and radiation alone may be adequate therapy in patients with early-stage disease?
Several recent trials using neoadjuvant chemotherapy and radiation followed by esophagectomy have demonstrated no evidence of tumor in up to 25% of resected specimens.

18. If there is no historic evidence of tumor after preoperative chemotherapy and radiation, why is surgical resection necessary?
Failure of our friends in pathology to find tumor does not mean that it is not there (see question 16). More than 50% of patients still die within 3 years from esophageal cancer.

BIBLIOGRAPHY

1. Brenner, Demeester: Surgical treatment for esophageal carcinoma. Gastroenterol Clin North Am 20:743–763, 1991.
2. Mayer R: Overview: The changing nature of esophageal cancer. Chest 103:404–405, 1993.
3. Muller J: Surgical therapy for esophageal cancer. Br J Surg 77:845–857, 1990.
4. Orringer M: Multimodality therapy for esophageal carcinoma—update. Chest 103:406–409, 1993.
5. Roth J: Surgery for cancer of the esophagus. Semin Oncol 21:4, 1994.
6. Sugarbaker O: Selecting the surgical approach to cancer of the esophagus. Chest 103:410–414, 1993.
7. Watson A: Operable esophageal cancer: Current results from the west. World J Surg 18:361–366, 1994.
8. Wright C: Evolution of treatment strategies for adenocarcinoma. Ann Thorac Surg 58:1574–1579, 1994.

39. DUODENAL ULCER DISEASE

Robert T. Rowland, M.D., and Benjamin O. Anderson, M.D.

1. Who gets duodenal ulcers?
Peptic ulcer disease of the stomach and duodenum afflicts more than 10 million people in the United States. The historical incidence is 3–4 times higher in men than women, but current evidence suggests little difference in gender distribution. Duodenal ulcers may appear at any age but occur most frequently between the ages of 20 and 60 years, with peak incidence in the fourth decade.

2. What causes duodenal ulcers?
The pathogenesis is not fully understood, but duodenal ulcers tend to be associated with acid hypersecretion. The mean basal and maximal acid outputs are 0.5–2 times greater compared with control patients. Ulcers, however, may occur in patients with normal acid secretion; only 40% of patients with duodenal ulcers hypersecrete. Furthermore, *Helicobacter pylori* is presently considered a major factor predisposing to the development of duodenal ulceration.

3. What are the stimuli for gastric acid secretion?
1. **Cephalic phase:** sight, smell, taste, or thought of food increases gastric acid secretion via vagal stimulation.
2. **Gastric phase:** distention of the gastric antrum and products of protein digestion stimulate gastrin release from the antral mucosa.
3. **Intestinal phase:** food in the small bowel releases enteroxyntin that increases acid release.

4. What are the normal rates of gastric acid secretion?
Basal acid output (BAO) is measured under fasting conditions and maximal acid output (MAO) is measured after histamine or pentagastrin stimulation. Normal BAO is 1.5–2.5 mEq/hr; MAO is normally 20–30 mEq/hr.

5. What physiologic abnormalities have been observed in patients with duodenal ulcer disease?

1. Increased number of parietal (acid-secreting) and chief cells
2. Increased sensitivity of parietal cells to gastrin stimulation
3. Increased gastrin response to a meal
4. Decreased inhibition of gastrin release in response to acidification of gastric contents
5. Increased rates of gastric emptying
6. Increased BAO to 3–3.5 mEq/hr and increased MAO to 30–40 mEq/hr

Not all of the above abnormalities are present in every patient with duodenal ulcers.

6. Are there any physiologic markers for patients at high risk for developing duodenal ulcers?

Acid hypersecretion has been associated with blood group O; people with blood group O have a 30–40% greater frequency of duodenal ulcer than people of other blood groups. About 75% of the population secrete the blood group antigens in gastric juice; the remaining 25% are nonsecretors. Nonsecretors are about one-half as likely to develop a duodenal ulcer as secretors. Specific leukocyte antigens (HLA-B5, B12, and BW35) are increased in patients with duodenal ulcers.

7. What other groups are at high risk?

Patients with multiple endocrine adenopathy, type I, have a 50–85% incidence of gastrinoma with severe ulcer diathesis. Deficiency of alpha$_1$-antitrypsin is associated with cirrhosis, pulmonary emphysema, and peptic ulcers. The frequency of peptic ulcers appears to be particularly high in patients who have emphysema.

8. What is *Helicobacter pylori*?

H. pylori is a gram-negative, multiflagellate, spiral bacterium found in the human gastric mucosa and is considered a pathogen in the development of both gastric and duodenal ulcers.

9. What is the association between *H. pylori* and duodenal ulcer disease?

H. pylori infection is strongly and consistently associated with duodenal ulceration in more than 90% of patients. Patients with *H. pylori*-associated chronic active gastritis have a 15-fold increased risk of developing a duodenal ulcer, whereas the risk rises to 50-fold in cases of duodenal infection. However, approximately 50% of the population is infected with *H. pylori*, and most do not develop duodenal ulcers.

10. What are the pathogenic mechanisms of *H. pylori*?

1. *H. pylori* infects the antral mucosa through a host of adhesion molecules and cytotoxins and alters gastric physiology, resulting in increased gastrin release and gastric acid secretion.
2. The increased bulboduodenal acid load results in gastric metaplasia.
3. Gastric metaplasia in the duodenal mucosa is colonized by *H. pylori*, resulting in chronic duodenitis.
4. Chronic duodenitis leads to duodenal ulcer formation and relapse.

11. How is *H. pylori* infection diagnosed?

Various tests are available for the diagnosis of *H. pylori*. **Histology** requires endoscopy and reveals a spiral bacterial rod adjacent to gastric epithelium. **Direct culture** is tedious and expensive and should be used only if an antibiotic-resistant organism is suspected. *H. pylori* produces a urease which is the basis for the **CLO test**. When urease catalyzes the breakdown of urea to ammonia and bicarbonate, the increased pH changes the color of a pH indicator. The CLO test requires antral tissue obtained endoscopically. **Serology** detects higher anti-*H. pylori* IgA and IgG antibody titers, using enzyme-linked immunosorbent assays (ELISA) without endoscopy.

12. What are the symptoms of a duodenal ulcer?
    1. **Burning pain** is the most common presenting symptom. The pain is well localized in the midepigastrium and often radiates to the back. Pain often occurs before meals or at night and is relieved by ingestion of food or antacids. The pain also may be episodic, interspersed by long periods of remission.
    2. **Nausea and vomiting** also may occur, even in the absence of obstruction.
    3. **Bleeding**.
    4. **Obstruction** may result from an inflammatory mass or pyloric spasm or secondary to repeated episodes of duodenal scarring and fibrosis. Obstruction usually results in nausea, vomiting, and anorexia.
    5. **Perforation** constitutes a surgical emergency and has an associated mortality rate of 5–10%. Ulcers located on the anterior duodenal surface are prone to perforation and may perforate without a significant history of duodenal ulcer disease.

13. Does the location of the ulcer dictate the likely presentation?
Yes. Posterior ulcers bleed by eroding into the gastroduodenal artery. Anterior ulcers may perforate the duodenal wall and present with an acute surgical abdomen and abdominal free air.

14. What is the appropriate medical treatment for duodenal ulcers?
    1. **Diet.** Barrier breakers (aspirin, NSAIDs) should be avoided. Alcohol and caffeine stimulate acid secretion and should be limited.
    2. **Antacids** are useful in neutralizing gastric pH and should be taken 1–3 hours after meals.
    3. **H₂-antagonists** decrease acid secretion by blocking histamine receptors on parietal cells.
    4. **Sucralfate** adheres to the ulcer base, providing a resistant coating to the actions of pepsin and acid digestion.
    5. **Bismuth compounds** also provide a coating action.
    6. **Cigarette smoking**, which has been associated with impaired ulcer healing and increased recurrence rates, should be discouraged.
    7. **Omeprazole** directly blocks acid production by inhibiting the hydrogen/potassium–adenosine triphosphatase proton pump in the gastric parietal cell.

15. What is the success rate of medical therapy?
With the above treatment strategies, approximately 75–95% of duodenal ulcers heal in 4–6 weeks. Recurrence is common, however, and 70% recur within 1 year of cessation of treatment.

16. How has medical treatment changed with *H. pylori* infection?
Treatment strategies are now aimed at the diagnosis and elimination of *H. pylori* infection. Multiple drug combinations have been used, but the optimal regimen is yet to be established. Currently, triple therapy—bismuth, tetracycline, and metronidazole—appears to give the best results; in combination with a histamine receptor antagonist, it provides a 90% cure rate. Patients in whom triple therapy fails may benefit from the addition of erythromycin, amoxicillin-omeprazole, or erythromycin-omeprazole.

17. What complications are associated with medical treatment?
Magnesium-containing antacids may cause diarrhea, whereas calcium-containing antacids may cause constipation. H₂-receptor antagonists may induce gynecomastia and changes in mental status as well as interfere with cytochrome oxidase-metabolized drugs (anticoagulants, diazepam, propranolol, and lidocaine). Omeprazole, through inhibition of gastric acid secretion, may cause marked hypergastrinemia.

18. When should serum gastrin levels be obtained?
Gastric analysis may be useful when severe ulcer diathesis leads to suspicion of Zollinger-Ellison syndrome. Serum gastrin levels should be obtained in patients who present with recurrent ulcers

after operation or multiple ulcers and in all patients with evidence of multiple endocrine neoplastic syndrome. Normal serum gastrin levels are less than 200 pg/ml, whereas in patients with Zollinger-Ellison syndrome they are usually above 500 pg/ml.

19. What is the secretin stimulation test?
Patients with borderline gastrin values (200–500 pg/ml) should have a secretin stimulation test. After intravenous administration of secretin (2 U/kg bolus), a rise in the serum gastrin level of ≥ 150 pg/ml within 15 minutes is diagnostic of Zollinger-Ellison syndrome.

20. How are duodenal ulcers diagnosed?
Barium study of the upper gastrointestinal tract may have a false-negative rate as high as 50%, particularly if superficial ulcerations are present. Esophagogastroduodenoscopy (EGD) has a 95% sensitivity and specificity and allows complete visualization of the entire upper GI tract.

21. What are the indications for operative treatment of duodenal ulcers?
Common indications for surgery include hemorrhage (> 6 units transfusion within 24 hours or, more precisely, two-thirds of the patient's blood volume calculated as 8% of body weight in kg), intestinal obstruction, and failure of medical management to control ulcer symptoms. Duodenal ulcer perforation is also an operative indication unless the patient presents more than 24–48 hours after the event and contrast (Gastrografin) study confirms a healed perforation.

22. What operations are used to treat duodenal ulcers?
  1. Truncal vagotomy and pyloroplasty or gastrojejunostomy
  2. Vagotomy and antrectomy with Billroth I or II (B-I or B-II) anastomosis
  3. Subtotal gastrectomy with B-I or B-II anastomosis
  4. Highly selective vagotomy
  5. Total gastrectomy

23. What are Billroth I and Billroth II anastomoses?
The Billroth I operation refers to an anastomosis between the duodenum and the gastric remnant (gastroduodenostomy), whereas the Billroth II is constructed by anastomosing a loop of jejunum to the gastric remnant (gastrojejunostomy). The Billroth I technique is more popular, but there is no conclusive evidence that the results are superior.

24. What are the rates of ulcer recurrence after surgical treatment?
Vagotomy and pyloroplasty—10%   Subtotal gastrectomy—1–2%
Vagatomy and antrectomy—2–3%   Total gastrectomy—< 1%
Highly selective vagotomy—10–15%

25. What is the mortality rate associated with surgical treatment?
Vagotomy and pyloroplasty—1%   Subtotal gastrectomy—1–2%
Vagatomy and antrectomy—1–3%   Total gastrectomy—2–5%
Highly selective vagotomy—0.1%

26. What is the treatment for a perforated duodenal ulcer?
Graham closure is commonly used and consists of closing the defect with an omental patch secured by seromuscular sutures on either side of the perforation. Stable patients may undergo an acid-reducing operation in addition to the omental patch closure. After closure, one-third remain asymptomatic, one-third have symptoms controlled by medical treatment, and the remaining one-third require definitive ulcer operation.

27. Who was Billroth?
Christian Albert Billroth (1829–1894) was an Austrian surgeon credited with performing the first gastric resection in 1881.

28. What are the early complications of surgery for duodenal ulcers?

Duodenal stump leakage may occur 3–6 days after antral resection and Billroth anastomosis. Treatment consists of prompt reoperation and controlled drainage of the leaking duodenal closure.

Gastric retention may result from edema at the anastomosis or atony of the stomach after vagotomy. Gastric retention usually resolves spontaneously in 3–4 weeks.

Bleeding may result from a suture line, a missed ulcer, or other gastric mucosal lesions. Bleeding usually ceases spontaneously, but endoscopy or reoperation may be necessary in some cases.

29. Where do ulcers recur after operation?

Ulcers recur in about 10% of patients treated by vagotomy and pyloroplasty or highly selective vagotomy and in 2–3% treated by vagotomy and antrectomy. Recurrent ulcers develop immediately adjacent to the anastomosis on the intestinal side (duodenum, jejunum).

30. What factors may account for recurrent ulceration?

Ulcers may recur because of inadequate gastric resection, incomplete vagotomy, inadequate drainage of the gastric remnant (stasis of gastric contents proximal to the anastomosis), or retained gastric antrum.

31. What is alkaline gastritis (bile reflux gastritis)?

Reflux of bile and pancreatic secretions into the stomach after a Billroth II anastomosis may cause marked gastric mucosal inflammation. The typical symptom is postprandial pain; the diagnosis often requires endoscopy and biopsy. Persistent severe pain is an indication for surgical reconstruction, which consists of Roux-en-Y gastrojejunostomy with a 40-cm efferent jejunal limb.

32. What is the dumping syndrome?

The dumping syndrome is a collection of symptoms after gastric resection. Although experienced by 10–20% of patients in the early postoperative period, it remains a long-term problem in only 1–2%. Symptoms fall into two categories: cardiovascular and gastrointestinal. Shortly after eating, the patient may experience palpitations, sweating, flushing, weakness, nausea, abdominal cramps, and syncope. The rapid entry of hyperosmolar material into the small bowel is responsible for the osmotic and glucose shifts that produce the symptoms. The dumping syndrome is typically relieved by eating small, dry, low-carbohydrate meals and restricting fluids to between meals. Anticholinergic drugs also may be of help in some patients. Rarely, further corrective operations may be needed to treat severe cases.

33. What is the afferent loop syndrome? How is it prevented?

Afferent loop syndrome refers to postprandial abdominal pain that is often relieved by bilious vomiting. The mechanism consists of a narrowing at the junction of the stomach and duodenal side of a Billroth II anastomosis. Biliary and pancreatic secretions build up within the afferent limb, causing pain. Pain is relieved when the contents are discharged from the afferent loop into the stomach, often resulting in vomiting and/or severe bile reflux. Prevention requires avoidance of a long or twisted afferent limb and construction of a patent anastomosis.

BIBLIOGRAPHY

1. Borody TJ, Brandl S, Andrews P, et al: High efficacy, low-dose triple therapy for *Helicobacter pylori*. Gastroenterology 102:A44, 1992.
2. Deakin M, Williams JG: Histamine H_2-receptor antagonists in peptic ulcer disease. Efficacy in healing peptic ulcers. Drugs 44:709, 1992.
3. Dooley CP, Cohen H: *Helicobacter pylori* infection. Gastroenterol Clin North Am 22:5–206, 1993.
4. Eagon JC, Miedema BW, Kelly KA: Postgastrectomy syndromes. Surg Clin North Am 72:445, 1992.

 5. Emas S, Eriksson B: Twelve-year follow-up of a prospective, randomized trial of selective vagotomy with pyloroplasty and selective proximal vagotomy with and without pyloroplasty for the treatment of duodenal, pyloric, and prepyloric ulcers. Am J Surg 164:4, 1992.
 6. Hunt RH: Peptic ulcer disease. Gastroenterol Clin North Am 19:101–140, 1990.
 7. Malfertheiner P, Dominguez-Munoz J: Rationale for eradication of *Helicobacter pylori* infection in duodenal ulcer disease. Clin Ther 15(Suppl B):37, 1993.
 8. Megraud F, Lamouliatte H: *Helicobacter pylori* and duodenal ulcer. Evidence suggesting causation. Dig Dis Sci 37:769, 1992.
 9. Miedema BW, Kelly KA: The Roux operation for postgastrectomy syndromes. Am J Surg 161:256, 1991.
10. Stable BE: Current surgical management of duodenal ulcers. Surg Clin North Am 72:335, 1992.

40. GASTRIC ULCERS AND GASTRIC CANCER

Randall S. Friese, M.D.

BENIGN GASTRIC ULCERS

1. What does a diagnosis of peptic ulcer disease (PUD) mean?

Peptic ulcer disease represents a heterogeneous group of chronic and recurrent disorders of the alimentary tract characterized by mucosal ulceration. Duodenal ulcer (DU) and gastric ulcer (GU), the most common forms of PUD, affect 10–15% of the population of the United States. The majority of patients (4–8 million) suffer from DU. Although the true incidence of GU is not known, it occurs less frequently than DU, with a higher incidence in women and the elderly.

2. How are gastric ulcers clinically classified?

Gastric ulcers are conventionally classified as type I (ulcer at the incisura or the most inferior portion of the lesser curve), type II (both gastric and duodenal ulcers), type III (prepyloric ulcer), and type IV (gastroesophageal junction/juxtacardial ulcer).

3. Is gastric ulcer disease caused by hypersecretion of acid?

Usually not. Gastric ulceration is believed to occur in the presence of normal rates of acid secretion. The cause is usually a focal defect in acid neutralization that allows acid diffusion into the underlying stomach mucosa; ulcer types II and III, however, may be associated with acid hypersecretion.

4. Describe the evaluation of a patient with peptic ulcer disease.

After a 4–6 week trial of antacid therapy, the patient with persistent pain should have endoscopy. If a gastric ulcer is identified, it should be biopsied at multiple sites to rule out malignancy.

5. What is *Helicobacter pylori*?

H. pylori is a motile, helical-shaped, urease-secreting organism that resides in the mucous layer of gastric epithelium and in the intracellular junctions of gastric mucus-secreting cells. The organism's urease-secreting capacity allows it to survive in the stomach's highly acidic environment through creation of an alkaline microenvironment by the splitting of urea into carbon dioxide and ammonia. This unique characteristic provides a rapid diagnostic tool for detecting *H. pylori* in biopsy samples. The rapid urease test is performed by adding urea to the biopsy sample; as the urease reaction takes place, the pH of the media increases, causing a color change. The test takes approximately 20 minutes. Other diagnostic tests involve histology, tissue culture, and serology.

6. Do all patients with *H. pylori* develop gastric ulcers?

No. In the United States *H. pylori* can be detected in the stomachs of 20–30% of asymptomatic people.

7. What is the incidence of *H. pylori* infection?
The prevalence of *H. pylori* infection is highly correlated with age. Approximately 10% of people younger than 20 years are infected, whereas over 50–60% of people older than 60 years may harbor the organism. In addition, the prevalence of *H. pylori* infection is higher in Hispanics and blacks than in whites.

8. How is *Helicobacter pylori* infection related to gastric ulcer disease?
H. pylori gastric colonization induces a nonspecific and nonerosive inflammation of the gastric mucosa called type B chronic active gastritis. This colonization and subsequent gastritis may be followed by mucosal damage leading to ulcer formation. Although strong evidence supports the involvement of *H. pylori* in the development of gastric ulceration, other factors, such as impaired mucosal defenses, may also be essential.

9. Is there a benefit to eradication of *H. pylori* in patients with gastric ulcer?
Although drug therapies aimed at eradicating *H. pylori* improve ulcer healing rates, the most compelling rationale for their use is the dramatic decrease in relapse rates after eradication of the organism. Several groups of investigators have described decreases in 1-year recurrence rates from 50% to < 10% with eradication of *H. pylori*.

10. What drug or combination of drugs is used to treat *H. pylori* infection?
Triple therapy is most effective; drug combinations include bismuth, metronidazole, and tetracycline or amoxicillin. In general, histamine (H2) blockers are added to speed ulcer healing and to decrease dyspeptic symptoms.

11. Can a gastric ulcer be malignant?
Yes. Gastric ulcers can be either benign or malignant, whereas duodenal ulcers are benign.

12. What treatment options are available for benign gastric ulcers?
Treatment options include mucosal protective agents (antacids and sucralfate), antisecretory agents (H_2 receptor antagonists), proton pump inhibition (omeprazole), and antimicrobial therapy (see question 9).

13. How is benign gastric ulcer evaluated?
Endoscopy (EGD) and biopsy (to rule out malignancy) are essential. Upper gastrointestinal radiologic studies may be helpful but are not diagnostic. A second endoscopy is usually performed 6–12 weeks after the initiation of medical therapy to evaluate the healing process.

14. What are the indications for operative therapy of benign gastric ulcers?
The indications for operative therapy are intractability, hemorrhage, perforation, and obstruction. Intractability is now a rare reason for operation because of relatively effective medication.

15. What surgical procedures are available for benign gastric ulcers?
The standard operative approach for gastric ulcer is hemigastrectomy or antrectomy without vagotomy. Recently, enthusiasm has increased for nonresective procedures, such as truncal vagotomy with drainage (pyloroplasty) or proximal gastric vagotomy (selective vagotomy). Nonresective procedures are associated with higher rates of recurrence, and the ulcer must be excised to confirm that it is histologically benign.

GASTRIC CARCINOMA

16. What is the incidence of gastric carcinoma?
The incidence of gastric carcinoma in the United States declined from 30/100,000 in 1930 to 15/100,000 in 1960 and presently remains at 5/100,000. Men are twice as likely to develop gas-

tric carcinoma as women. Of interest, the incidence remains high in several other developed countries, such as Chile (40/100,000), Japan (50/100,000), and Germany (25/100,000). Despite the declining incidence, the 5-year survival rate of patients with gastric carcinoma (10%) has remained relatively unchanged over the past 30 years.

17. What is the cause of gastric carcinoma?
The numerous causes of gastric carcinoma include diet (nitrates, nitrites, and cured or pickled foods), environmental factors (smoke, dust, cigarettes, and alcohol), chronic gastritis (atrophic and hypertrophic gastritis, gastric ulcers, achlorhydria, pernicious anemia, and prior gastric resection), and genetic factors (blood group A).

18. What are the histologic types of gastric carcinoma?
Almost all gastric carcinomas are adenocarcinomas. Carcinoids and sarcomas of the stomach occur in less than 1% of cases, and squamous carcinomas are extremely rare. Adenocarcinomas are further classified as intestinal or diffuse.

19. Is pernicious anemia a causal factor in gastric carcinoma?
Probably. However, it is estimated that 5–10% of patients with pernicious anemia develop gastric carcinoma despite adequate vitamin B_{12} therapy.

20. Are screening tests available for detecting gastric carcinoma?
Yes. Screening techniques are used in countries with a high incidence of gastric cancer. Their use in countries with relatively low rates of disease, such as the United States, is not cost-effective.

21. What factors are used to determine prognosis for gastric carcinoma?
Prognostic factors include (1) stage—notably lymph node involvement; (2) type of tumor—superficial/polypoid (better) vs. ulcerating/scirrhous (poorer); (3) histologic class—intestinal (better) vs. diffuse (poorer); (4) location in stomach—distal (better) vs. proximal (poorer); and (5) tumor size.

22. What treatment options are available for gastric carcinoma?
Surgical resection offers the only chance of cure for gastric carcinoma.

23. How do the principles of resection differ for curative and palliative therapy?
Curative therapy. For *distal lesions* a subtotal gastrectomy with 4–6 cm proximal margins, omentectomy, and lymph node dissection should be performed. Because distal carcinomas are known to spread into the duodenum, the extent of distal resection should include 1–3 cm of duodenum. For *proximal lesions* esophagogastrectomy with removal of the proximal stomach and distal esophagus (5-cm tumor-free margin) and lymph node dissection are necessary. A pyloroplasty also should be done to prevent gastric retention.

Palliative therapy. When operation for cure is not possible, a palliative resection often provides relief from symptoms and perhaps prolongs acceptable quality of life. In general, the morbidity of a total gastrectomy for palliation is too high and therefore not warranted.

24. Is radiation therapy of benefit in gastric carcinoma?
Preoperative, intraoperative, and postoperative radiation have not proved to be of value in the therapy of gastric adenocarcinoma. In some instances, however, radiation may provide pain relief and control bleeding from ulcerating gastric cancers. Radiation therapy, on the other hand, is a valuable tool in the therapy of gastric lymphoma, with cure rates as high as 40%.

25. Is chemotherapy of benefit in gastric carcinoma?
Many combinations of chemotherapeutic agents have been tried in the treatment of gastric cancer with little to no benefit. Japanese researchers have reported beneficial results in the treatment of gastric carcinoma by a combination of radical surgery with adjuvant chemotherapy and radiation.

These findings have not been reproduced in the United States. Presently, no evidence indicates that either radiation or chemotherapy improves survival rates in patients with gastric carcinoma.

26. What is dumping syndrome?

Dumping syndrome is a physiologic disturbance that follows removal of the pylorus during gastrectomy. Dumping results from the destruction or bypass of the pyloric sphincter, which allows rapid passage of food into the small intestine. This abrupt osmotic load pulls fluid into the bowel lumen with resultant hypovolemia and symptoms of flushing or fainting and hypotension. Symptoms can be controlled by eating smaller and more frequent meals. Other postgastrectomy or postvagotomy syndromes include alkaline reflux gastritis, postvagotomy diarrhea, postsurgical gastroparesis, malabsorption syndromes, bezoar formation, and small gastric remnant syndrome. The most frequent and significant problem after truncal vagotomy is diarrhea.

27. Is there an association between *H. pylori* and gastric cancer?

In many sites chronic irritation leads to malignant tissue degeneration. For instance, reflux esophagitis is associated with esophageal carcinoma. The distinct association between gastric carcinoma and chronic or atrophic gastritis is well established. Thus, *H. pylori* colonization and smoldering infection may play a role in the development of gastric cancer.

28. What is Sister Mary Joseph's sign?

Dr. William Mayo's long-time surgical assistant, Sister Mary Joseph, noted that patients with a hard nodule at the umbilicus and an intraabdominal malignancy (particularly gastric cancer) did not fare well. Thus, the association of metastases to the umbilicus with intraabdominal cancer was made.

BIBLIOGRAPHY

1. Adam Y, Efron G: Trends and controversies in the management of carcinoma of the stomach. Surg Gynecol Obstet 189:371, 1989.
2. Ateshkadi A, Lam N, Johnson C: *Helicobacter pylori* and peptic ulcer disease. Clin Pharm 12:34, 1993.
3. Breaux J, Bringaze W, Chappins C, et al: Adenocarcinoma of the stomach: A review of 35 years and 1,710 cases. World J Surg 77:1330, 1990.
4. Dulchavsky SA, Fromm D: Benign gastric ulcer. In Cameron JL (ed): Current Surgical Therapy, 4th ed. Baltimore, B.C. Decker, 1992.
5. Efron G: Gastric cancer. In Cameron JL (ed): Current Surgical Therapy, 4th ed. Baltimore, B.C. Decker, 1992.
6. Interdisciplinary Group for Ulcer Study: Sucralfate, ranitidine, and no treatment in gastric ulcer management—a multicenter, prospective, randomized, 24 month follow-up with a study of risk factors of relapse. Digestion 53(1–2):72, 1992.
7. Sung J: Antibacterial treatment of gastric ulcers associated with *Helicobacter pylori*. N Engl J Med 332:139, 1995.
8. Ziller SA, Netchvolodoff CV: Uncomplicated peptic ulcer disease. Postgrad Med 93(4):126, 1993.

41. SMALL BOWEL OBSTRUCTION

J. Brad Ray, M.D., and Robert C. McIntyre, Jr., M.D.

1. Name the three mechanisms for the development of small bowel obstruction. Give examples of each.

    1. Obturation of the bowel lumen (e.g., gallstone ileus, bezoars, foreign bodies, and worms)

    2. Mural disease with encroachment on the bowel lumen (e.g., inflammatory conditions, such as regional enteritis; carcinoma; traumatic or radiation strictures; hematomas)

    3. Extrinsic lesions (e.g., adhesions, hernias, carcinomatosis, intraperitoneal abscesses)

2. What are the most common causes of small bowel obstruction?
1. Adhesions from prior abdominal procedures (70%)
2. Incarcerated or strangulated hernias (10%)
3. Neoplasms (5%)

These three causes account for approximately 85% of all cases of small bowel obstruction.

3. What are the most common presenting symptoms?
1. **Abdominal pain** begins as a diffuse, poorly localized, intermittent cramping that coincides with waves of peristalsis as the bowel tries to force contents past the obstruction.
2. **Vomiting** is more frequent, profuse, and bilious with proximal obstructions; it is less frequent and feculent in distal obstructions.
3. **Obstipation** is the failure to pass flatus and feces.

4. What are the most common physical findings on presentation?
The most common findings include mild, diffuse abdominal tenderness; high-pitched, tinkling bowel sounds; and an old abdominal incision. Common systemic manifestations include low-grade fever, dehydration, and low urine output. Severe, localized tenderness or signs of peritoneal irritation indicate complications of bowel obstruction, such as ischemic or perforated bowel.

5. What is the single best test to establish the diagnosis?
A three-way radiographic series of the abdomen includes a posteroanterior chest film and upright and supine abdominal films. Findings consistent with a small bowel obstruction include (1) distended loops of small bowel with air-fluid levels arranged in stepladder pattern; (2) absence of distal colonic or rectal gas; (3) elevated hemidiaphragms due to bowel distention; (4) a "ground-glass" appearance suggestive of peritoneal fluid; and (5) free air (best seen on the chest film), which is an ominous sign of bowel perforation.

6. Which laboratory abnormalities are usually present?
A complete blood count, chemistry panel, and urinalysis should be done to assess for (1) a normal or slightly elevated white blood cell count, (2) hyponatremia, (3) hypokalemia, (4) hypochloridemia, (5) metabolic alkalosis, (6) prerenal azotemia (increased blood urea nitrogen and creatinine), (7) hyperamylasemia, and (8) increased urine specific gravity.

7. What are the routes of fluid loss in small bowel obstruction?
Intravascular fluid is lost to (1) vomiting, (2) intraluminal pooling, (3) bowel wall edema, and (4) intraperitoneal accumulation of fluid from the edematous bowel wall.

8. Name the three types of obstruction based on bowel viability.
1. **Simple obstruction:** the lumen is obstructed, but the blood supply is not compromised.
2. **Strangulated obstruction:** twisting of the mesentery results in vascular compromise of the involved bowel.
3. **Closed-loop obstruction:** the segment is obstructed at two points, vascularity is compromised, and the involved loop cannot decompress itself proximally; the result is massive distention of an isolated segment of bowel with high risk of perforation.

9. What steps should be taken in the initial treatment of a small bowel obstruction?
1. Intravenous fluid resuscitation is done to correct dehydration as well as electrolyte abnormalities.
2. A Foley catheter is placed to monitor urine output and to guide resuscitation.
3. Nasogastric suction is used to decompress proximal bowel distention.
4. Timely surgical intervention is scheduled.

10. How can a partial obstruction be differentiated from a complete obstruction?
The most common important clinical finding is the continued passage of flatus or feces. Air in the colon or rectum on abdominal radiograph suggests partial obstruction. Upper GI contrast studies, ultrasound, and computed tomography are currently under investigation for the diagnosis of partial vs. complete obstruction (see controversies).

11. List the differential diagnosis for patients with a presumed mechanical small bowel obstruction.
1. **Paralytic ileus.** *History:* recent operation, trauma, or sepsis; abdominal pain is not prominent. *Physical examination:* absence of bowel sounds. *Radiographs:* a three-way series shows both small and large bowel distention with air/fluid levels.
2. **Mesenteric vascular occlusion.** *History:* an elderly patient with recent myocardial infarction or atrial fibrillation; sudden, severe abdominal pain. *Physical examination:* abdominal tenderness out of proportion to physical findings. *Laboratory tests:* markedly elevated white blood cell count; hyperamylasemia; unexplained, persistent metabolic acidosis.
3. **Large bowel obstruction.** *History and physical examination:* marked abdominal distention before significant symptoms appear; vomiting is a late feature. *Radiographs:* three-way series shows distended, gas-filled colon and absence of air in rectum.

12. What factors should be considered in the timing of surgical intervention?
1. Localized abdominal pain, fever, tachycardia, focal tenderness, leukocytosis, hyperamylasemia, and metabolic acidosis suggest bowel ischemia. However, studies have failed to confirm these signs as sensitive or specific for threatened bowel. In their absence, it is safe to manage the patient nonoperatively in the early period.
2. The old adage, "never let the sun set or rise on a bowel obstruction," is less true today. In the absence of the above signs and symptoms of threatened bowel, nonoperative management is relatively safe for up to 5 days. Failure to resolve the obstruction within this time is an appropriate indication for surgical intervention.
3. Resuscitation to ensure cardiovascular stability, adequate pulmonary function, and adequate urine output must be done for the patient to tolerate general anesthesia and laparotomy for bowel obstruction.
4. Nonoperative management is more valuable in patients with multiple previous episodes of bowel obstruction, previous radiation therapy, or known intraabdominal metastatic cancer.

13. List the surgical options at the time of laparotomy.
- Lysis of adhesions
- Reduction and repair of hernias
- Resection of obstructing lesions with primary anastomosis
- Resection of compromised or dead bowel with primary anastomosis
- Bypass of obstructing lesions
- Placement of a long intestinal tube to minimize risk of recurrent obstruction (see controversies)

14. What are the best criteria of bowel viability at laparotomy?
The best criteria are color, peristalsis, and arterial pulsations. Other methods, all with variable reports of accuracy, include fluorescein dye, surface oximetry, Doppler studies, and nicking the serosa to gauge bleeding.

15. What is the mortality rate for surgical treatment of small bowel obstruction?
Modern, timely treatment has reduced the mortality rate from 50% three decades ago to < 1% in patients undergoing surgery within 24 hours of presentation and not requiring bowel resection. The mortality rate for strangulated hernias remains approximately 25%.

16. What is the risk of recurrent obstruction after laparotomy?
Many authors estimate the lifetime risk of developing an obstruction secondary to adhesions after laparotomy at approximately 5%. After operative treatment of an initial adhesive obstruction, approximately 12% of patients develop a second obstruction.

17. Can adhesion formation be prevented?
No. Adhesion formation may be due to rough handling, ischemia, intraperitoneal sepsis, blood in the peritoneal cavity, and foreign bodies (such as mesh); nothing has been shown to prevent or significantly reduce adhesion formation. Experimental approaches to the prevention of adhesions include (1) interference with the apposition of damaged peritoneal surfaces; (2) prevention of the initial inflammatory response by blocking the production of eicosanoids, oxygen free radicals, or inflammatory cells; (3) dissolution or removal of fibrinous exudate from the peritoneal cavity; (4) inhibition of collagen formation; and (5) stimulation of motility with prokinetic agents.

18. Does small bowel obstruction occur after laparoscopic procedures?
Yes. Small bowel obstruction may result from herniation through 10-mm or larger trocar slits that do not have fascial closure. Preliminary data suggest that laparoscopic procedures may cause fewer adhesions than the open counterpart. It is unclear whether laparoscopic operations decrease the risk of bowel obstruction compared with laparotomy.

CONTROVERSIES

19. Upper gastrointestinal contrast radiographs.
Barium contrast material given orally or via a nasogastric tube may be used to differentiate partial from complete bowel obstruction and to define the cause of the obstruction. Water-soluble contrast may be therapeutic in partial small bowel obstruction.

20. Ultrasonography and computed tomography.
Ultrasonography and computed tomography are currently under investigation as methods to differentiate partial from complete small bowel obstruction. Their use is still investigational.

21. Long tubes to treat or prevent small bowel obstruction.
Long tubes passed transpylorically immediately above the obstruction do not decompress the bowel more effectively than nasogastric tubes. Because long tubes require more time and effort for proper placement, their use for bowel decompression has been abandoned in favor of the nasogastric tube.

Long tubes placed at the time of surgery have been used to stent the bowel and to prevent recurrent obstruction in high-risk patients. Theoretically they allow the bowel to become plicated in gentle curves as new adhesions form. The long-term efficacy of long tubes has not been definitively demonstrated.

BIBLIOGRAPHY

1. Assalia A, Schein M, Kopelman D, et al: Therapeutic effect of oral Gastrografin in adhesive, partial small bowel obstruction: A prospective, randomized trial. Surgery 115:433–437, 1994.
2. Menzies D, Ellis H: Intestinal obstruction from adhesions—how big is the problem? Ann R Coll Surg Engl 72:60–63, 1990.
3. Pickleman J, Lee RM: The management of patients with suspected early postoperative small bowel obstruction. Ann Surg 210:216–219, 1993.
4. Seror D, Feigin E, Szold A, et al: How conservatively can postoperative small bowel obstruction be treated? Am J Surg 165:121–126, 1993.
5. Tittel A, Schippers E, Anurov M: Postoperative adhesions—laparoscopy vs. laparotomy. Surg Endosc 7:A138, 1993.

42. INTESTINAL ISCHEMIA

Brian G. Halloran, M.D., and B. Timothy Baxter, M.D.

1. What is the arterial blood supply to the gut?
The intraperitoneal portion of the gut receives its blood supply from the celiac artery, superior mesenteric artery (SMA), and inferior mesenteric artery (IMA), which perfuse the foregut, midgut, and hindgut, respectively. The foregut includes the stomach and duodenum, the midgut extends from the proximal jejunum to the proximal descending colon, and the remainder of the intraperitoneal colon constitutes the hindgut.

2. What are the major collaterals that may develop in response to gradual occlusion of one of these vessels?
Between the celiac artery and SMA, the superior and inferior pancreaticoduodenal arteries are the major collateral vessels. The middle colic branch of the SMA and the left colic branch of the IMA communicate through the meandering mesenteric artery, also called the arc of Riolin. The marginal artery of Drummond, a more peripheral and less important collateral vessel, is formed by branches of the SMA and IMA.

3. What are the arterial causes of intestinal ischemia?
Compromise of one of the major vessels to the gut may result from thrombotic or embolic occlusion or extrinsic compression, as occurs in a strangulated hernia. Microvascular impairment of circulation may result from vasculitis or arterial spasm (nonocclusive mesenteric ischemia), which occurs, paradoxically, in response to systemic hypoperfusion. Prolonged distention of the bowel wall also impedes local blood flow and may result in ischemia.

4. Will acute occlusion of one of the three major arteries cause ischemia? What about gradual occlusion secondary to atherosclerotic disease?
Sudden occlusion of the SMA from an embolus is the most common cause of acute intestinal ischemia and may result in infarction of the midgut because of the absence of well-developed collaterals. When single-vessel thrombosis follows the progression of atherosclerotic occlusive disease, ischemia is unlikely because of the development of a rich collateral network before occlusion.

5. What are the clinical features of patients with chronic mesenteric ischemia?
Chronic intestinal ischemia, the end stage of atherosclerotic occlusive disease, usually involves all three of the visceral vessels. Weight loss is the most consistent sign of mesenteric ischemia. Patients gradually, and sometimes unknowingly, become afraid to eat (food fear) because of postprandial pain (intestinal angina). Nonspecific abdominal pain and diarrhea also may be features of the disease. In the absence of weight loss, chronic intestinal ischemia is unlikely. Conversely, in patients with severe atherosclerosis and weight loss of unknown etiology, mesenteric ischemia should be strongly considered.

6. How should patients with suspected chronic mesenteric ischemia be evaluated?
Duplex scanning noninvasively provides important physiologic information about the celiac and superior mesenteric arteries and should be the initial study. When surgery is contemplated and duplex scan findings are positive or equivocal, angiography is performed. Because chronic occlusive disease most often affects the ostia of the SMA and celiac, the lateral view of the aorta is the most informative imaging study.

7. What diagnostic triad is found with acute SMA embolus?

Sudden onset of severe abdominal pain, bowel evacuation (vomiting or diarrhea), and a history of cardiac disease, often with previous arterial emboli.

8. Does acidosis usually accompany acute intestinal ischemia?

No. Acidosis is a late finding in less than 25% of patients and is a poor prognostic indicator. Although the white blood cell count is elevated in the majority of patients, no laboratory studies are specific, and the diagnosis must be pursued on the basis of clinical suspicion alone.

9. When acute intestinal ischemia is suspected, what study is diagnostic?

Emergent arteriography is diagnostic. Again it is important to obtain both anteroposterior and lateral views of the aorta to visualize the visceral vessels.

10. What are the causes of nonocclusive mesenteric ischemia? How is it diagnosed and managed?

Nonocclusive mesenteric ischemia is initiated by systemic hypoperfusion and compounded by intense vasoconstriction within the mesenteric vascular bed. Vasospasm in the absence of organic occlusion is demonstrated angiographically. Predisposing factors include cardiac, renal, and hepatic failure as well as major abdominal or thoracic operations. Although infusion of vasodilators through the angiogram catheter can counteract local vasospasm, survival depends on reversal of the low output state, which is possible in < 20% of patients.

11. Can mesenteric ischemia result from venous occlusion?

Yes. Mesenteric venous thrombosis can result from hypercoagulable states such as polycythemia. The diagnosis can be made by contrast-enhanced CT scan.

12. How do the operative findings differ in patients with atherosclerotic occlusion and SMA embolism?

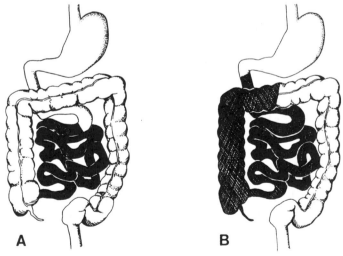

Because an SMA embolus usually lodges beyond the proximal jejunal and middle colic arteries, these segments are spared *(A)*, whereas thrombotic occlusion occurs at the ostia, where the atherosclerotic narrowing is most severe, causing ischemia of the entire midgut *(B)*.

13. What is the appropriate surgical management of an SMA embolus?

Embolectomy, assessment of bowel viability 30 minutes after reperfusion, and resection of infarcted bowel. Postoperative anticoagulation is essential to reduce the risk of further embolization.

14. What is the appropriate management of visceral ischemia from thrombotic occlusion?
Mesenteric ischemia from thrombotic occlusion is the end stage of progressive atherosclerotic occlusion. Therefore, thrombectomy alone is not sufficient; bypass or endarterectomy of the proximal diseased vessel is necessary. Again, bowel viability is evaluated after reperfusion, and a decision is made about the need for resection.

15. Does any intraoperative test help to assess bowel viability?
Yes. Both systemic intravenous infusion of fluorescein and intraoperative Doppler examination of the bowel may be helpful, but ultimately the decision is based on clinical judgment.

16. How much small intestine is required to sustain adequate nutrition? Is the ileocecal valve important?
Adequate nutrition requires 50–100 cm of small intestine. The ileocecal valve appears to be important in experimental studies.

17. When bowel viability remains in question and massive resection is necessary to remove all questionable bowel, what should be done?
A second-look operation should be undertaken in 12–24 hours to reassess bowel viability and to resect infarcted bowel. Some of the segments in question may become clearly viable during this period; salvaged small bowel may be critical to avoid dependence on parenteral nutrition.

18. Should the second-look operation be aborted if the patient improves clinically?
Never. The decision is made in the operating room based on the findings at surgery. No clinical parameters within the ensuing 12–24 hours accurately indicate the status of the bowel in question.

19. What is the mortality rate for acute mesenteric ischemia?
Although the prognosis of patients presenting with embolic occlusion is somewhat better because the presentation is more dramatic, the diagnosis is often not made before infarction. The result is a high mortality rate (60–90%), regardless of the etiology.

BIBLIOGRAPHY

1. Ballard JL, Stone WM, Hallett JW, et al: A critical analysis of adjuvant techniques used to assess bowel viability in acute mesenteric ischemia. Ann Surg 59:309–311, 1993.
2. Flinn WR, Rizzo RJ, Park JS, Sandager GP: Duplex scanning for assessment of mesenteric ischemia. Surg Clin North Am 70:99–107, 1990.
3. Hallett JW Jr, James ME, Ahlquist DA, et al: Recent trends in the diagnosis and management of chronic intestinal ischemia. Ann Vasc Surg 4:126–132, 1990.
4. Kurland B, Brandt LJ, Delany HM: Diagnostic tests for intestinal ischemia. Surg Clin North Am 72:85–105, 1992.
5. Stoney RJ, Cunningham CG: Acute mesenteric ischemia. Surgery 114:489–490, 1993.
6. Taylor LM: Management of visceral ischemia syndromes. In Rutherford RB (ed): Vascular Surgery, 4th ed. Philadelphia, W.B. Saunders, 1995.

43. DIVERTICULAR DISEASE OF THE COLON

W. Stuart Johnston, M.D., and Lawrence W. Norton, M.D.

1. What is a colonic diverticulum?
A colonic diverticulum is an outpouching of mucosa and submucosa through the muscular layers of the bowel wall. It is devoid of a muscular covering. Its formation may be related either to

weakness of the bowel wall at the sites of vessel perforation or to increased intraluminal pressure caused by low dietary fiber and constipation.

2. What is the difference between diverticulosis and diverticulitis?
Diverticulosis refers to colonic diverticula without associated inflammation. Diverticulitis refers to diverticula associated with inflammation and infection. Only 10–15% of patients with diverticulosis develop diverticulitis.

3. How does a diverticulum cause pain?
Pain is apparently the result of perforation of the diverticulum. The resulting leakage may be scant and contained within pericolic fat or extensive, involving the mesentery, other organs, or peritoneal cavity. Pain is usually located in the left lower quadrant.

4. Where in the colon are diverticula usually located?
In the United States, 95% of all diverticula occur in the left colon, primarily in the sigmoid colon. Diverticula, however, may occur anywhere in the colon. In Japan and China right colon diverticula are more common.

5. At what age is diverticulitis most common?
Most patients with diverticulitis are in the sixth or seventh decade. Patients younger than 50 who develop diverticulitis tend to have more complications. Younger patients are more likely than older patients to have right colon diverticulitis.

6. What strategy may decrease the risk of diverticulitis in patients with diverticula?
A diet high in fiber appears to reduce the risk of diverticulitis.

7. What is the best imaging test for diagnosing acute diverticulitis?
Contrast enema was the diagnostic standard for many years, but CT scan is now advocated by many as the best initial imaging study. CT scan also appears to be the initial exam for diagnosing most local complications of diverticulitis.

8. What complications may result from perforation of a colonic diverticulum?

Inflammatory phlegmon or abscess in the bowel mesentery	Intraabdominal abscess
	Internal fistula
Peritonitis	Bowel obstruction

9. Can diverticular disease cause bleeding?
Yes. Diverticulosis is one of the most common causes of lower GI bleeding. Bleeding from diverticulitis is uncommon.

10. How can the site of diverticular bleeding be localized?
The most accurate means of localization is angiography performed via the inferior mesenteric artery and, if necessary, the superior mesenteric artery. Tagged red blood cell studies are less useful. Colonoscopy is rarely helpful.

11. When should an operation be performed for a bleeding colonic diverticulum?
Replacement of 5–6 units of blood within 24 hours and rebleeding during hospitalization are indications for emergency resection of the segment of colon containing a bleeding diverticulum.

12. If bleeding is life-threatening but cannot be localized within the colon, what treatment is required?
Subtotal colectomy with ileostomy and closure of the sigmoid colon at the peritoneal reflection (Hartmann's operation).

13. What three procedures may be used when perforation of the diverticulum results in an abscess? Which has the lowest operative mortality rate?

1. Diverting colostomy and abscess drainage (first of 3 stages)

2. Resection of involved colon with proximal colostomy and distal mucous fistula or closure (first of 2 stages)

3. Resection with primary anastomosis (1 stage)

Operative mortality is lowest after resection and proximal colostomy for fecal diversion. Despite reports of success with the one-stage procedure, most surgeons favor a two-stage approach for perforated diverticulitis.

14. What is the clinical evidence of a vesicocolic or ureterocolic fistula after diverticular perforation?

Pneumaturia, fecaluria, and chronic urinary tract infections (especially polymicrobial).

15. What procedure is required to repair a vesicocolic fistula?

A staged procedure was the standard until recently. Now most patients can be treated with a single procedure that includes sigmoid resection, colonic anastomosis, and primary repair of bladder defect with absorbable suture. A Foley catheter is usually left in place for 7–10 days after surgery.

BIBLIOGRAPHY

1. Birnbaum BA, Balthazar EJ: CT of appendicitis and diverticulitis. Radiol Clin North Am 32:885–898, 1994.
2. Cho KC, Morehouse HT, Alterman DD, et al: Sigmoid diverticulitis: Diagnostic role of CT—comparison with barium enema studies. Radiology 176:111–115, 1990.
3. Elfrink RJ, Miedema BW: Colonic diverticula. Postgrad Med 92:97–105, 1992.
4. Freeman SR, McNally PR: Diverticulitis. Med Clin North Am 77:1149–1167, 1993.
5. Murray JJ, Schoetz DJ, Coller JA, et al: Intraoperative colonic lavage and primary anastomosis in nonelective colon resection. Dis Colon Rectum 34:527–531, 1991.
6. Roberts PL, Veidenheimer MC: Current management of diverticulitis. Adv Surg 27:189–208, 1994.
7. Roberts PL, Abel M, et al: Practice parameters for sigmoid diverticulitis—supporting documentation. Dis Colon Rectum 38:126–132, 1995.
8. Rothenberger DA, Wiltz O: Surgery for complicated diverticulitis. Surg Clin North Am 73:975–992, 1993.
9. Schoetz DJ: Uncomplicated diverticulitis. Surg Clin North Am 73:965–974, 1993.

44. ACUTE LARGE BOWEL OBSTRUCTION

Elizabeth C. Brew, M.D.

1. What are the mechanical causes of large bowel obstruction?

The three most common mechanical causes are carcinoma (50%), volvulus (15%), and diverticular disease (10%). Less common causes include hernias, intussusception, benign tumors, and fecal impaction.

2. How is the diagnosis made?

1. The patient complains of crampy abdominal pain, distention, and obstipation. Nausea and vomiting occur later in large bowel obstruction and may be feculent in nature. Physical examination reveals abdominal distention and high-pitched bowel sounds with rushes. Symptoms may progress to silence and localized tenderness, which are signs of peritonitis or sepsis and require immediate operative attention.

2. Flat and upright plain abdominal films reveal gas in the dilated colon with haustral markings. An upright chest film may show free air under the diaphragm if a perforation has occurred.

3. How is the diagnosis confirmed?
Plain abdominal films are usually sufficient to confirm a diagnosis. However, a barium enema is confirmatory and further delineates the level and nature of an obstruction. A volvulus can be identified by a "bird's beak" narrowing. A stricture also can be demonstrated with the use of a contrast enema. Sigmoidoscopy or colonoscopy is an essential part of the evaluation, because it allows visualization of the colon and may be therapeutic in the case of a sigmoid volvulus.

4. When is surgery performed?
Surgery is performed early in colon obstruction. Danger signs are quiet abdomen, right lower quadrant tenderness, and increasing pain. The patient's cardiopulmonary status should be assessed and optimized. It is essential to correct dehydration and electrolyte imbalances preoperatively with intravenous fluids. Nasogastric suction prevents further distention. Antibiotics are also necessary.

5. Why is tenderness in the right lower quadrant important?
The cecum is the area that is most likely to perforate. When the cecum reaches 15 cm at its widest diameter, the tension on the wall is so great that decompression is essential to prevent perforation. The larger diameter of the cecum causes more tension of the cecal wall at the same intraluminal pressure (law of Laplace).

6. Which operation should be performed?
The standard (and safest) procedure for a large bowel obstruction traditionally has been a decompressing colostomy. However, after careful assessment of the patient's condition, viability of the bowel, location of the obstruction, and absence of intraabdominal contamination may allow a primary anastomosis. An **obstructing carcinoma** may be resected satisfactorily under emergency conditions in 90% of patients. **Volvulus** should be reduced or resected. Reduction can be achieved nonoperatively by sigmoidoscopy or by hydrostatic decompression with a contrast enema. The recurrence rate of volvulus after simple nonoperative reduction is approximately 50%. Surgical therapy includes operative detorsion alone and detorsion with colopexy or resection. **Diverticular disease** can be resected; however, a primary anastomosis may not be possible because of infection.

7. Where is the obstructing cancer usually located?
The majority of obstructing colorectal carcinomas occur in the splenic flexure, descending colon, and hepatic flexure. In contrast, lesions of the right colon usually present with occult bleeding. Cecal and rectal cancers are uncommon causes of obstruction.

8. Where is the volvulus located?
Volvulus is an abnormal rotation of the colon on an axis formed by its mesentery and occurs in either the sigmoid colon (75%) or the cecum (25%). **Sigmoid volvulus** occurs in the older population when chronic constipation causes the sigmoid colon to elongate and become redundant. The recommended surgical therapy is sigmoid resection. Right colon or **cecal volvulus** requires a hypermobile cecum as a result of incomplete embryologic fixation of the ascending colon. Colonoscopic nonoperative treatment has not been as successful with cecal volvulus as with sigmoid volvulus; therefore, most therapy is surgical. A simple cecoplexy is the best method to prevent recurrent volvulus.

9. What are the nonmechanical causes of large bowel obstruction?
Toxic megacolon and paralytic ileus.

10. What is Ogilvie's syndrome?
Ogilvie's syndrome is paralytic (adynamic) ileus or pseudoobstruction (i.e., enormous dilatation of the colon without a mechanical distal obstructing lesion). Patients present with a massively dilated abdomen and a small amount of pain. Nonoperative management is the therapy of choice. Colonoscopy is both diagnostic and therapeutic in patients with colons larger than 10 cm in di-

ameter. The risk of cecal perforation is high, and decompression of the colon should be attempted. If surgical intervention is necessary a tube cecostomy is recommended.

11. What is toxic megacolon?

Toxic megacolon is dilatation of the entire colon secondary to acute ulcerative colitis. The disease is manifested by acute onset of abdominal pain, distention, and sepsis. Initial therapy includes intravenous fluid resuscitation, nasogastric suction, and broad-spectrum antibiotics. If symptoms do not resolve within a few hours, the patient requires an operation to avoid perforation. Surgical therapy most often consists of an emergency colostomy with formation of an ileostomy.

BIBLIOGRAPHY

1. Buechter KJ, Boustany C, Caillouette R, et al: Surgical management of the acutely obstructed colon: A review of 127 cases. Am J Surg 156:163, 1988.
2. Gosche JR, Sharpe JN, Larson GM: Colonoscopic decompression for pseudo-obstruction of the colon. Am Surg 55:111, 1989.
3. Sariego J, Matsumoto T, Kerstein MD: Colonoscopically guided tube decompression in Oglivie's syndrome. Dis Colon Rectum 34:720, 1991.

45. INFLAMMATORY BOWEL DISEASE

Gilbert Hermann, M.D.

1. What two clinical entities encompass the diagnosis of inflammatory bowel disease?

Crohn's disease and ulcerative colitis, the latter being either acute or chronic.

2. While there is often an overlap between these two diseases, they can usually be distinguished by clinical, radiologic, and pathologic criteria. What are some major clinical differences?

Rectal bleeding is unusual in Crohn's disease but common in chronic ulcerative colitis. An abdominal mass and anal complications (fissure, fistula) are more common findings in Crohn's disease.

3. What are some major radiologic differences?

Terminal ileal involvement, skip areas, internal fistulas, and thumb printing are all rare or absent in chronic ulcerative colitis but common in Crohn's disease.

4. What are some major morphologic differences?

Granulomas in the intestinal wall and adjacent lymph nodes are absent in ulcerative colitis but occur in 60% of patients with Crohn's disease.

5. Whereas Crohn's disease has been documented to affect the gastrointestinal tract from the pharynx to the anus, what are the most common clinical patterns of gastrointestinal involvement?

Small-bowel-type only, 28%; both ileum and colon (ileocolitis), 41%; and colon only, 27%. This latter goes by several names, among those being Crohn's colitis and granulomatous colitis.

6. Crohn's colitis and ulcerative colitis are often difficult to distinguish clinically. What are some major differences that one can note on colonoscopy?

The colonic appearance of Crohn's disease is that of focal, predominantly right-sided disease. The mucosa is cobblestone in appearance with transverse ulcerations in affected areas. Biopsies reveal transmural disease with focal granulomas. On colonoscopy, chronic ulcerative colitis usually appears as a diffuse disease. However, if only a portion of the colon is involved, it is on the left side and almost always involves the rectum. Pathologic changes involve primarily the mucosa and submucosa.

7. What are the major indications for surgery in Crohn's disease?
It depends on the site of involvement. Enteroenteral fistulas (controversial), abscess, and intestinal obstruction are the most common indications for small intestinal and ileocolic types. Perianal disease and medical failure as well as ileocolic fistulas and abscess formation are the most common indications for surgery in the colonic type.

8. How does this contrast with surgical indications in chronic ulcerative colitis?
Medical intractability (including failure to thrive in children, diarrhea, weight loss, and abdominal pain), toxic megacolon with or without perforation, and concern about the development of colonic cancer (controversial) are the main indications.

9. What is the surgical procedure for the treatment of ulcerative colitis?
Total colectomy with ileoanal pouch anastomosis is the currently accepted standard procedure. A standard Brooke ileostomy or Kock pouch can be used for special circumstances. Ileorectal anastomosis has been advocated by some (controversial).

10. What are the acceptable surgical procedures for the treatment of complications of Crohn's disease?
Complications requiring surgery are usually corrected by removing all areas of bowel involved in the complication. There has been increasing experience with strictureplasty as opposed to resection in selected cases of small bowel obstruction (controversial). When resection is necessary, grossly clear margins are satisfactory. Skip areas are left alone unless they are directly adjacent to resected intestine.

11. What should the patient be told to expect regarding recurrence of the inflammatory bowel disease following surgery?
With chronic ulcerative colitis surgery is definitive and curative. With Crohn's disease, however, the aim of surgery is to treat the complications, i.e., obstruction, sepsis, etc. Recurrence can be expected in a high percentage of cases if the patient is followed long enough. The incidence of small bowel recurrence following total colectomy for Crohn's colitis is controversial.

CONTROVERSIES

12. All patients with enteroenteral fistulas secondary to Crohn's disease should have surgery when the fistula is discovered.
For: These patients do poorly, will develop further intraperitoneal septic complications and will always eventually need surgery.
Against: Studies have indicated that many patients with enteroenteral fistulas do well without operative treatment provided they remain asymptomatic.

13. All patients with documented chronic ulcerative colitis for over 10–15 years, whether active or not, should have a colectomy to avoid the risk of carcinoma of the colon.
For: The incidence of carcinoma of the colon overall is 3–5%, which is 10–15 times higher than that for the general population. In addition, the cancers tend to be multifocal and are at a more advanced stage when diagnosed.
Against: Using biopsy techniques, only those patients whose colons show dysplastic changes need have a colectomy if the disease is quiescent.

14. Ileorectal anastomosis is an acceptable operation following colectomy for ulcerative colitis.

For: The patients have reasonably normal bowel habits and avoid the problems and complications associated with other procedures.

Against: At least 50% of these patients need to be reoperated upon for recurrence of disease. Also, the remaining rectum can be a site for the development of cancer.

15. Standard (Brooke) ileostomy is a good way to handle the terminal ileum following total colectomy for chronic ulcerative colitis.

For: Complication rate is very low. Over 90% of the patients studied lead very satisfactory lives.

Against: There are definite psycho-social-sexual problems associated with the use of external appliances. This is particularly true in the teenage group, among whom chronic ulcerative colitis is quite common.

16. The Kock pouch is a good procedure to use following colectomy for chronic ulcerative colitis.

For: It avoids the use of an external appliance and is quite easy to manage.

Against: Approximately 20–30% of all patients who have a Kock pouch need to have a revision because of slippage of the valve mechanism allowing the pouch to become incontinent.

17. An ileoanal anastomosis is a good operation following colectomy for chronic ulcerative colitis.

For: It allows the patient to avoid any external appliances or ostomies. This is, of course, very well accepted by the patients. This operation is probably the most commonly performed surgery following colectomy at this time.

Against: It is more difficult technically to construct, and, thus, the complication rate is higher. The average number of bowel movements is at least four to six a day, and there may soilage at night.

18. Strictureplasty is an acceptable procedure for small bowel obstruction in Crohn's disease secondary to fibrotic stricture.

For: It preserves maximum length of small bowel in a disease prone to recurrence.

Against: Surgical morbidity may be higher and there may recurrent stricture at the site of the strictureplasty.

BIBLIOGRAPHY

1. Azon ATR: Cancer surveillance in ulcerative colitis—a time for re-appraisal. Gut 35:587–589, 1994.
2. Block GE, Michelassi F: Surgical management for Crohn's disease. Adv Surg 26:307–322, 1993.
3. Chevalier JM, et al: Colectomy and ileorectal anastomosis in patients with Crohn's disease. Br J Surg 81:1379–1381, 1994.
4. Cornell WR, et al: Lower gastrointestinal malignancy in Crohn's disease. Gut 35:347–352, 1994.
5. Grotz RL, Pemberton JH: The ileal pouch operation for ulcerative colitis. Surg Clin North Am 73:909–930, 1993.
6. McLeod RS: Chronic ulcerative colitis—traditional surgical techniques. Surg Clin North Am 73:891–908, 1993.
7. Spencer MP, et al: Strictureplasty for obstructive Crohn's disease—The Mayo experience. Mayo Clin Proc 69:63–66, 1994.
8. Strong SA, Fazio YW: Crohn's disease of the colon, rectum and anus. Surg Clin North Am 73:933–963, 1993.
9. Tjandra JJ, Fazio YW: Surgery for Crohn's disease. Int Surg 77:9–14, 1992.

46. UPPER GASTROINTESTINAL BLEEDING

Lawrence W. Norton, M.D.

1. What is upper gastrointestinal (UGI) bleeding?

Bleeding from lesions of the GI tract proximal to the ligament of Treitz (junction between the duodenum and the jejunum) that leads to hematemesis, hematochezia, or melena.

2. What are the most frequent causes of UGI bleeding?

Acute gastritis (alcohol, drugs, stress)	40%
Duodenal ulcer	17%
Gastric ulcer	15%
Mallory-Weiss tear	11%
Esophageal or gastric varices	8%

Note: The frequency of these lesions varies among different populations. For instance, among alcoholic patients the incidence of bleeding esophageal varices is greater, whereas acute gastritis remains the most common source of bleeding across populations.

3. What is the first step in managing patients with UGI bleeding?

Therapy must precede diagnostic procedures such as endoscopy. A large-bore needle or catheter is placed in a peripheral vein to withdraw blood for hematocrit, type and cross-match, and liver function tests and to begin infusion of crystalloid solution (saline or Ringer's lactate).

4. What is the role of a nasogastric tube in patients with hematemesis?

The primary role of a nasogastric tube is to monitor the presence of blood in the stomach. This may be the only way to detect cessation or recurrence of bleeding. Large-bore tubes (Ewald) allow clot to be aspirated, with or without saline irrigation, but are awkward to manage.

5. How can the source of bleeding be identified?

Endoscopic examination of the esophagus, stomach, and proximal duodenum (esophagogastro-duodenoscopy [EGD]), even when performed during active bleeding, identifies a bleeding site in 85–90% of patients.

6. What endoscopic techniques can be used to control bleeding?

- Electrocoagulation with a unipolar or bipolar cautery
- Heat probe
- Laser (yttrium-aluminum-garnet [YAG] or argon)
- Direct injection of bleeding vessels with sclerosing agents or vasoconstrictors
- Sclerotherapy or rubber banding of esophageal varices

7. What is the success rate of therapeutic endoscopy in stopping hemorrhage?

Success varies with different lesions. Bleeding from acute gastritis is controlled or resolves spontaneously in 90% of patients. Peptic ulcer bleeding is less frequently controlled (80%), because larger vessels are bleeding. Mallory-Weiss tear hemorrhage responds in 95% of patients. Variceal bleeding is stopped by sclerotherapy or rubber banding in over 90% of patients, but rebleeding is frequent (40%).

8. What other nonoperative techniques can stop bleeding from gastritis or ulcers?

If a bleeding site can be visualized angiographically, the feeding vessel(s) can be constricted in some patients by intraarterial infusion of vasopressin. Alternatively, the vessel(s) can be occluded by angiographic embolization.

9. What proportion of patients with upper GI bleeding fail to respond to conservative (nonoperative) therapy?
10%.

10. What are the indications for operative intervention?
1. Persistent hypotension with ongoing bleeding
2. Replacement of 2500 ml of blood during the first 24 hours (typically, 5 units or two-thirds of the patient's blood volume)
3. Replacement of 1500 ml of blood during the second 24 hours
4. Rebleeding through an initial hospitalization while on maximal medical therapy

11. What operations are useful to stop bleeding from acute gastritis?
Truncal vagotomy arrests bleeding from alcohol- or drug-induced acute gastritis in most patients. Pyloroplasty or gastroenterostomy is added because vagotomy may impair gastric emptying. Gastric resection is required rarely.

12. What operations are useful to stop bleeding from peptic ulcers?
Duodenal ulcer bleeding usually requires suture ligation of the bleeding vessel followed by vagotomy and pyloroplasty (in higher-risk patients) or vagotomy and antrectomy (in lower-risk patients). Highly selective vagotomy is an elective procedure seldom performed for the emergent control of UGI bleeding. Gastric ulcer bleeding is best stopped by excising the ulcer either as a local procedure or as part of a subtotal gastrectomy. Vagotomy and pyloroplasty after ligation of a bleeder are usually effective for an ulcer at the esophagogastric junction.

13. What emergent operation can stop bleeding from esophageal varices in a patient with cirrhosis?
When variceal bleeding cannot be stopped by nonoperative means (sclerotherapy, rubber banding, transcutaneous intrahepatic portosystemic shunting [TIPS], or Sengstaken-Blakemore tube), an operation to decrease portal venous pressure is required emergently. The usual procedure is portacaval shunt or mesocaval shunt using an interposition graft. Rarely, devascularization of the proximal stomach and distal esophagus (modified Sugiura procedure) is done.

14. What is the mortality rate of bleeding esophageal varices?
Nearly 60% of patients die within 1 year after the first bleed from esophageal varices.

15. What is the rebleeding rate after operative control of UGI bleeding?
10%.

CONTROVERSIES

16. Should all patients with UGI bleeding undergo immediate diagnostic endoscopy?
For: Endoscopy is a relatively safe (complication rate: 0.25%) and accurate (85–90%) means of detecting a bleeding site. Information about the location and type of the bleeding lesions helps the surgeon to decide what operative approach is most appropriate.
Against: Emergency endoscopy in patients with massive bleeding risks aspiration and respiratory compromise. Several randomized trials fail to show a survival benefit with early endoscopy in patients with major UGI bleeding.

17. Should gastric lavage be performed with iced saline?
For: Iced saline lavage theoretically causes local gastric mucosal hypothermia and vasoconstriction, which may stop small vessel bleeding.
Against: Studies show no advantage with use of iced saline vs. isothermic saline.

BIBLIOGRAPHY

1. Branick FJ, Boey J, Fok PJ, et al: Bleeding duodenal ulcer. Ann Surg 211:411, 1990.
2. Cook DJ, Guyatt GH, Salena BJ, et al: Endoscopic therapy for acute nonvariceal upper gastrointestinal hemorrhage: A meta-analysis. Gastroenterology 102:139, 1992.
3. Gomes AS, Lois JF, McCoy RD: Angiographic treatment of gastrointestinal hemorrhage:Comparison of vasopressin infusion and embolization. AJR 146:1031, 1986.
4. Hunt PS: Bleeding gastroduodenal ulcer: Selection of patients for surgery. World J Surg 11:289, 1987.
5. Miller AR, Farnell MB, Kelly K, et al: Impact of therapeutic endoscopy on the treatment of bleeding duodenal ulcers: 1980–1990. World J Surg 19:89, 1995.
6. O'Connor KW, Lehman G, Yune H, et al: Comparison of three nonsurgical treatments for bleeding esophageal varices. Gastroenterology 96:899, 1989.
7. Warren WD, Henderson JM, Millikin WJ, et al: Distal splenorenal shunt versus endoscopic sclerotherapy for long-term management of variceal bleeding: A preliminary report of a prospective randomized trial. Ann Surg 30:454, 1986.

47. LOWER GASTROINTESTINAL BLEEDING

Kathleen Liscum, M.D.

1. Describe the treatment of a patient who presents with lower gastrointestinal bleeding.
Treatment begins with the ABCs (airways, breathing, circulation). Venous access should be established immediately by placing two large-bore catheters in the upper extremities. Blood should be analyzed for hemoglobin, hematocrit, and type and cross-match. A Foley catheter should be placed to help monitor volume status.

2. What is the next step in evaluating the patient?
A nasogastric tube should be placed to rule out an upper gastrointestinal source. If the aspirate is bilious, the examiner can be fairly certain that the source is distal to the ligament of Treitz. However, if the aspirate reveals no bilious fluid, the patient may have a bleeding source in the duodenum with a competent pylorus.

3. What are the two most common causes of massive lower gastrointestinal bleeding?
Diverticular hemorrhage (diverticulosis) and bleeding vascular ectasias are the two most common causes. Historically diverticular disease was thought to be the most common cause of lower gastrointestinal bleeding, but vascular ectasias are now responsible for an increasing number of cases.

4. Name several other processes that may be associated with passage of blood per rectum.

Colon cancer	Inflammatory bowel disease
Polyps	Anorectal disorders (hemorrhoids, fissure)
Ischemic colitis	Meckel's diverticulum
Infectious colitis	

5. After a good history and physical exam, what is the first step toward identifying the specific site of bleeding?
Anoscopy and rigid proctosigmoidoscopy should be done first to rule out anorectal disease and an extraperitoneal source.

6. Name four options available to localize lower gastrointestinal bleeding.

Tagged red blood cell scan	Angiography
Sulfur colloid scan	Colonoscopy

7. Discuss the differences between sulfur colloid scan and tagged red blood cell scan.

The **sulfur colloid scan** can be accomplished quickly and detects bleeding as minimal as 0.1 ml/minute. The radiolabeled sulfur colloid is cleared quickly by the liver and spleen, which may obscure the bleeding site if it is located in the hepatic or splenic flexure. The test is complete within 20 minutes of administration of the radionuclide.

The **tagged red blood cell scan** requires a 30–60 minute delay while the red cells are labeled. The test detects bleeding as slow as 0.5 ml/minute. Because the tagged cells stay in the patient's system, it is also helpful in identifying the source when the patient is bleeding intermittently. The study takes at least 2 hours to complete.

8. What is the role of angiography in the evaluation?

Angiography detects bleeding rates of 0.5–1.0 ml/minute. When a bleeding site is identified, the angiographic appearance may provide further insight into the cause of the bleeding. Diverticular bleeding is often seen as extravasation of contrast, whereas vascular ectasias may be identified by a vascular tuft or early filling vein.

9. What therapeutic options are available with angiography?

Two options are available: (1) infusion of pitressin into a selected vessel and (2) embolization of the bleeding vessel.

10. Which patients should have angiographic embolization of the bleeding site?

Most surgeons believe that embolization should be reserved for patients who are poor operative risks. A 15% complication rate is associated with the procedure. Patients may perforate or develop a stricture as a result of bowel wall ischemia.

11. What is the role of vasopressin infusion?

Vasopressin should be used as a temporizing measure. Control of the bleeding with vasopressin allows time for resuscitation and essentially converts an emergent case into an urgent one. Vasopressin occasionally may be used as the only treatment for diverticular bleeding. If the patient has a repeated episode of bleeding after weaning from vasopressin, the surgeon must decide between embolization and surgery.

12. In what percentage of patients does lower gastrointestinal hemorrhage spontaneously resolve?

Spontaneous resolution occurs in 75% of patients with vascular ectasias and 90% of patients with diverticular bleeding.

13. What are the generally accepted indications for operative intervention?

Most surgeons believe that an operation is indicated if the patient has received 6 units of blood (two-thirds of the patient's blood volume in 24 hours) without resolution of bleeding. Any patient who continues to bleed or has recurrent bleeding after vasopression or embolization should undergo resection.

14. What is the role of blind subtotal colectomy in the management of patients with massive lower gastrointestinal bleeding?

Blind subtotal colectomy is limited to the small group of patients in whom a specific bleeding source cannot be identified. The procedure is associated with a 16% mortality rate. Younger patients tend to tolerate the procedure better than elderly patients. Older patients often suffer with severe diarrhea, urgency, and incontinence. However, blind segmental colectomy is associated with an even higher mortality rate (39%) and a 54% rebleeding rate.

15. What is the most common cause of lower GI hemorrhage in the pediatric population?

Meckel's diverticulum.

BIBLIOGRAPHY

1. Bar AH, DeLaurentis DA, Parry CE, et al: Angiography in the management of massive lower gastrointestinal tract hemorrhage. Surg Gynecol Obstet 150:226, 1980.
2. Boley SJ, Brandt LJ: Vascular ectasias of the colon 1986. Dig Dis Sci 31:26S–42S, 1986.
3. Matolo NM, Link DP: Selective embolization for control of gastrointestinal hemorrhage. Am J Surg 138:840, 1979.
4. Treat MR, Forde KA: Colonoscopy, technetium scanning, and angiography in active rectal bleeding—an algorithm for their combined use. Surg Gastroenterol 2:135–138, 1983.
5. Wright HK, Pelliccia O, Higgins EF Jr, et al: Controlled, semielective segmental resection for massive colonic hemorrhage. Am J Surg 139:535–538, 1980.

48. COLORECTAL CARCINOMA

Kathleen Liscum, M.D.

1. What are the top three causes of cancer deaths in the United States?
Lung, breast or prostate, and colon cancer.

2. List the common presenting symptoms of a patient with colorectal cancer.

Intermittent rectal bleeding	Constipation
Vague abdominal pain	Tenesmus
Fatigue secondary to anemia	Perineal pain
Change in bowel habits	

3. What options are available to evaluate patients with guaiac-positive stool?
To evaluate the entire colon and rectum one may perform a barium enema and proctoscopy or colonoscopy. Colonoscopy is approximately 10 times more expensive, but it is also more sensitive for lesions < 1 cm.

4. List the major risk factors for colorectal cancer.
Adenomatous polyps
Family history of colorectal cancer
Age over 40
Chronic ulcerative colitis
Crohn's colitis
Personal history of colon cancer
Exposure to pelvic radiation for prostate or cervical cancer
Familial polyposis
Hamartomatous polyps (Peutz-Jeghers syndrome), inflammatory polyps, and hyperplastic polyps are not considered premalignant.

5. What are the current screening recommendations of the American Cancer Society for colorectal cancers?
A yearly digital rectal exam is recommended for all patients 40 and older. For patients over 50 a yearly digital rectal exam with occult blood testing is suggested. In addition, patients over 50 should have flexible sigmoidoscopy every 3–5 years.

6. In what part of the colon and rectum are most cancers found?
Historically a higher incidence of cancers has been found in the rectum and left colon. However, over the past 50 years there has been a gradual shift toward an increased incidence of right colon cancers. This change in patterns may reflect improvement in early detection.

7. Surgical options for colorectal cancer depend on tumor location. What operation should be performed for a lesion 25 cm from the anal verge?
Sigmoid colectomy.

8. What operation should be performed for a lesion 9 cm from the anal verge?
Low anterior resection (LAR).

9. What operation should be performed for a lesion 4 cm from the anal verge?
Abdominoperineal resection (APR).

10. What is the significance of adenomatous polyps in the colon?
Patients with adenomatous polyps are 6 times more likely to develop colorectal cancer than patients without polyps. Evidence suggests that all colon cancers arise from adenomatous polyps. The adenoma-carcinoma sequence describes this transformational process. Patients with familial adenomatous polyps (FAP) have > 100 polyps that cover the colonic wall. If such patients go untreated, without exception they develop adenocarcinoma of the colon by the age of 40.

11. How does the surgeon prepare the colon for operation?
Bowel preparation includes both mechanical cleansing and appropriate antimicrobial prophylaxis. This combination has resulted in significant decrease in morbidity and mortality from colon surgery. Mechanical cleansing is accomplished by lavage with polyethylene glycol (Go-Lytely) or a combination of cathartics and enemas (Fleet's Prep).

Antimicrobial prophylaxis should cover the expected aerobic and anaerobic flora of the gut. Significant controversy exists over whether the antibiotics should be given enterally (e.g., neomycin, 1 gm, and metronidazole, 1 gm, 3 times orally at 4-hour intervals on the evening before surgery) or parenterally (e.g., cefotetan, 2 gm intravenously within 1 hour before surgery). Many clinicians give both to obtain intraluminal and systemic effects.

12. What is Dukes' staging system?
In 1932 Dukes described a staging system for rectal cancer:

  . Dukes A: Tumor confined to bowel wall
   Dukes B: Tumor invading through the bowel wall
   Dukes C: Tumor cells found in the regional lymph nodes

Since his original article this classification has been modified several times. One of the most commonly used modifications is the inclusion of Dukes D stage, which correlates with distant metastases.

13. Which patients with colorectal cancer require postoperative adjuvant therapy?
Patients with colon cancer and lymph node involvement (Dukes C) should receive chemotherapy postoperatively to treat micrometastases. Two large studies have documented a survival advantage for such patients. However, no studies have documented a survival advantage for patients with Dukes B disease who are treated with chemotherapy.

Patients with rectal cancer and a significant chance of local recurrence (Dukes B and C) should be treated with radiation therapy, which may be given preoperatively, postoperatively, or with a combined "sandwich" technique.

BIBLIOGRAPHY

1. Fisher B, Wolmark N, Rockette H, et al: Postoperative adjuvant chemotherapy or radiation therapy for rectal cancer: Results from NSABP protocol R-01. J Natl Cancer Inst 80:21–29, 1988.
2. Fuchs CS, Giovannucci EL, Colditz GA, et al: A prospective study of family history and the risk of colorectal cancer. N Engl J Med 331:1669–1694, 1994.
3. Ghahremani GG, Dowlatshahi K: Colorectal carcinomas: Diagnostic complications of their changing frequency and anastomotic distribution. World J Surg 13:321–325, 1989.

4. Jass JR: Do all colorectal carcinomas arise in pre-existing adenomas? World J Surg 13:45–51, 1989.
5. Moertel CG, Fleming TR, MacDonald JS, et al: Levamisole and fluorouracil for adjuvant therapy of resected colon carcinoma. N Engl J Med 322:352–358, 1990.
6. Toribara NW, Sleisenger MH: Screening for colorectal cancer. N Engl J Med 332:861–867, 1995.
7. Wolmark N, Fisher B, Rockette H, et al: Postoperative adjuvant chemotherapy or BCG for colon cancer:
   Results from the NSABP protocol C-01. J Natl Cancer Inst 80:30–36, 1988.

49. COLORECTAL POLYPS

John H. Sun, M.D., and Greg Van Stiegmann, M.D.

1. What is a polyp?

A polyp is an elevation of the mucosal surface, usually consisting of a rounded projection into the
lumen of the colon or rectum. The word "polyp" has Greek derivation and means "many feet."
Polyps occur throughout the gastrointestinal tract but are most common in the colon and rectum.

2. What is the difference between a sessile and a pedunculated polyp?

A pedunculated polyp is one whose head is attached by a stalk to the mucosa of the colon or
rectum. The stalk is usually covered with normal mucosa. The term "sessile" refers to a polyp
resting on a broad base. In either type, the muscularis mucosa is the important landmark for differentiation of invasive from noninvasive carcinoma. Lymphatics and vascular channels do not
extend across the muscularis mucosa; hence, carcinoma developing on the mucosal side of this
border is considered carcinoma in situ (also referred to as severe atypia or dysplasia). Such lesions do not metastasize.

3. Which polyps have malignant potential?

Adenomatous polyps of the colon and rectum are recognized for their potential as precursors of
cancer. Three types of adenomatous polyps are recognized histologically: tubular adenoma, villotubular adenoma, and villous adenoma. Polyps containing more than 75% tubular (glandular)
elements are called **tubular**; those containing more than 75% villous elements are called **villous**.
When more than 25% of the polyp consists of both tubular and villous components, it is called
villotubular. Adenomatous polyps are thought to occur as a result of failure of the colonic epithelium to suppress DNA synthesis, resulting in a proliferative lesion that accumulates in the
colonic mucosa, forming a clinical polyp. Polypoid cancers may represent degeneration of larger
adenomatous polyps.

4. Do carcinoid polyps have malignant potential?

Carcinoid tumors of the rectum may present clinically as elevations of the mucosa. These lesions
grow in the submucosa as nodules and represent cancer of substantial malignant potential if
larger than 2 cm in diameter.

5. Which polyps have no malignant potential?

Hyperplastic (metaplastic) polyps are the most common polyps in the colon and rectum. These
are usually small (1–5 mm) and constitute over 90% of the polyps in the colon and rectum that
are smaller than 3 mm. Unlike adenomatous polyps, hyperplastic polyps are formed by a failure
of normally matured mucosal cells to spread over the mucosal lumen. These cells accumulate at
the intestinal surface of the colon, forming a polypoid lesion. **Hamartomas** are abnormal collections of normal tissue. Such hamartomas have excess proliferation of the muscularis mucosa;
others consist of excess connective tissue. **Inflammatory polyps** are commonly seen in diseases
such as ulcerative colitis, granulomatous colitis (Crohn's disease), and schistosomiasis. These

polyps represent islands of healing or healed mucosa, are not premalignant, and parallel the severity of the underlying inflammatory process. **Lipomas** may present as do carcinoids, with submucosal growth and a nodular lump projecting the mucosal lumen. Occasionally lipomas may also occur in polypoid form with a head and stalk. Lipomas have no significant malignant potential.

6. At what age do polyps occur?
Adenomatous polyps of the colon and rectum occur infrequently under age 30. The incidence increases with age, with some autopsy series reporting a high incidence (70%) in patients over 45. This figure is based on careful postmortem examination under magnification, however, and hardly represents the true clinical incidence. A reasonable figure for polyps of clinical incidence is 25% in patients over age 60.

7. How often are colorectal polyps multiple?
Approximately 10% of patients will harbor more than one adenomatous polyp at the time an initial polyp is discovered. Another 25% will develop additional adenomatous polyps in the following 4-year period.

8. Where do most colorectal polyps occur?
The majority of colorectal polyps (two-thirds) occur in the rectum, sigmoid colon, and descending colon. The remaining third are distributed between the right and transverse colons.

9. What is a juvenile polyp?
Juvenile polyps occur in the colon and rectum of infants, children, and adolescents. Histologically, they consist of large mucus-filled glands with excess connective tissue. Some believe these polyps develop in response to inflammation, while others conclude they represent variations of hamartomas. The common presenting symptom of juvenile polyps is rectal bleeding. Abdominal pain resulting from intussusception may also occur. These polyps may be treated conservatively and frequently undergo autoamputation.

10. Which clinical syndromes are associated with colorectal polyps?
Familial polyposis coli (FPC) is inherited as an autosomal dominant trait characterized by multiple adenomatous polyps throughout the colon and rectum. Diagnosis is made by observing at least 100 adenomatous polyps in the colon; the average is over 1,000 polyps. Patients with FPC often have a family history of the disease or of rectal cancer. Those lacking a family history but found to harbor multiple adenomatous polyps may represent a mutation, and subsequent generations are expected to be at risk. Bleeding, diarrhea, and abdominal pain are common presenting features. These patients have a nearly 100% incidence of cancer if left untreated.

Gardner's syndrome is inherited as an autosomal dominant trait. This syndrome consists of osteomas of the skull and mandible with multiple epidermoid cysts and soft-tissue tumors of the skin in addition to multiple adnenomatous polyps of the colon. The risk of cancer in patients with Gardner's syndrome is equal to that of patients with FPC.

Peutz-Jeghers syndrome consists of multiple hamartomatous polyps throughout the entire gastrointestinal tract. Brownish-black melanotic spots are seen on the lips and inside the oral cavity as well as on the dorsum of the fingers and toes. Patients with this disease are not at high risk for malignant change.

Turcot syndrome is a rare autosomal recessive trait consisting of central nervous system tumors and multiple adenomatous colon polyps. Treatment is the same as for PFC.

11. What are nonneoplastic polyps?
Hyperplastic polyps, Peutz-Jeghers polyposis, benign lymphoid polyps, and juvenile polyps have a very low risk for cancer and require no special follow-up.

12. What are the proper treatment and timing of treatment for these syndromes?
Polyps develop in patients with familial polyposis and Gardner's syndrome at or after puberty. Nearly all who will develop polyps have them by young adulthood. Because of the high risk of cancer, the current recommended treatment is panproctocolectomy with rectal mucosectomy and ileoanal anastomosis. Patients with Peutz-Jeghers syndrome do not merit a prophylactic colectomy.

13. What is the relationship between cancer risk and the size and histologic type of the adenomatous polyp?
Polyps less than 1 cm have a cancer risk of 1–10%, 1- to 2-cm polyps have a cancer risk of 7–10%, and polyps greater than 2 cm have a cancer risk of 35–53%. Sixty percent of villous adenomatous polyps are greater than 2 cm, whereas 77% of tubular adenomatous polyps are less than 1 cm in diameter at the time of discovery. Tubular adenomatous polyps have less malignant potential than villous adenomatous polyps in all sizes. Tubulovillous adenomatous polyps have an intermediate-to-low cancer risk in all sizes.

14. How is the diagnosis of a colorectal polyp made?
Colorectal adenomatous polyps seldom produce symptoms until they enlarge. Bleeding is the most common symptom and is usually occult. Screening for colon polyps with fecal occult blood tests has a 40% specificity (true negative) but only a 30% sensitivity (true positive).

Colonoscopy and flexible sigmoidoscopy provide the most sensitive tests for detecting colonic polyps. Colonoscopy is the gold standard; however, it is costly, often uncomfortable, and has small but significant risks. Flexible sigmoidoscopes, which are 60 cm long, will reach about two-thirds of colorectal polyps. The sensitivity and specificity are operator-dependent; however, in the hands of an experienced endoscopist, the detection rate should approach 98%. Barium enema (also an operator-dependent examination) is very accurate for polyps that are 5 mm or larger if performed with the double-air contrast technique. Problems in interpretation most often arise from the inability to differentiate a polyp from a small piece of fecal material adherent to the mucosa.

We recommend colonoscopic examination of patients suspected of having polyps or at high risk for same. Patients in whom colorectal (adenomatous) polyps have been detected and removed are at higher risk (approximately two- to three-fold) and should undergo endoscopic examination of the colon at least every 2–3 years.

15. Which polyps should the colonoscopist remove?
Virtually all polyps discovered at colonoscopy or sigmoidoscopy that are larger than 3 mm should be removed. Removal is accomplished with a diathermy snare device so that the pedunculated polyp is transected at the base of the stalk. The polyp then is either removed en masse with the endoscope or aspirated through the suction channel and recovered from the suction device. Histologic examination of all polyps is imperative, and each polyp should be submitted and labeled separately with specific information regarding the site from which it has been removed.

16. What is the success rate of colonoscopic polypectomy?
Virtually all polyps smaller than 2.5 cm in diameter that are pedunculated can be removed endoscopically. Larger ones or those with a very short stalk and broad base may be excised using special endoscopic techniques; however, great caution must be employed to avoid undue risk of perforation. Broad-based and sessile polyps generally cannot be removed endoscopically. Biopsies from broad-based polyps such as villous adenomas must be viewed with caution. Unless total removal of the lesion is accomplished, the presence or absence of cancer cannot be ascertained.

17. What are the complications of endoscopic polypectomy?
Perforation during endoscopic polyp removal occurs with a frequency of 1% or less. Bleeding may occur more often; however, most bleeding following polypectomy is self-limited. Persistent bleeding requires reexamination and an attempt at electrocoagulation of the bleeding polyp stalk. Laparotomy for control of hemorrhage is seldom required.

18. What is the proper treatment of a villous adenoma of the rectum?

Villous adenomas of the middle and upper third of the rectum are often large and involve a substantial portion of the circumference of the bowel. These lesions are best treated with a low anterior resection. Lesions in the lower rectum may be excised locally provided that a clear margin of surrounding normal mucosa is obtained. Discovery of invasive carcinoma in the locally resected specimen or a villous lesion too large for local removal may mandate an abdominal perineal resection. Some villous lesions may lend themselves to a posterior sacral approach, in which the rectum is entered following excision of the coccyx or division of the sphincter muscles. Careful attention to detail preserves normal rectal function in these patients and allows wide local excision of certain lesions. Smaller villous lesions in high-risk patients may also be treated with electrocautery or laser ablation.

19. Is endoscopic removal of a polyp that contains carcinoma considered adequate treatment?

Polyps with clear-cut carcinoma in situ are adequately treated by endoscopic polypectomy. In addition, most agree that a well-differentiated invasive carcinoma that has no sign of vascular or lymphatic invasion and is confined to the head of the polyp can be adequately treated by endoscopic removal.

20. What are the indications for colon resection following removal of a polyp?

Indications for colon resection following endoscopic polyp removal include (1) evidence of lymphatic or vascular invasion; (2) poorly differentiated invasive cancer; (3) incomplete removal of an adenoma or a carcinoma; and (4) sessile adenomas with or without invasive carcinoma.

21. What is the natural history of familial polyposis?

In a review of over 1,000 cases of familial polyposis, the mean age of diagnosis of familial polyposis was 34, the mean age of diagnosis of colorectal cancer was 40, and the mean age at death was 43. It is recommended that patients with familial polyposis have colon resections by age 25.

22. What are the options for surgical treatment of familial polyposis?

Treatment options include total proctocolectomy with permanent ileostomy, proctocolectomy with continent ileostomy (Kock pouch), abdominal colectomy and rectal preservation, abdominal colectomy and ileorectal anastomosis, and ileal pouch-anal anastomosis.

BIBLIOGRAPHY

1. Collins JA, Snow CF: Gastrointestinal polyps. Sci Am Med 13(4):1–6, 1986.
2. Cooper HS: Surgical pathology of endoscopically removed malignant polyps of the colon and rectum. Am J Surg Pathol 7:613–623, 1983.
3. Ghazi A, Grossman M: Complications of colonoscopy and polypectomy. Surg Clin North Am 62:889–896, 1982.
4. Hill MJ, Morson BC, Bussey HJR: Etiology of adenoma-carcinoma sequence in large bowel. Lancet 1:245–247, 1978.
5. Iwama T: The impact of familial adenomatous polyposis (FAP) on the tumorigenesis and mortality: Its rational treatment. Ann Surg 217:101, 1993.
6. Kohler LW, Pemberton JH, et al: Quality of life after proctocolectomy: A comparison of Brooke ileostomy, Kock pouch, and ileal pouch-anal anastomosis. Gastroenterology 101:679–684, 1991.
7. Leavitt J, Klein I, Kendricks F, et al: Skin tags: A cutaneous marker for colonic polyps. Ann Intern Med 98:928–930, 1983.
8. Macrae FA, St. John DJB: Relationship between patterns of bleeding and Hemoccult sensitivity in patients with colorectal cancers or adenomas. Gastroenterology 82:891–989, 1982.
9. Shinya H, Cooperman A, Wolff WI: A rationale for the endoscopic management of colonic polyps. Surg Clin North Am 62:861–867, 1982.
10. Webb WA, McDaniel L, Jones L: Experience with 1,000 colonoscopic polypectomies. Ann Surg 201:626, 1985.
11. Yashiro K, Nagasako K, Sato S, et al: Follow-up after polypectomy of colorectal adenomas. The importance of total colonoscopy. Surg Endosc 3(2):87–91, 1989.

50. ANAL DISEASE

John H. Sun, M.D.

HEMORRHOIDS

1. What are hemorrhoids?

Hemorrhoids are vascularized (venous) fibromuscular columns that line the internal wall of the anal canal. The major columns are located in the right anterior, right posterior, and left lateral positions.

2. How are internal and external hemorrhoids different?

External hemorrhoids occur below the dentate line as part of the external hemorrhoidal venous plexus. They are highly innervated and covered by modified squamous epithelium. Internal hemorrhoids are insensate, above the dentate line, and supplied by the superior and middle hemorrhoidal venous plexus. They are usually covered by transitional or columnar epithelium.

3. How are internal hemorrhoids classified?

First-degree hemorrhoids present with painless bleeding noticed after defecation. **Second-degree** hemorrhoids have a prolapsing component that spontaneously reduces after defecation. **Third-degree** hemorrhoids have a prolapsing component that needs manual reduction after defecation. **Fourth-degree** hemorrhoids exhibit irreducible prolapse.

4. What causes hemorrhoids?

Many theories address the cause of hemorrhoids. Burkitt believed that the low-fiber, high-fat diet of developed nations was associated with hemorrhoids. Manometric studies have identified higher resting anal pressures with symptomatic hemorrhoids. The lack of bulk in the diet causes engorgement and secondary prolapse of hemorrhoidal vascular cushions with straining on defecation.

5. Describe the treatment of internal hemorrhoids.

First-degree hemorrhoids are treated by conservative measures, including dietary manipulation (fiber supplements), which decreases constipation and straining, and good anal hygiene. Second- and third-degree hemorrhoids may be treated with rubber-band ligation, sclerotherapy, infrared photocoagulation, and hemorrhoidectomy. Fourth-degree hemorrhoids are treated with hemorrhoidectomy. Cryotherapy, electrocoagulation, lateral internal sphincterotomy, Lord's dilation, and laser hemorrhoidectomy may play limited roles.

6. Describe the treatment of external hemorrhoids.

External hemorrhoids do not pose a problem until thrombosis is encountered. Then they pose a big problem. A painful lump near the anal verge signifies a thrombosed hemorrhoid. Simple evacuation should not be performed because of the high recidivism. Excision with local anesthesia is the procedure of choice.

ANAL FISSURE

7. What is an anal fissure? How is it diagnosed?

An anal fissure is a linear defect in the anal mucosa that begins distal to the dentate line and may terminate around the anal verge. Characteristically, the patient is asymptomatic until the beginning of a bowel movement. The pain and bleeding may be exacerbated with each bowel movement. Diagnosis is made by the characteristic history and by finding a linear tear on the posterior or anterior midline on physical examination.

8. What causes anal fissures?
The cause of most fissures is unknown. Chronic episodic diarrhea may decrease the diameter of the anus, and subsequent formed stools may cause a tear. Constipation may produce changes in the consistency and size of stool, leading to tearing of the distal rectum and anus. Anal fissures are often seen in the postpartum period and associated with inflammatory bowel disease. A hypertrophic internal sphincter may show an exaggerated response to stretch that perpetuates the fissure.

9. When is an operation indicated?
An operation is indicated for recurrences, nonhealing fissures, severe acute fissures, stenotic fissures, and fissures associated with abscess or fistula formation. Acute anal fissures should be treated with conservative treatment by dietary fiber supplementation and application of steroid creams.

10. How are fissures managed?
Treatment focuses on the interruption of the function of the internal sphincter. Manual dilation of the sphincter has been replaced by precise dilatation with a rectosigmoid balloon. Sphincterotomy in the midlateral position is a good option for fissures and may be achieved by a closed or open procedure. The internal sphincter is transected from the intersphincteric groove to the dentate line, with care to avoid injury to the external sphincter.

ANORECTAL ABSCESS AND FISTULA

11. How are fistulas and abscesses related in the anorectum?
One-half of all anorectal abscesses are associated with anal fistulas. An abscess is formed secondary to an infection of the crypt of Moragni at the dentate line. The infection may spread from the intersphincteric space and propagate outside the external sphincter or even above the levator muscles.

12. What is Goodsall's rule?
The relationship between the anal opening and the course of the fistulous tract is predicted by Goodsall's rule. If the fistula exists in the posterior half of the rectum, the tract curves toward the posterior midline. If the fistula exists in the anterior half of the rectum, the tract takes a straight radial course to the dentate line. This rule is accurate in 95% of fistulas.

13. Describe the management of perirectal abscess.
Perirectal abscesses should be incised and drained. Antibiotics are indicated only in immunocompromised patients and patients with diabetes and concomitant systemic response. The abscess cavity should be lightly packed with fine mesh gauze and frequently changed. Often the abscess cavity is a site of a fistulous tract.

14. What is a seton?
A seton is a suture placed through the fistulous tract. It promotes a fibrotic reaction and encourages healing, minimizing the risk of incontinence. A seton can be placed to transect the sphincter muscle gradually in two or three stages, converting a high fistula into a low fistula.

ANAL CANAL CARCINOMA

15. What is the cause of anal canal cancers?
Patients who present with anal canal cancers have a long history of anorectal disease. One-half of such patients have had problems with condyloma, chronic fistulas, and fissures. Other associated diseases include perirectal abscess, hemorrhoids, immunocompromised states, and pruritus ani.

16. How are anal cancers diagnosed?
Most patients complain of mild but persistent bleeding, sometimes associated with tenesmus, pain, and discharge. Careful examination of the anal verge, anal canal, and transition zone reveals the lesion responsible for the bleeding. A full-thickness biopsy is performed for pathologic diagnosis.

17. What is the transition zone?

The transition zone is an 8–12-mm area proximal to the dentate line that contains cuboidal cells much like the lining of the urinary tract. This zone, which may be a remnant of the cloacal membrane, gives rise to cloacogenic cancers. It also acts as an area separating the squamous epithelium from the columnar epithelium of the rectum.

18. How are anal canal cancers staged?

Anal canal cancer is staged by primary tumor, regional nodes, and metastasis (TNM system).

Ti	Preinvasive tumor
T1	< 2 cm
T2	2–4 cm
T3	> 4 cm in diameter; freely mobile with no evidence of invasion
T4a	Invades vagina
T4b	Invades other organs
N	Nodal status
M	Distant metastasis

19. What is the treatment for anal canal cancer?

Before the mid 1970s the treatment for anal canal cancers obligated a formal abdominoperineal resection. The 5-year survival rate was 50%. Many other, more radical procedures did not improve the survival rate. In 1974 Nigro and colleagues reported the results of a preoperative chemotherapy and irradiation trial (neoadjuvant therapy). They were surprised to find that most patients no longer had evidence of tumor. Today a 5-year survival rate > 80% can be expected with a combination of radiation therapy (up to 4500 cGy) and chemotherapy (5-fluorouracil and mitomycin-C).

PRURITUS ANI

20. What is pruritus ani? What is its cause?

Pruritus ani is irritation of the anal area that causes an irresistible urge to scratch. It is often caused by excessive cleaning of the anal area. Any condition that may increase the moisture around the anus exacerbates the irritation. Consumption of certain beverages, such as alcohol, milk, citrus fruit juices, and drinks containing caffeine, may aggravate the condition. Infections and allergies also may play a role in pruritus ani.

21. How is pruritus ani treated?

1. Minimize trauma to the affected area; avoid soaps and use baby wipes.
2. Avoid moisture in the anal region; apply cotton or gauze to keep the area dry.
3. Apply an antibacterial ointment to act as a moisture barrier and to avoid infections.
4. Avoid excessive consumption of fluids; drinking more than 6 glasses of fluid daily has no health benefit.

BIBLIOGRAPHY

1. Bauer JJ, Sher ME, et al: Transvaginal approach for repair of rectovaginal fistulae complicating Crohn's disease. Ann Surg 213:151–158, 1991.
2. Bleday R, Pena JP, et al: Symptomatic hemorrhoids: Current incidence and complications of operative therapy. Dis Colon Rectum 35:477–481, 1992.
3. Nigro ND: The force of change in the management of squamous-cell cancer of the anal canal. Dis Colon Rectum 34:482–486, 1991.
4. Pescatori M, Interisano A, et al: Management of perianal Crohn's disease: Results of a multicenter study in Italy. Dis Colon Rectum 38:121–124, 1995.
5. Romano G, Rotodano G, et al: A critical appraisal of pathogenesis and morbidity of surgical treatment of chronic anal fissure. J Am Coll Surg 178:600–604, 1994.

51. INGUINAL HERNIA

James Bascom, M.D.

1. "Groin" hernia refers to what three hernias?
Direct and indirect inguinal hernias and femoral hernias.

2. Francois Poupart, a French surgeon and anatomist (1616–1708), described a ligament that bears his name. What is the anatomic name of the Poupart ligament?
Inguinal ligament, which is a key element in most groin hernia repairs.

3. Franz K. Hesselbach, a German surgeon and anatomist (1759–1816), described a triangle that is the common site of direct hernias. What are the anatomic margins of Hesselbach's triangle?
The triangle is defined inferiorly by the inguinal ligament, superiorly by the inferior epigastric vessels, and medially by the rectus fascia. The floor of the triangle is formed by the transversalis fascia. The original description used Cooper's ligament as the inferior limit, but because of the common use of the anterior approach to hernias the more apparent inguinal ligament was substituted as the inferior limit of the triangle. With the increasing use of preperitoneal approaches to hernia repair, Cooper's ligament is again much more apparent and useful as an anatomic touchstone.

4. Sir Astley Paston Cooper, an English surgeon and anatomist (1768–1841), described a ligament bearing his name. What is the anatomic name for the ligament and the proper name of Cooper's ligament repair?
The anatomic name of Cooper's ligament is iliopectineal ligament. The McVay repair was popularized by Chester McVay (1911–1987). With Barry Anson, professor of anatomy at Northwestern University, McVay provided the modern description of the groin anatomy.

5. Antonio de Gimbernat, a Spanish surgeon and anatomist (1734–1816), had his interesting name attached to the lacunar ligament, which marks the medial margin of a groin area opening. What is the opening? What hernia protrudes into this opening?
The femoral hernia protrudes into the femoral canal.

6. Indirect inguinal hernia (particularly in children) and hydrocele are associated with what congenital abnormality?
Persistence of an open processus vaginalis, in the case of a hernia, allows descent of bowel into the inguinal canal. With fluid accumulation, partial obstruction presents as a hydrocele of the spermatic cord.

7. What are the diagnostic criteria for hernia in an infant or child?
1. Inguinal, scrotal, or labial lump that may or may not be reducible.
2. History of a lump seen by a health care provider.
3. History of a lump seen by the mother.
4. The "silk sign" (the feeling of rubbing together two surfaces of silk cloth when gently rubbing together the two surfaces of a hernia sac).
5. An incarceration sometimes felt on rectal exam.

8. What can be done to reduce an incarcerated hernia in an infant or child?
The four-point program is easier said than done, but worth the effort:
1. Sedate the patient.
2. Place the patient in the Trendelenburg position.

3. Apply a cold pack (over petrolatum gauze to avoid skin injury) in inguinal area.
4. In the absence of spontaneous reduction—and if the patient is quiet—use gentle manipulation.

9. How often can incarcerations be successfully reduced? What next?

About 80% of incarcerated hernias can be reduced in children; in adults the percentage is lower. Despite the fact that 80–90% of inguinal hernias occur in boys, most incarcerations occur in girls. The hernia should be repaired electively within a few days after incarceration. The 20% of hernias that are still incarcerated are operated immediately.

10. What is a Bassini repair?

The Bassini repair sutures together the conjoined tendon and the inguinal ligament up to the internal ring. This classic procedure, introduced in 1887 at the Italian Society of Surgery in Genoa, revolutionized hernia repair. Until recently it has been the standard of repair. After graduation from medical school and while fighting for Italian independence, Edoardo Bassini (1844–1924) was bayoneted in the groin and as a prisoner was hospitalized for months with a fecal fistula.

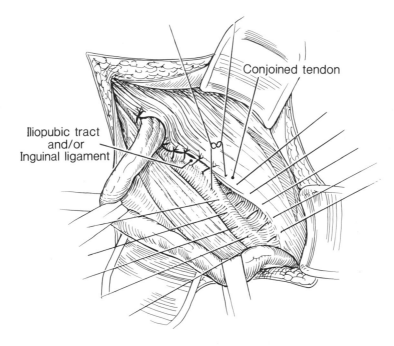

Conjoined tendon

Iliopubic tract and/or Inguinal ligament

The standard right inguinal hernia repair using the conjoined tendon and inguinal ligament.

11. What is the recurrence rate with indirect and direct hernias that have been repaired with classic Bassini repair technique?

Over a follow-up period of 50 years, the recurrence rate of adult indirect hernias is 5–10%; of direct hernias, 15–30%.

12. Describe a McVay hernia repair.

The line of interrupted sutures starts at the pubic tubercle and joins the tendinous arch of the transversus abdominis muscle to Cooper's ligament up to the femoral canal. At this point 2 or 3 transitional sutures are placed from Cooper's ligament to the anterior femoral fascia, effectively closing the medial extreme of the femoral canal. The final set of sutures joins the transversus abdominis arch and the anterior femoral fascia. The stitches usually incorporate the inguinal ligament at the upper limit of the repair, the site of the new internal inguinal ring and cord structures. About 15 years ago, McVay described laying in a mesh patch and stitching it, at its periphery, to the same anatomic structures. This application of mesh closely resembles the Lichtenstein repair (see question 17), except that it uses Cooper's ligament.

13. For what types of hernia is the McVay Cooper's ligament repair most useful?
Femoral and direct hernias.

14. What is the Shouldice repair?
The Shouldice repair, popularized at the Shouldice clinic near Toronto, imbricates or overlays the transversalis fascia and conjoined tendon with 4 continuous lines, using 2 fine-wire sutures. The suture tract runs from the pubic tubercle to a new internal ring. Care is taken with the inferior epigastric vessels. The result is layered approximation of the conjoined tendon to the inguinal ligament tract.

15. What is the reported recurrence rate for the Shouldice repair?
1%—the lowest reported rate for nonmesh repairs of inguinal hernias in adults.

16. For what type of groin hernia is the Shouldice repair not appropriate?
Femoral hernia.

17. Describe the Lichtenstein repair.
The Lichtenstein repair consists of a sutured patch of polypropylene mesh (Marlex, C.R. Bard, Inc., Covington, GA) that covers Hesselbach's triangle and the indirect hernia area. It is considered a tension-free repair because the mesh is sutured in place without pulling ligaments or tissues together as in all other repairs. The mesh is divided at its upper end to wrap closely around the spermatic cord and its associated structures in the normal position of the internal inguinal canal. The Lichtenstein procedure is rapidly becoming the most widely used repair of adult inguinal hernia. The reported recurrence rate is <1%.

18. What are the advantages of using the Marlex mesh?
Central to acceptance and success of the Lichtenstein hernia repair has been the development of and experience with the Marlex mesh. The monofilament mesh is strong, inert, and resistant to infection. The interstices are rapidly and completely infiltrated with fibroblasts, and the mesh is not subject to deterioration, rejection, or fragmentation.

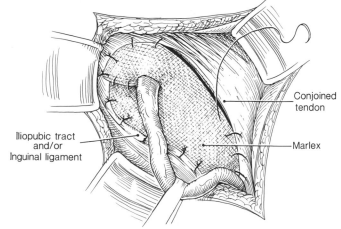

The Marlex mesh repair of a right inguinal hernia. Note that the same structures are used but not brought together; thus the name of "tension-free" repair.

19. For what groin area is the Lichtenstein repair not appropriate?
Femoral hernia.

20. What repair is acceptable for the femoral hernia?
Several different repairs can be used. Mesh in the form of a plug can be inserted and fixed in place. A McVay Cooper's ligament repair can be done. A preperitoneal approach to the hernia can be used to suture or plug the defect. A suture repair or a sartorius facial flap applied from below the inguinal ligament in a femoral approach also may be used. The preperitoneal approach is increasingly used for complicated inguinal and femoral hernias.

21. What is the preperitoneal or Stoppa procedure?
The preperitoneal or Stoppa procedure is a groin hernia repair on the internal side of the abdominal wall between the peritoneum and fascial surfaces that do not open into the peritoneal cavity. The anatomic landmarks are very different and initially quite challenging to the surgeon accustomed to the external abdominal wall approach. The technique is suited for recurrent hernias in which scarring and obliterated anatomy increase the risk of cord injury and recurrence. Other problems such as large hernias and femoral hernias are corrected with this approach. Conceptually the laparoscopic hernia repair uses the same approach.

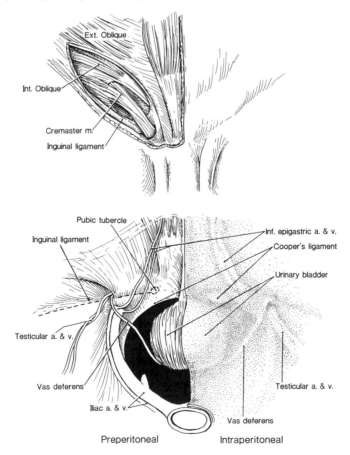

The different appearance and landmarks are seen in the anterior view (above) and the posterior view (below) of the inguinal/femoral area. In the posterior view the importance of the inferior epigastric vessels, bladder, and Cooper's ligament as anatomic landmarks is apparent.

22. Where are the spaces of Retzius and Bogros? Why are they increasingly important?
Retzius' space is between the pubis and the urinary bladder. **Bogros' space** is between the peritoneum and the fascias and muscle planes on the posterior aspect of the abdominal wall below the umbilicus and down to Cooper's ligaments. Laterally the space goes to the iliac spines. In either the open Stoppa procedure or the laparoscopic preperitoneal repair, the spaces of Retzius and Bogros are developed for mesh placement and surgical exposure.

23. How tight around the spermatic cord should a surgically fashioned, internal inguinal ring be?
About 5 mm, which is less than a fingertip and more than a forceps tip.

24. What is the common fascial defect of larger indirect and all direct inguinal hernias?
Weakness or attenuation of the transversalis fascia.

25. On examination the femoral hernia may be confused with what other inguinal hernia?
The femoral hernia may be confused with a direct inguinal hernia because of the tendency of the femoral hernia to present at the lateral edge of the inguinal ligament.

26. What is the difference between an incarcerated and a strangulated hernia?
    Incarcerated: structures in the hernia sac still have a good blood supply but are stuck in the sac because of adhesions or a narrow neck of the hernia sac.
    Strangulated: herniated structures, such as bowel or omentum, have lost their blood supply because of anatomic constriction at the neck of the hernia. The herniated, ischemic tissue is therefore in various stages of gangrenous changes. Strangulated hernias are surgical emergencies.

27. What is the operation for an uncomplicated indirect infant hernia?
High ligation of the sac.

28. What is the operation for an uncomplicated indirect hernia in young adults?
The appropriate operation consists of high ligation and possibly 1 or 2 stitches in the transversalis fascia to tighten the internal ring. This is the basic Marcy technique, developed by Henry Orlando Marcy (1837–1924); it is smaller and more anatomically focused than the Bassini repair.

29. What is the operation for an uncomplicated but sizable direct hernia in elderly adults?
Traditionally, the Bassini or McVay repair was chosen. More recently, because of the low recurrence rate, the Shouldice or Lichtenstein repair is favored.

30. What organ systems should be reviewed with particular care in the work-up of patients with hernia (especially elderly patients with recent onset of hernia)?
The gastrointestinal, urinary, and pulmonary systems should be reviewed with particular care. One is looking for causes of chronic strain or sudden forces that may have induced the hernia. Straining at stooling or urinating, unusual coughing, or difficulty with breathing, if corrected, may be of great value to the patient and reduce the chance of recurrent hernia.

31. What is a sliding hernia?
A sliding hernia is formed when a retroperitoneal organ protrudes (herniates) outside the abdominal cavity in such a manner that the organ itself and a peritoneal surface constitute the hernia sac.

32. What organs can be found in sliding hernias?

Colon	Bladder
Cecum	Fallopian tubes
Appendix	Uterus (rare)
Ovary	

33. What are common operative and postoperative complications of hernia repairs?
Intraoperative complications
- Injury to spermatic cord, especially in children
- Injury to spermatic vessels, resulting in atrophy or acute necrosis of testes
- Injury to ilioinguinal nerve, genitofemoral nerve, and lateral femoral cutaneous nerve. (The lateral femoral cutaneous nerve is uniquely vulnerable in laparoscopic and properitoneal procedures.)
- Injury to the femoral vessels

Postoperative complications
- Infection—high risk in children with diaper rash and patients with bowel injury or necrosis
- Hematoma—should resolve in time
- Nerve injury—the nerve is not always divided and with time may improve. If pain persists, try xylocaine block for both diagnosis and treatment. If a nerve block is not successful, one may consider reexploration to free the nerve from scar or to excise a postsurgical neuroma.

34. What are the common sites of hernia recurrence?
Direct hernias often recur at the pubic tubercle. Indirect hernias recur at the internal ring. The cause is usually related to poorly placed or insufficient stitches. Other possible causes include infection, poor tissue, poor collagen formation, or too much tension at the surgical suture line. A single line of repair under moderate tension probably will fail in a significant number of patients, regardless of adequacy of repair or healing process. Tension is almost always bad in surgery.

35. How long should the patient avoid heavy lifting after a hernia repair?
The standard advice for decades has been 6 weeks. The current advice varies from no limitation with the Lichtenstein or preperitoneal repairs to 6 weeks for a Bassini repair. The self-limitation of pain is an excellent guide.

CONTROVERSIES

36. Anatomic issues.
At issue is the **iliopubic tract**, which is central to the Anson/McVay anatomic description of the inguinal area and featured in the McVay Cooper's ligament repair. Although the McVay repair is used in England, the iliopubic tract is not referred to or described in English anatomic texts.

The term **conjoined tendon**, although commonly used, is considered by many to be anatomically inaccurate and misleading. The internal oblique and transversus abdominis muscles that make up the conjoined tendon are obvious and can be used surgically either alone or together. The tendinous edge of the transversus abdominis muscle and the tendinous edge of the internal oblique muscle start at their insertion on the pubic tubercle and course laterally and superiorly to the medial edge of the internal ring. At this point the tendinous elements diminish, leaving only muscle tissues, and continue laterally and superiorly to their origins.

Whether the lacunar ligament or the iliopubic tract defines the medial border of the femoral canal is controversial. The compromise position is that in the normal unstretched state the iliopubic tract is the border, whereas in the presence of hernia (stretched state) the lacunar ligament (Gimbernat's ligament) is the border. At surgery it is enough to say that a palpable, visible curved ligament is present and used in some femoral repairs.

37. Surgical issues.
The controversy over implanting mesh, as in the Lichtenstein repair, has been resolved in favor of mesh. Another controversy concerns the use of the laparoscope for hernia repair. A further issue is intraabdominal or preperitoneal placement of mesh. At present, most surgeons accept laparoscopic repair as an alternative for preperitoneal hernia repair. The indications for a preperitoneal approach for hernia repair are still being defined, although the preperitoneal approach is acceptable

for repair of recurrent hernias and unusually large or difficult hernias. The preperitoneal approach is used with increasing frequency for repair of femoral hernias.

The repair should be appropriate to the circumstance of the hernia. Thus, hernia location and size as well as the patient's age, general condition, and recurrence status should be factored into the strategy of repair.

BIBLIOGRAPHY

1. Cobb R: Inguinal hernias. In Morris PJ, Malt RA (eds): Oxford Textbook of Surgery. Oxford, Oxford University Press, pp 1399–1404.
2. Grosfeld JL: Groin hernia in infants and children. In Nyhus LM, Condon RE (eds): Hernia, 4th ed. Philadelphia, J.B. Lippincott, 1995.
3. Lichtenstein IL: The tension-free hernioplasty. Am J Surg 157:188–193, 1989.
4. McVay CB, Anson BJ: Inguinal and femoral hernioplasty. Surg Gynecol Obstet 88:473, 1949.
5. Nyhuus LM, Condon RE (eds): Hernia, 4th ed. Philadelphia, J.B. Lippincott, 1995.
6. Panos RG, Beck DE, Maresh JE,Harford FJ: Preliminary results of a prospective randomized study of Cooper's ligament versus Shouldice herniorrhaphy technique. Surg Gynecol Obstet 175:315–318, 1992.
7. Schapp HM, van de Pavoordt HDWM, Bast TJ: The preperitoneal approach in the repair of recurrent inguinal hernias. Surg Gynecol Obstet 174:460–464, 1992.
8. Stoppa RE: The preperitoneal approach and prosthetic repair of groin hernias. In Nyhus LM, Condon RE (eds): Hernia, 4th ed. Philadelphia, J.B. Lippincott, 1995.
9. Zimmerman LM, Anson BJ (eds): Anatomy and Surgery of Hernia. Baltimore, Williams & Wilkins, 1953.

IV. Endocrine Surgery

52. HYPERPARATHYROIDISM

Robert C. McIntyre, Jr., M.D., and R. Dale Liechty, M.D.

1. What is the prevalence of hyperparathyroidism?

There are approximately 100,000 new cases of hyperparathyroidism (HPT) annually in the United States. Primary HPT occurs in 1 in 500 women over 40 years old and in 1 in 2000 men.

2. What are the symptoms of hyperparathyroidism?

Primary HPT is associated with "painful bones, renal stones, abdominal groans, and psychic moans." The three most common symptoms are fatigue, depression, and constipation.

Classic Symptoms and Signs of Hyperparathyroidism

Bones: arthralgia, osteoporosis, fractures
Stones: renal stones, renal insufficiency, polyuria, polydipsia
Abdominal groans: pancreatitis, peptic ulcer disease, constipation
Psychic moans: fatigue, weakness, depression

With the widespread use of multiphase biochemical screening tests, many patients are found to have hypercalcemia without symptoms.

3. What are the leading causes of hypercalcemia?

The most common cause of hypercalcemia in hospitalized patients is metastatic bone disease. HPT is the most common cause of hypercalcemia among outpatients and the second most common cause in the hospital setting. Primary HPT and malignancy account for 90% of cases of hypercalcemia.

Differential Diagnosis of Hypercalcemia

Endocrine	Increased intake
Hyperparathyroidism	Milk alkali syndrome
Hyperthyroidism	Vitamin D intoxication
Addison's disease	Granulomatous disease
Malignancy	Sarcoidosis
Bone metastasis	Tuberculosis
Paraneoplastic syndrome	Miscellaneous
Solid tumors (squamous cell carcinoma	Familial hypocalciuric hypercalcemia
of the lung)	Thiazides
Hematologic malignancy (myeloma, leukemia,	Lithium
lymphoma)	

4. What is the essential laboratory evaluation for hyperparathyroidism?

Elevated serum calcium (> 10.3 mg/dl) should be assessed at least twice. Hypercalcemia must be associated with elevation of parathyroid hormone (intact). Serum phosphate levels are low in nearly 80% of patients, whereas serum chloride is increased in 40%. A chloride-to-phosphate ratio > 33 suggests primary HPT. Increased alkaline phosphatase levels are uncommon and occur only in the setting of advanced bone disease. A 24-hour urine collection for calcium excretion should be done to exclude benign familial hypocalciuric hypercalcemia (FHH). In patients with primary HPT, the 24-hour urine calcium is > 200 mg/day vs. < 100 mg/day in FHH.

5. Describe the embryology and anatomy of the parathyroid glands.
The upper parathyroid glands arise from the dorsal part of the fourth brachial pouch along with the lateral lobes of the thyroid. The lower parathyroid glands arise from the dorsal part of the third brachial pouch, along with the thymus. The average weight of a normal gland is 35–50 mg. In most cases, the upper parathyroid gland lies on the posterior portion of the upper one-half of the thyroid, cephalad to the inferior thyroid artery and posterior to the recurrent laryngeal nerve. The normal lower parathyroid gland is found on the lateral or posterior surface of the lower pole of the thyroid gland. Four glands are present in 89% of patients, 5 in 8%, 6 in 3%, and less than 4 in 0%.

Because the upper parathyroid glands do not migrate a great distance, their location is more constant. The most common ectopic sites of the upper glands are posterior to the esophagus or in the posterior superior mediastinum. The lower parathyroid glands are more commonly ectopic and may lie within the thyrothymic ligament, thymus, mediastinum (but outside the thymus), carotid sheath, thyroid, and upper neck in the undescended position.

6. What are the indications for parathyroidectomy?
All patients with symptomatic HPT or with serum calcium 1–1.5 mg/dl above normal should undergo parathyroidectomy. The treatment of asymptomatic patients with minimal elevation (10.3–11.0 mg/dl) of serum calcium is controversial. Close medical supervision of nonsurgical patients (every 6–12 months) should include bone density, renal function studies, and serum calcium evaluation. The cost of parathyroidectomy is equivalent to medical follow-up at 5–6 years.

7. What localization studies are available? When are they indicated?
Experienced radiologists may localize parathyroid tumors in as many as 75–85% of cases. Noninvasive localization studies include technetium-99m–sestamibi or technetium-99m–thallium scintigraphy, ultrasound, computed tomography, and magnetic resonance imaging. Invasive localization procedures include arteriography and venous sampling. The tests are most accurate with a single abnormal parathyroid gland. Localization procedures in cases of hyperplasia may be misleading.

Because experienced surgeons are successful in 95% of cases, localization studies are not routinely indicated. Localization studies should be done before all reoperative parathyroidectomies for persistent or recurrent HPT or in patients with previous thyroid surgery. Other indications include patients with a short, obese neck and poor-risk, elderly patients.

8. What is the pathology of primary HPT?
Primary HPT is due to a single adenoma in 83% of cases, hyperplasia in 12%, double adenoma in 4%, and carcinoma in 1%. In familial HPT and the multiple endocrine neoplasia syndromes (MEN I and MEN II), hyperplasia is the rule.

9. Outline the surgical strategy of an initial exploration for primary HPT.
A meticulously dry, blood-free operative field must be maintained at all times. Tissue in the region of the recurrent laryngeal nerve should not be clamped or divided until the nerve is definitively identified. A bilateral operation should be the rule. It is difficult to differentiate an adenomatous gland from hyperplasia on the basis of the appearance of 1–2 glands. Therefore, the surgeon must identify all four parathyroid glands. If a solitary adenoma and three normal glands are found, the adenoma is removed and one of the normal glands biopsied. Frozen section examination confirms that the tissue is parathyroid. Enlargement of four glands (hyperplasia) indicates subtotal parathyroidectomy, which leaves approximately 50 mg of well-vascularized parathyroid

tissue. The remnant should be marked with a nonabsorbable suture or staple. Thymectomy eliminates the possibility of thymic supernumerary glands. If more than one enlarged gland is found in association with normal-appearing glands (double adenoma), all abnormal glands should be removed with frozen section confirmation of parathyroid tissue. The glands left in situ should be marked as above. For patients with MEN I or II (hyperplasia), we recommend total parathyroidectomy and thymectomy with autotransplantation of 50 mg of tissue into the forearm.

10. What should one do if an adenoma is not found in the usual locations?
If an adenoma cannot be found in the usual locations, each normal gland should be biopsied and marked. Do not remove normal parathyroid glands. If three normal glands are identified and the fourth cannot be located, the surgeon should determine whether the missing gland is an upper or lower parathyroid. If the missing gland is an upper one, it often falls posterior to the esophagus or into the posterior superior mediastinum. The common mistake in this situation is that the dissection is not carried posterior enough to the prevertebral fascia. On the other hand, if the missing gland is a lower one, its location is more varied. First, the thyrothymic ligament should be inspected for ectopic parathyroid glands. The thymus can then be resected through the neck incision. If the adenoma is still not found, the area around the hyoid bone should be dissected to search for an undescended parathyroid. Next, the carotid sheath should be opened. In addition, the area lateral to the jugular vein should be explored. Finally, the thyroid lobe on the side of the missing parathyroid should be palpated for nodules. If a nodule is palpated, it should be excised and examined by frozen section; it may be an intrathyroidal parathyroid. If no nodule is palpated, a blind thyroid lobectomy should be performed.

A sternotomy should not be done as part of the initial exploration. If the above maneuvers are unsuccessful in revealing a parathyroid adenoma, the surgeon should stop. A diagram of the location of the identified glands should be made for future reference. Persistent hypercalcemia indicates the need for localization procedures.

11. What is the outcome of surgery for primary HPT?
The expected cure rate for experienced surgeons should be 95% in patients undergoing an initial exploration for primary HPT. After parathyroidectomy, bone density and renal function improve in 60–80% of symptomatic patients. Even in asymptomatic patients urinary calcium and deoxypyridinoline levels decrease. Patients have fewer episodes of nephrolithiasis, gout, and peptic ulcer disease. Parathyroidectomy also appears to improve longevity in patients with primary HPT.

12. What are the complications of parathyroidectomy?
Permanent recurrent laryngeal nerve injury occurs in < 1% of patients; however, temporary nerve paresis occurs in 3%. Hungry bone syndrome may lead to temporary hypocalcemia in up to 40% of patients, but permanent hypoparathyroidism occurs in only 3% of cases. An elevated preoperative alkaline phosphatase level may predict which patients are likely to experience postoperative hypocalcemia.

13. What physical signs of hypocalcemia should be assessed in patients after surgery?
Chvostek's sign is spasm of the facial muscles due to tapping the facial nerve trunk. Trousseau's sign is carpal spasm elicited by occlusion of the brachial artery for 3 minutes with a blood pressure cuff.

14. How should patients with hypocalcemia be treated?
Patients with tetany due to hypoparathyroidism require emergency treatment with intravenous calcium to prevent laryngeal stridor and convulsions; 10–20 ml of 10% calcium gluconate (90 mg elemental calcium/10 ml) should be given over 1–2 minutes until symptoms resolve. Maintaining calcium levels of 7.5–9 mg/dl is adequate. Oral calcium should be started as soon as possible in the form of calcium carbonate (Tums or Oscal) at 1–5 gm/day in divided doses. Calcium citrate is preferred for patients with renal lithiasis, because the citrate may be prophylactic against renal

lithiasis. In most patients, vitamin D preparations increase intestinal absorption of calcium and may be given as calcitriol (Rocaltrol), 0.25–5 μg/day.

15. What are the definitions of persistent and recurrent hyperparathyroidism?
Operative success is defined by long-term normocalcemia. Persistent HPT is defined as hypercalcemia within 6 months of surgery, whereas recurrent HPT is hypercalcemia after 6 months.

16. What is the strategy for management of patients with persistent or recurrent hyperparathyroidism?
First, the patient should be reevaluated to ensure that the hypercalcemia is due to primary HPT and not some other cause. Patients should be evaluated for familial hypocalciuric hypercalcemia, which does not warrant reoperation. Next, the patient should be evaluated to ensure that the severity of HPT warrants repeat treatment. The previous operative notes and pathology reports should be reviewed to assist in planning repeat therapy. Localization studies should be used extensively. Before reexploration, vocal cord function should be assessed in all patients.

Repeat cervical exploration is done through the previous incision. Because the strap muscles are usually adherent to the thyroid, a lateral approach through the plane between the sternocleidomastoid and strap muscles may be used instead of the usual medial approach. With positive localization studies or retrospective determination of the side of the missing adenoma, the dissection may be limited if an adenoma is found.

An alternative to repeat exploration is angiographic ablation of parathyroid tissue. Especially useful for mediastinal adenomas, it avoids a median sternotomy. It is done by delivering ionic contrast through an arterial catheter wedged into the feeding vessel.

17. Who performed the first parathyroidectomy?
In 1925 Felix Mendl performed the first successful parathyroidectomy at the Hochenegg Clinic in Vienna. His patient was Albert, a 34-year-old tram car conductor who could not work because of severe osteitis fibrosa cystica.

18. Who was Captain Martell?
An officer in the U.S. Merchant Marine, Captain Martell was the first patient to undergo surgery for primary HPT in the U.S. Captain Martell had progressive HPT that reduced his height from 6 feet to a kyphotic 5 feet 6 inches. After 7 operations the adenoma was finally removed from the mediastinum; however, the captain died of chronic renal failure.

BIBLIOGRAPHY
1. Clark OH: Asymptomatic hyperparathyroidism: Is parathyroidectomy indicated. Surgery 116:947–953, 1994.
2. Irvin GL, Prudhomme DL, Desario GT, et al: A new approach to parathyroidectomy. Ann Surg 219:574–581, 1994.
3. Kaplan EL, Yashiro T, Salti G: Primary hyperparathyroidism in the 1990's. Choice of surgical procedures for this disease. Ann Surg 215:300–317, 1992.
4. Liechty RD, Weil R: Parathyroid anatomy in hyperplasia. Arch Surg 127:813–816, 1992.
5. McIntyre RC Jr, Kumpe DA, Liechty RD: Re-exploration and angiographic ablation for persistent and recurrent hyperparathyroidism. Arch Surg 129:499–505, 1994.
6. Roe SM, Burns RP, Graham LD, et al: Cost-effectiveness of preoperative localization studies in primary hyperparathyroid disease. Ann Surg 219:582–586, 1994.
7. Shaha AR, LaRosa CA, Jaffe BM: Parathyroid localization prior to primary exploration. Am J Surg 166:289–293, 1993.
8. Wei JP, Burke GJ, Mansberger AR: Preoperative imaging of abnormal parathyroid glands in patients with hyperparathyroid disease using combination Tc-99m-pertechnetate and Tc-99m-sestamibi radionuclide scans. Ann Surg 219:568–573, 1994.

53. HYPERTHYROIDISM

Robert C. McIntyre, Jr., M.D.

1. What are the symptoms and signs of hyperthyroidism?

The principal symptoms of hyperthyroidism include nervousness, fatigue, palpitations, exertional dyspnea, weight loss, heat intolerance, irritability, tremor, muscle weakness, decreased menstrual flow in women, sleep disturbance, increased perspiration, increased frequency of bowel movements, change in appetite, photophobia, eye irritation, diplopia, change in visual acuity, and thyroid enlargement. Physical examination should include assessment of weight and height, pulse, cardiac rhythm, blood pressure, thyroid enlargement, proximal muscle weakness, tremor, ophthalmopathy, and skin (for pretibial myxedema).

2. What are the causes of hyperthyroidism?

The most common form of hyperthyroidism is **Graves' disease** (90%), which is due to production of thyrotropin receptor-stimulating antibodies. Ten percent of hyperthyroidism among middle-aged and elderly patients is due to **Plummer's disease** (toxic nodular goiter), which is caused by nodules that function independently of the normal feedback regulation.

Less common forms of hyperthyroidism include **thyroiditis** (subacute, silent, postpartum), in which inflammation leads to an increase in the release of thyroxine and triiodothyronine. **Iatrogenic hyperthyroidism** is due to excessive administration of thyroxine or triiodothyronine.

Rare causes of hyperthyroidism include neonatal hyperthyroidism, pituitary thyrotropin-secreting tumor, exogenous iodine, and factitious disease. Very rare causes are thyroid cancer, choriocarcinoma, hydatidiform mole, embryonal testicular carcinoma, and struma ovarii.

3. How should hyperthyroidism be investigated?

When hyperthyroidism is suspected, the diagnosis should be confirmed by measurement of thyrotropin and total or free thyroxine. Hyperthyroidism is confirmed by a low level of serum thyrotropin and high level of serum thyroxine. If the serum thyroxine level is normal, a high level of serum triiodothyronine indicates triiodothyronine toxicosis; a normal level of triiodothyronine excludes hyperthyroidism. A normal level of serum thyrotropin almost always excludes hyperthyroidism, except for the rare patient with a thyrotropin-producing pituitary tumor.

Serum total thyroxine may be increased in the setting of increased serum thyroid-binding globulin. This finding occurs in pregnant women, patients on estrogen therapy, and patients with an inherited increase in thyroid-binding globulin.

Toxic nodular goiter is confirmed by a radionuclide scan that shows uptake into a single thyroid nodule or patchy uptake into more than one hyperfunctioning nodule. Scintigraphy reveals low or absent uptake of radioiodine in thyroiditis.

4. What are the three treatment options?

Antithyroid drugs, radioiodine, and surgery.

5. What drugs are useful for the treatment of hyperthyroidism? What are their mechanisms of action?

Carbimazole, methimazole (the active metabolite of carbimazole), and propylthiouracil (PTU) are the mainstays of treatment. The goal of treatment is remission of Graves' disease or achievement of euthyroidism before treatment with radioiodine or surgery. All three drugs inhibit the organification of iodine and coupling of iodothyronines. PTU also inhibits the peripheral monodeiodination of thyroxine to triiodothyronine. All three drugs reduce the serum concentration of thyrotropin receptor antibodies and increase suppressor T-cell activity; thus, they may have an immunosuppressive action. Treatment is started with 10–20 mg/day of methimazole or 75–100 mg of PTU 3 times/day. The dose may be reduced after 4–6 weeks of treatment as the patient shows clinical and biochemical improvement. Therapy is usually maintained for 1–2 years. Patients must be monitored for side effects, which include rash, pruritus, agranulocytosis, hepatitis, cholestatic jaundice, and lupus-like syndrome.

Beta-adrenergic antagonists ameliorate the signs and symptoms of the disease. They should not be used alone except for short periods prior to radioiodine or surgical therapy. Nadolol (80 mg/day) or atenolol (50–100 mg/day) is the most commonly used agent.

Iodine given as Lugol's solution (5% iodine and 10% potassium iodide in water, 0.1–0.3 ml/day) or potassium iodide (60 mg 3 times/day) inhibits the release of thyroid hormone for a short period before its benefit is lost. It is useful for short-term therapy in preparation for surgery, after radioiodine therapy to hasten the fall in hormone levels, and for thyroid storm.

6. What is the outcome of drug treatment?

Long-term remission of Grave's hyperthyroidism during antithyroid drug therapy occurs in 10–75% of patients. Relapse is most common in the first 6 months after cessation of treatment but may occur years later.

7. What are the indications and objectives of radioiodine therapy?

Radioiodine is the most common form of therapy. It is the treatment of choice for recurrence after antithyroid drug therapy. The objective of radioiodine therapy is to destroy enough thyroid tissue to cure hyperthyroidism yet preserve enough to avoid hypothyroidism.

8. What is the regimen of radioiodine treatment?

The usual dose of radioiodine is 5–10 cm. If hyperthyroidism is not cured, the dose should be repeated in 6 months. Some prefer to use a higher initial dose (15 mCi). Most patients are pretreated with antithyroid drug therapy. Drugs should be discontinued 3–4 days before radioiodine and resumed 3–4 days after therapy.

Pregnancy is an absolute contraindication. Women of childbearing age should be evaluated with a pregnancy test before treatment and should avoid pregnancy for 6 months after treatment. Evidence indicates that radioiodine may exacerbate ophthalmopathy. Thus, some recommend drug therapy until the eye disease improves.

9. What is the outcome of radioiodine treatment?

Euthyroidism is not achieved for months after treatment. Once euthyroidism is achieved, recurrence of hyperthyroidism is rare. Hypothyroidism, the only serious side effect, is dose-dependent; it occurs at the rate of 2–3% per year, affects essentially 50% of patients at 10 years, and is nearly universal at 25 years.

10. What are the indications for thyroidectomy in the treatment of hyperthyroidism?

Thyroidectomy is the treatment of choice for (1) pregnant women who are difficult to treat medically, (2) patients with large goiter and low radioiodine uptake, (3) children, (4) noncompliant patients, (5) patients with nodules suspected to be cancer, (6) patients with compression of the trachea or esophagus, (7) patients with ophthalmopathy, and (8) cosmetic concerns.

11. How should patients be prepared for surgery?

All patients with hyperthyroidism should be rendered euthyroid before surgery. Patients may be treated with methimazole alone, a beta-adrenergic antagonist alone, or either drug in combination with potassium iodine.

12. What is the extent of thyroidectomy?

The two surgical options for Graves' disease are bilateral subtotal thyroidectomy or unilateral total lobectomy with contralateral subtotal lobectomy. In either case the goal of therapy is to preserve 4–8 gm of well-vascularized thyroid tissue. In Plummer's disease, lobectomy or partial thyroidectomy for unilateral lesions and contralateral subtotal thyroidectomy for multiple lesions render the patient euthyroid.

13. What is the incidence of hypothyroidism after surgery?
Permanent hypothyroidism occurs in 5% of patients within the first year and in 30% at 25 years.

14. What is the appropriate treatment for toxic nodular goiter?
Hyperthyrodism due to toxic nodular goiter is permanent and without spontaneous remission; antithyroid drugs are not appropriate long-term therapy. Radioiodine is the most common form of therapy. Larger doses (10–50 cm) minimize the risk of persistent hyperthyroidism; such patients tend to be older and to have prominent cardiovascular symptoms of hyperthyroidism.

15. What is the appropriate treatment for hyperthyroidism due to thyroiditis?
Subacute thyroiditis should be suspected if the patient has pain and tenderness in the thyroid region. The hyperthyroidism is usually mild and of short duration (weeks). Patients are treated with a beta-adrenergic antagonist and salicylate or glucocorticoid. Hypothyroidism may occur but is usually not permanent.

16. What is the appropriate treatment for thyroid storm?
Thyrotoxic crisis is treated with an antithyroid drug (PTU, 100 mg orally or rectally every 6 hours). Potassium iodine (orally or intravenously) may be given in combination with PTU. Beta-adrenergic antagonist (propranolol, 2–5 mg intravenously every 4 hours) may control the cardiovascular manifestations of the crisis.

17. Who performed the first thyroidectomy?
Johann von Mikulicz-Radecki performed the first thyroidectomy in 1885.

18. What surgeon won the Nobel prize for his work with thyroid disease?
Theodor Kocher won the Nobel prize in medicine in 1909. His achievements were related to the treatment of hyperthyroidism and its correction through surgery. He was successful in reducing the high mortality of thyroidectomy to less than 1%. His most significant achievement was in describing postoperative hypothyroidism as **cachexia strumipriva**.

BIBLIOGRAPHY
1. Franklyn JA, Daykin J, Drolc Z, et al: Long-term follow-up of treatment of thyrotoxicosis by three different methods. Clin Endocrinol (Oxf) 34:71–76, 1991.
2. Franklyn JA: The management of hyperthyroidism. N Engl J Med 330:1731–1737, 1994.
3. Patwardhan NA, Moroni M, Rao S, et al: Surgery still has a role in Grave's hyperthyroidism. Surgery 114:1108–1113, 1993.
4. Singer PA, Cooper DS, Levy EG, et al: Treatment guidelines for patients with hyperthyroidism and hypothyroidism. JAMA 27:808–812, 1995.
5. Surks MI, Chopra IJ, Mariash CN, et al: American Thyroid Association guidelines for use of laboratory tests in thyroid disorders. JAMA 263:1529–1532, 1990.

54. THYROID NODULES AND CANCER

Robert C. McIntyre, Jr., M.D., and R. Dale Liechty, M.D.

1. What is the incidence of thyroid nodules and cancer?
The prevalence of thyroid nodules varies with age, sex, and history of radiation to the neck. The frequency of thyroid nodules increases throughout life. Nodules are about 4 times more common in women than in men. After exposure to radiation, nodules develop at an annual rate of approximately 2%, reaching a peak at 25 years. Nodules are 10 times more frequent in glands examined by ultrasound, at surgery, or at autopsy. Less than 50% of thyroid nodules that appear solitary on physical exam are truly solitary.

Approximately 12,000 new cases of thyroid cancer are reported each year in the United States; 1,000 deaths/year in the U.S. are due to thyroid cancer. Up to 35% of thyroid glands examined at autopsy contain occult papillary cancer (< 1.5 cm).

2. What is the importance of the distinction between solitary and multiple thyroid nodules?
Multiple thyroid nodules are considered benign unless some finding suggests carcinoma (hardness, rapid growth, enlarged lymph nodes, laryngeal nerve paralysis). Solitary thyroid nodules are more likely to be malignant.

3. What is the differential diagnosis of thyroid nodules?

Differential Diagnosis of Thyroid Nodules

Adenoma	Cyst
Macrofollicular (colloid)	Nodular goiter with a dominant nodule
Microfollicular (fetal)	Other
Embryonal	Inflammatory diseases (i.e., Hashimoto's
Hürthle-cell	thyroiditis)
Carcinoma	Developmental abnormalities
Papillary	
Follicular	
Medullary	
Anaplastic	
Lymphoma	

4. What features of the history and physical exam indicate a higher risk of cancer?
Nodules occurring at the extremes of age are more likely to be cancerous, particularly in males. Rapid tumor growth and local invasion raise the possibility of malignancy, but these symptoms are rare. A history of radiation exposure increases the frequency of both benign and malignant nodules. A family history of medullary or papillary thyroid cancer or familial polyposis (Gardner's syndrome) increases the risk of cancer.

Cancer is more often found in patients with firm, solitary nodules than in patients with multiple nodules. Fixation to adjacent structures, vocal cord paralysis, and enlarged lymph nodes are also associated with an increased risk of malignancy.

5. What is the proper laboratory evaluation of a patient with a thyroid nodule?
The only biochemical test that is routinely needed is assessment of the serum concentration of thyroid stimulating-hormone (TSH) to identify patients with unsuspected thyrotoxicosis. Serum calcitonin should be measured in patients with suspected medullary thyroid carcinoma. In patients with known medullary carcinoma, assessment of serum calcium and a 24-hour urine test

for catecholamines and their metabolic products should be done to exclude multiple endocrine neoplasia before thyroidectomy.

6. Which single test best predicts the need for surgical intervention?
The single best test to predict the need for surgery is fine-needle aspiration (FNA). Provided that an adequate specimen is obtained, there are three possible results: benign, suspicious, and malignant. The reported accuracy ranges from 70–97%, depending on the experience of the person performing the biopsy and the cytologist interpreting it. FNA is most reliable for the diagnosis of papillary carcinoma and medullary and anaplastic cancer. It is least reliable in distinguishing benign from malignant follicular and Hürthle-cell neoplasms. The overall accuracy exceeds 95% in experienced hands. When FNA reveals cancer, it is 99% correct (1% false-positive rate); when the FNA specimen is benign, cancer is present in 4% (4% false-negative rate). On the other hand, when the FNA is suspicious, 20–30% of nodules are malignant.

7. What other tests may be useful in the evaluation of a thyroid nodule?
Thyroid radionuclide studies with isotopes of either iodine (more common) or technetium are often performed but cannot reliably differentiate malignant from benign nodules. Scans may be useful in patients with indeterminate FNA results, because hyperfunctioning nodules are almost always benign.

Ultrasound categorizes nodules as cystic, solid, or mixed and is the best measure of the size of a nodule. Ultrasound is also useful to determine the presence of other nodules in patients with a solitary nodule on physical exam. It is particularly useful to follow the size of a nodule. Like radionuclide scans, ultrasound cannot distinguish malignant from benign nodules.

8. Should a solitary thyroid nodule be suppressed with thyroxine for 3–6 months to determine if it is benign or malignant?
Most nodules change very little over the short term. In one series of 74 patients with colloid nodules, 13% became smaller, 22% disappeared, 46% did not change, and 19% enlarged. Studies of thyroxine therapy suggest that treatment is not superior to placebo in patients with solitary nodules; most nodules do not change in size, 15–35% decrease in size, and a few increase in size. On the other hand, thyroxine therapy has been reported to decrease the size of malignant nodules. FNA remains the single best test to determine the need for surgery.

9. What are the types and distribution of thyroid cancer?
Papillary 70%   Medullary 5%
Follicular 15–20%   Anaplastic and lymphoma 5%

10. What are the axioms of thyroid surgery?
Clark noted the following axioms:
   1. A meticulously dry operative field must be maintained.
   2. Tissue in the region of the recurrent laryngeal nerve should not be cut or clamped until the nerve is definitively identified.
   3. Every parathyroid gland should be treated as if it were the last functioning gland.
   4. If malignancy is suspected, the operation should be done as if the lesion were cancer.

11. What is the minimal extent of thyroidectomy for a solitary thyroid nodule?
The goal of surgery is to remove all foci of neoplastic tissue and any palpable cervical adenopathy. With the exception of small lesions in the thyroid isthmus, the minimal procedure for suspected malignancy should be lobectomy, including the isthmus. Enucleation is to be avoided. Frozen section is accurate for papillary, medullary, and anaplastic carcinoma. Frozen section is no more accurate than FNA for follicular and Hürthle-cell carcinoma. Functioning toxic nodules may be resected by a partial lobectomy, because they are usually benign. If the lesion is large, a lobectomy is preferred.

12. What is the most common form of thyroiditis in nodules?
The most common inflammatory disorders of thyroid nodules include Hashimoto's thyroiditis, subacute thyroiditis, and Reidel struma (rare). These conditions usually do not require surgery. Thyroidectomy is indicated for local symptoms or when cancer cannot be excluded.

13. What is the surgical therapy for thyroid carcinoma?
Thyroid carcinoma should be treated by near total or total thyroidectomy except in young patients with small, well-differentiated tumors ($\leq$ 2 cm) and no evidence of lymph node or extrathyroidal disease. In such cases, lobectomy with resection of the isthmus is adequate therapy. Total thyroidectomy eliminates multifocal cancer in the thyroid, allows postoperative radioiodine for diagnosis and therapy of metastatic disease, and improves the accuracy of serum thyroglobulin as a marker for persistent or recurrent disease. Enlarged cervical lymph nodes should be removed and examined by frozen section. If metastatic cancer is identified, a central neck dissection is performed. A central neck dissection is mandatory for patients with medullary carcinoma. If nodes are palpable in the lateral neck, a modified neck dissection should be done by extending the Kocher collar incision laterally to the anterior border of the trapezius muscle (McFee extension). "Berry-picking" results in an increased regional recurrence rate and should be avoided.

14. What is the arterial supply and venous drainage of the thyroid?
The blood supply to the thyroid gland comes from the superior and inferior thyroid arteries. Occasionally, a midline thyroid ima artery arises from the aortic arch. The superior thyroid artery is the first branch of the external carotid artery. The inferior thyroid artery arises from the thyrocervical trunk. The three major veins are the superior, middle, and inferior thyroid veins. The superior and middle thyroid veins drain into the internal jugular vein, whereas the inferior vein drains into the innominate vein.

15. Describe the anatomy of the recurrent laryngeal nerves.
The right recurrent laryngeal nerve (RLN) arises from the vagus and loops around the right subclavian artery. The left vagus nerve gives off the left RLN, which loops around the aorta. The RLNs run obliquely through the neck, usually in the tracheoesophageal groove. The nerves are more lateral low in the neck and course medially as they ascend. The right nerve runs more obliquely than the left. Occasionally the RLN may branch before entering the larynx, more commonly on the left side. The motor fibers are usually in the most medial branch. In 1% of cases the right RLN is not recurrent and enters the neck from a lateral and superior direction.

16. What defect results from injury to the RLN?
Injury to a single RLN results in a paralyzed vocal cord, which causes a weak, hoarse voice. Injury to both nerves, which causes paralysis of both cords and obstruction of airflow, necessitates a tracheostomy. RLN injury occurs in 1–2% of thyroidectomies.

17. Describe the anatomy of the superior laryngeal nerve and the defect that occurs when it is injured.
The superior laryngeal nerve gives off the external laryngeal nerve, which runs medial to the superior pole vessels to enter the cricothyroid muscle. This motor nerve increases tension of the vocal cords, allowing for high notes (Amelita Galla Curci nerve). The internal laryngeal nerve provides the sensory innervation to the posterior pharynx. It lies superior to the thyroid cartilage. Injury to the nerve leads to a weak, low voice that lacks resonance. Patients may also have problems with aspiration.

18. What is the other major complication of thyroidectomy?
Permanent hypoparathyroidism occurs in 1–2% of thyroidectomies.

19. What is the postoperative therapy for well-differentiated thyroid carcinoma?
Patients with certain risk factors should be treated with postoperative radioiodine (I-131). The high-risk factors include distant disease at presentation, older age (> 45 years old), male gender, and direct local invasion. All patients with well-differentiated thyroid cancer should be treated with levothyroxine (Synthroid), 0.2–0.5 µU/ml, to suppress serum TSH levels. Good evidence indicates that this postoperative therapy decreases recurrence of carcinoma; however, reduced recurrence does not appear to convey a survival advantage.

20. How should a patient be followed after therapy for well-differentiated thyroid carcinoma?
In young, low-risk patients, physical examination of the neck is done every 6 months for 2 years and then yearly thereafter. In high-risk patients, close follow-up includes assessment of serum thyroglobulin levels in addition to repeat neck examination. As useful as serum thyroglobulin levels are in follow-up, they need to be combined with diagnostic radioiodine scans for detection of recurrent disease.

Patients with recurrent cervical disease by palpation or ultrasound should have repeat surgery if the procedure can be performed with low morbidity. Recurrent distant disease should be treated with radioiodine if the metastases absorb iodine.

BIBLIOGRAPHY

1. Cady B, Rossi R: An expanded view of risk-group definition in differentiated thyroid carcinoma. Surgery 104:947–953, 1988.
2. Hay ID, Grant OS, Taylor WF, McConahey WM: Ipsilateral lobectomy versus bilateral lobar resection in papillary thyroid carcinoma: A retrospective analysis of surgical outcome using a novel prognostic scoring system. Surgery 102:1088–1095, 1987.
3. Maxon HR, Smith HS: Radioiodine 131 in the diagnosis and treatment of metastatic well differentiated thyroid cancer. Endocrinol Metab Clin North Am 19:685–718, 1990.
4. Mazzaferri EL: Papillary thyroid carcinoma: Factors influencing prognosis and current therapy. Semin Oncol 14:315–332, 1987.
5. Mazzaferri EL: Management of solitary thyroid nodule. N Engl J Med 328:553–559, 1993.
6. Ozta M, Suzuki S, Miyamoto T, et al: Serum thyroglobulin in the follow-up of patients with treated differentiated thyroid cancer. J Clin Endocrinol Metab 79:98–105, 1994.
7. Ridgway EC: Clinical evaluation of solitary thyroid nodules. In Braverman LE, Utiger RD (eds): Werner and Ingbar's the Thyroid: A Fundamental and Clinical Text, 6th ed. Philadelphia, J.B. Lippincott, 1991, pp 1197–1203.

55. SURGICAL HYPERTENSION

Thomas A. Whitehill, M.D.

1. What are the surgically correctable causes of hypertension?
Renovascular hypertension
Pheochromocytoma
Cushing's syndrome
Primary hyperaldosteronism (Conn's syndrome)
Coarctation of the aorta
Unilateral renal parenchymal disease
The overall incidence of surgical hypertension is 6–8% of all hypertensive individuals.

2. Which is the most common?
Renovascular hypertension. Although the overall frequency of renovascular hypertension among patients with elevated diastolic blood pressure is < 1%, moderate or severe diastolic hypertension

may be caused by renal artery occlusive disease in as many as 5–25% of cases. Pheochromo-cytoma, hyperaldosteronism, Cushing's disease, and coarctation of the aorta each account for around 0.1% of all hypertensive patients.

3. What are the most common causes of renovascular hypertension?

Atherosclerosis is the most common cause (70%); it affects men twice as often as women. The second most common is fibromuscular dysplasia (20–25%), which invariably affects women; of the many pathologic subtypes, the most common is medial fibrodysplasia (85%). Third is devel-opmental renal artery stenosis (5–10%), which often is associated with neurofibromatosis and abdominal aortic coarctation.

4. What clinical criteria support the pursuit of investigative studies for suspected reno-vascular hypertension?

Renovascular hypertension has no pathognomonic clinical characteristics. The following find-ings strongly suggest the presence of an underlying renal artery stenotic lesion:

  1. Systolic or diastolic bruits of the upper abdomen or flank
  2. Initial presentation of diastolic blood pressure > 115 mmHg or a sudden worsening of presumed preexisting essential hypertension
  3. Hypertension in very young patients or in women < 50 years of age
  4. Rapid onset of severe hypertension after age 50
  5. Malignant hypertension
  6. Hypertension resistant to usual medical regimens
  7. Deterioration of renal function after initiation of antihypertensive agents (especially an-giotensin converting enzyme [ACE] inhibitors)

5. What is the best test to diagnose renovascular hypertension?

Aortography or selective renal arteriography is the most accurate preoperative means by which renal artery disease can be defined anatomically. In many instances, the hemodynamic and functional importance of a lesion may be demonstrated by the existence of collateral vessels cir-cumventing stenosis.

Complementary functional studies to document the presence of renin-dependent hypertension should be undertaken in patients with renal artery disease of equivocal significance. Simultaneous **selective transcatheter sampling** of venous blood from both renal veins and the inferior vena cava is the most reliable. **Renal vein-renin ratios** (RVRR) and **renal-systemic renin index** (RSRI) are useful in assessing the importance of unilateral disease and bilateral disease, respectively.

Hypertensive urography, **isotopic renography**, and **split renal function studies** are not sufficiently sensitive or specific to be considered good diagnostic tests for renovascular hyperten-sion. **Duplex ultrasonography** holds strong promise for the future.

6. What is the renin-angiotensin-aldosterone axis?

Renin is released from the juxtaglomerular apparatus of the kidney in response to changes in renal cortical afferent arteriolar perfusion pressure (as little as a 10-mmHg gradient across a renal artery stenosis triggers release of renin). Renin acts locally and in the systemic circulation on renin substrate, a nonvasoactive alpha$_2$-globulin produced in the liver (also known as an-giotensinogen or hypertensinogen) to form angiotensin I. Angiotensin I undergoes enzymatic cleavage by ACE in the pulmonary circulation to produce angiotensin II, a potent vasopressor re-sponsible for the vasoconstrictive element of renovascular hypertension. Conversion of an-giotensin I to angiotensin II is about 90% complete with one passage through the lungs. Angiotensin II also increases adrenal gland production of aldosterone, with subsequent retention of sodium and water; this process establishes the volume element of renovascular hypertension.

7. How do ACE inhibitors work?

ACE is a peptidyl dipeptidase that catalyzes the conversion of angiotensin I to angiotensin II. Direct inhibition of ACE decreases concentrations of angiotensin II and leads to decreased vasopressor activity and aldosterone secretion. Removal of angiotensin II-negative feedback on renin secretion leads to increased plasma renin activity.

In clinical studies in hypertensive patients with unilateral or bilateral renal artery stenosis, increases in blood urea nitrogen and serum creatinine are observed in 20% of patients receiving ACE inhibitors. This observation often uncovers clinically unsuspected renovascular hypertension.

8. Should renovascular hypertension be treated medically or surgically?

Although prospective randomized studies comparing drug and interventional therapy have not been published, most clinicians favor surgical treatment and percutaneous transluminal renal angioplasty (PTRA) over drug therapy in managing patients with renovascular hypertension.

9. When should renovascular hypertension be treated with PTRA?

Fibromuscular dysplastic stenoses can be dilated with balloon catheters in nearly 90% of cases. Percutaneous dilation is best avoided in complex dysplastic disease with segmental vessel involvement, as seen in 20% of cases, because of the risk of dissection and thrombosis.

PTRA of atherosclerotic stenosis is often unsuccessful because of an inability to dilate spillover plaque from extensive aortic disease. This factor accounts for the limited (about 60%) initial success of PTRA for atherosclerotic lesions and an overall 1-year benefit rate of only 40% due to recurrence of stenotic disease, especially with ostial lesions.

Ostial lesions associated with developmental aortic anomalies or neurofibromatosis represent hypoplastic vessels with considerable elasticity that also are less likely to be successfully dilated.

10. What findings in the history and physical examination should lead to suspicion of pheochromocytoma?

Pheochromocytomas are tumors primarily of the adrenal medulla. They are classified as functioning when they produce catecholamines, always autonomously and usually in great excess. The predictable clinical effect of increased endogenous catecholamine outpouring is (1) sustained hypertension; (2) sustained hypertension with episodes of increased blood pressure, tachycardia, or flushing; or (3) in rare cases, normotension with infrequent and unpredictable episodes of hypertension.

11. How is the diagnosis of pheochromocytoma established?

Diagnosis is best confirmed by 24-hour urine collection for excreted catecholamines, metanephrines, and vanillylmandelic acid (VMA). The best test to confirm the diagnosis of pheochromocytoma is debated; some consider the metanephrine level to be the most precise (85%). It has been argued that plasma catecholamines are the most precise and specific test, but given the variability of results in individual patients and in many assays, the current approach should continue to emphasize the use of urinary catecholamines. Of patients with pheochromocytoma, 80% have at least one urinary metabolite greater than twice the normal value. The diagnosis of pheochromocytoma should be followed by studies to localize the tumor.

12. What is the best test to localize pheochromocytoma?

For most patients with a sporadic nonfamilial pheochromocytoma, simple CT identifies the lesion in the adrenal gland, especially if it is larger than 1 cm. Extraadrenal lesions should be sought only if a lesion is not found on CT scan. MRI is complementary to CT. Although CT is better for detecting the lesion, MRI is better for distinguishing one type of lesion from another.

The most appropriate test to localize solitary lesions or multiple lesions or metastases is ^{131}I-metaiodobenzylguanidine (MIBG), a norepinephrine analog. MIBG labels catecholamine precursors and is concentrated in adrenergic storage vesicles; the false-negative rate is < 5% and the false-positive rate is 1–2%. Another scintigraphic radiopharmaceutical, [131]I-6β-iodomethyl-19-norcholesterol (NP-59), a cholesterol analog, can distinguish adrenocortical hyperplasia from functioning adenomas or carcinomas. It accurately localizes the adrenal cortex and any functioning tumors.

13. Describe the acute antihypertensive treatment in patients with pheochromocytoma.
Hypertension from pheochromocytoma is caused by vascular smooth alpha$_1$-receptor activation, which results in vasoconstriction. Thus, the best acute treatment is intravenous administration of the alpha$_1$-blocker, phentolamine. Sodium nitroprusside is also a reasonable choice. Beta blockers should be avoided initially, because they cause both unopposed peripheral alpha$_1$-receptor stimulation and decreased cardiac output.

14. How is primary hyperaldosteronism (Conn's syndrome) diagnosed?
Conn's syndrome, which is caused by autonomous mineralocorticoid hypersecretion, is characterized by hypertension, hypokalemia, hypernatremia, metabolic alkalosis, and periodic muscle weakness and paralysis, often due to an aldosterone-secreting adenoma. Hypoinsulinemia and hyperglycemia may also result from hypokalemia-induced reduction of β-cell insulin release. The syndrome is now identified by the combined findings of hypokalemia, suppressed plasma renin activity despite sodium restriction, and high urinary and plasma aldosterone levels after sodium repletion in hypertensive patients.

15. Why does Cushing's syndrome cause hypertension?
Patients with Cushing's syndrome have hypercortisolism or excessive amounts of glucocorticoids. In the cardiovascular system, glucocorticoids appear to produce an increased chronotropic and inotropic effect on the heart, along with increased peripheral vascular resistance. Receptors in the distal renal tubules respond to glucocorticoids by inducing increased tubular resorption of sodium. These receptors belong to a different class from receptors that mediate the more potent actions of aldosterone.

16. What findings suggest aortic coarctation?
Coarctation of the aorta is suggested in patients who have a lower blood pressure in the legs than in the arms; they also have notably decreased or absent femoral pulses. Rib notching may be evident on chest radiograph in patients with longstanding, hemodynamically significant coarctation. Bruits may be heard over the chest wall. Adults may have an ongoing history of congestive heart failure. Life expectancy with untreated aortic coarctation is 35 years.

17. How does aortic coarctation cause hypertension?
No single cause has been identified. Mechanical obstruction of ventricular ejection is one component, leading to elevation of arterial pressure. Hypoperfusion of the kidneys, with resulting activation of the renin-angiotensin-aldosterone axis, probably contributes to some degree. Abnormal aortic compliance, variable capacity of collateral vessels, and abnormal setting of baroreceptors also have been implicated in the pathogenesis of hypertension.

BIBLIOGRAPHY

1. Blumenfeld JD, Sealey JE, Schlussel Y, et al: Diagnosis and therapy of primary hyperaldosteronism. Ann Intern Med 121:877–885, 1994.
2. Hansen KJ, Starr SM, Sands RE, et al: Contemporary surgical management of renovascular disease. J Vasc Surg 16:319–331, 1992.
3. Lairmore TC, Ball DW, Baylin, et al: Management of pheochromocytomas in patients with multiple endocrine neoplasia type 2 syndromes. Ann Surg 217:595–603, 1993.
4. Lamki LH, Haynie TP: Role of adrenal imaging in surgical management. J Surg Oncol 43:139–147, 1990.
5. Pommier RF, Brennan MF: Management of adrenal neoplasms. Curr Probl Surg 28:659–739, 1991.
6. Pommier RF, Vetto JT, Billingly K, et al: Comparison of adrenal and extra-adrenal pheochromocytoma. Surgery 114:1160–1166, 1993.
7. Sealy WC: Paradoxical hypertension after repair of coarctation of the aorta: A review of its causes. Ann Thorac Surg 50:323–329, 1990.
8. Sheps SG, Jiang NS, Klee GC, et al: Recent developments in the diagnosis and treatment of pheochromocytoma. Mayo Clin Proc 65:877–885, 1994.
9. Stanley JC: The evolution of surgery for renovascular disease. Cardiovasc Surg 2:195–202, 1994.

V. Breast Surgery

---

56. BREAST MASSES

Benjamin O. Anderson, M.D., and Roger E. Moe, M.D.

---

1. What makes up the normal breast?

The breast is a secretory gland composed of fibroglandular tissue housed within an envelope of subcutaneous fat and skin. Fibroglandular tissue is a composite of dense fibrous stroma and functional glandular lobules and ducts. The stroma supports the array of lobules that produce milk and the network of branching ducts that carry milk from the distant lobules to the nipple. The fibrous framework rather than the glandular epithelium provides the palpably firm, sometimes lumpy breast consistency. The surface of the fibroglandular tissue forms fluted ridges that feel like waves on a lake. Such normal surface irregularities, called Cooper's ligaments, are particularly evident on palpation in thin patients with abundant or dense fibroglandular tissue. Interposed between the fibroglandular tissue and skin is a layer of hundreds of subcutaneous fat globules. In obese patients, these fat lumps may become so prominent that they are confused on palpation with the underlying fibroglandular tissue. Fibroglandular tissue responds to hormonal cycling and involutes at menopause. As the involuting fibroglandular tissue becomes replaced by fat after menopause, its decreased density makes the breast less radiopaque and easier to evaluate on mammography.

2. What are the goals of breast examination? What features should be evaluated?

In simple terms, the goal of physical examination of the breast is to detect abnormal tissue. The examiner looks for visual changes that suggest pathology, assesses the overall consistency and texture of the fibroglandular tissue, and then palpates for irregularities or masses that contrast with the general pattern of fibroglandular architecture. In general, abnormal tissue **lacks uniformity** in comparison with surrounding tissue and/or **lacks symmetry** in comparison with the opposite breast. Abnormalities detected by examination are further evaluated by diagnostic modalities, including imaging and/or biopsy. The ultimate proof or disproof of malignancy requires microscopic examination of the glandular epithelium within the tissue of concern.

3. How should a breast examination by performed?

Multiple approaches to breast examination are used with success. In addition to palpation of the breast, a complete examination includes inspection and palpation of the axillae, supraclavicular fossae, and nipples with the patient in the upright position. Each nipple is compressed between the fingertips to detect thickening that resembles a bee-bee or piece of twine. Manually induced nipple discharge is common and normal. When the patient sits with hands on hips, the shoulder girdle muscles become relaxed; this position facilitates axillary palpation. In this position, with the examiner standing behind the patient, a bimanual examination of the axilla may reveal subtle axillary adenopathy. With one hand over the patient's shoulder toward the junction of the first rib and clavicle and the other hand reaching under the arm up into the axilla, the hands are brought together to appreciate more fully the tissue posterior to the edge of the pectoralis major. The patient may then be shifted to the supine position with arms raised above the head. This position flattens the breast and facilitates palpation of breast parenchyma using both hands.

4. What features should be looked for on visual inspection of the breast?

Breast masses within the fibroglandular stroma displace and deform normal tissues. Such displacement may cause dimpling of the skin, nipple retraction or deviation, or, in advanced cancer, frank skin edema, erythema, ulceration, or foreshortening of the breast. A red shiny color at the end of the nipple may be a sign of Paget's carcinoma. By contrast, a red scaly area on the areola but not on the nipple is a sign of eczema, a benign skin disorder. Redness of the breast distributed 360° around the areola may be a sign of inflammatory carcinoma. Redness confined to a sector on one side of the areola is more likely to be mastitis, a benign inflammatory process.

5. What is a dominant mass in the breast?

Breast fibroglandular tissue in premenopausal women tends to have a uniform, wavelike surface of ridges that when particularly prominent, is sometimes described as lumpy. These ridges represent normal breast architecture. A dominant mass is an area in the breast parenchyma that is protuberant, palpably thicker, or simply firmer compared with the surrounding fibroglandular tissue. Such masses may be benign lesions (e.g., round or knobby fibroadenomas, nondescript patches of benign proliferative changes, rounded fluid-filled cysts) or cancers. Breast ultrasound often helps to distinguish malignant from benign lesions.

6. Does the feel or quality of a lump in the breast help in the diagnosis?

Only to a degree. Discrete, smooth nodules like a marble are more likely to be benign than contracted, hard, ill-defined, and thickened areas. However, there is a large degree of variability, and examination alone can be misleading. Simultaneous bilateral mirror-image palpation is valuable to compare one breast with the other and to assess asymmetry.

7. Is a tender mass more likely to be benign?

Yes—but the association is in no way definitive. Some breast cancers present as a new internal pulling, tugging, burning, or itching and occasionally are frankly painful. Breast symptoms should not be ignored.

8. Is palpable adenopathy a reliable indicator of nodal spread from breast cancer?

No. One-third of invasive breast cancers with palpable adenopathy prove to be node-negative (without nodal metastases), and one-third of cancers with palpably normal axillae prove to have nodal metastases on microscopic examination.

9. Is it reasonable to monitor a breast nodule over one menstrual period?

Yes—if the nodule seems likely to be benign. However, a time limit for observation should be set from the beginning. A diagram and actual caliper measurements are important for accuracy. It is a reasonable axiom not to dismiss any persistent lump before the diagnosis is cleared.

10. Are any diagnostic modalities helpful in assessing breast lumps?

Mammography and ultrasound are key tools for breast evaluation. Mammography gives information about the remainder of the ipsilateral breast as well as the contralateral breast. Ultrasound differentiates cysts from solid masses and helps to characterize the nature of dominant masses in dense breast parenchyma. Other studies, such as MRI and nuclear medicine ("Mibi") scanning, are promising but expensive tests that remain investigational.

11. What is the approach to a mammographic abnormality that is not palpable?

If a lesion has a low probability of representing malignancy by radiographic criteria, it may be followed closely with serial mammography. If the radiographic findings raise the suspicion of cancer or if the lesion enlarges during observation, it should be biopsied. Microcalcifications, the earliest mammographic findings of cancer, are tiny white dots of calcium that appear like clustered pinpoints on a radiograph. Microcalcifications often but not always warrant biopsy. The shape, number, and tendency to group determine the likelihood of malignancy.

12. Does a negative mammogram negate the need for biopsy of a palpable mass?
Absolutely not. Among the palpable cancers, 15% are missed by mammography. In particular, invasive lobular carcinoma (in contrast to invasive ductal carcinoma) tends to grow in sheets rather than as rounded masses, inducing subtle mammographic changes until the cancer is fairly extensive. **Do not dismiss a palpable abnormality as benign simply on the basis of a normal mammogram**. An abnormal lump requires a diagnosis.

13. What are the recognized risk factors for carcinoma of the breast?
A family history of breast cancer, particularly bilateral cancers, in multiple first-degree relatives (mother, sister, or daughter) is the strongest risk factor for breast cancer, because it suggests a genetic predisposition for the disease. Ovarian cancers also may occur in the same families. A woman with a family history of breast-ovarian cancer who has inherited a mutated copy of the BrCa-1 gene has an 86% chance of developing breast cancer by the age of 80. Lesser risk factors appear to be hormonally related, such as early menarche and late initiation of childbearing. However, **most women who develop breast cancer have no identifiable risk factors for the disease other than female gender.**

14. If a cyst is aspirated and disappears, is it safe to assume that the cyst is benign?
Yes—if it does not chronically recur. On the other hand, if a cyst is aspirated and the palpable mass does not fully disappear, it needs to be evaluated further. Cytologic examination of clear or straw-colored cyst fluid has not been found to be helpful and does not need to be requested. Dark brown or black aspirated fluid may be old blood, which may arise from a malignancy. If a hemoccult test of dark-colored aspirated fluid is positive for blood, the fluid should be sent for cytology to evaluate for the presence of malignant cells.

15. What particular findings suggest that a biopsy is necessary?
In general, any patient who has an unexplained abnormality on physical examination or mammography should be considered a candidate for biopsy. The exception is patients with mammographic lesions that (1) have low probability for malignancy by radiographic criteria and (2) appear unchanged from prior mammograms or ultrasound studies. Stable, low-probability lesions may be carefully observed by serial mammography or ultrasound.

16. Are there different ways to biopsy a breast mass?
Yes. A mass may be biopsied by surgical excision or sampled by needle biopsy. The standard excisional biopsy removes the entire lesion, gives the pathologist the largest amount of tissue, and is the most accurate diagnostic technique. Needle biopsy also may be helpful in work-up and management of cancers, but its ability is limited because it represents a sampling technique. A positive malignant diagnosis by needle biopsy is helpful because it allows the patient to be fully informed before major surgery and to participate in operative selection (see question 9 in chapter 57). A negative diagnosis by needle sampling can be problematic, because it cannot definitively rule out cancer in the unbiopsied tissue.

17. What types of needle biopsies are used?
   Fine-needle aspiration (FNA) of breast masses is a simple technique performed in the clinic or the radiology suite to obtain a cellular smear (cytology) from a lesion of concern. A positive FNA cytology is highly accurate for cancer. However, because the histologic architecture is generally not seen on a smear, FNA usually cannot distinguish invasive from noninvasive (in situ) cancers (see question 4 in chapter 57).
   Core-needle biopsy, by contrast, removes a core of intact tissue through a 14-gauge needle. It is more accurate than FNA in distinguishing invasive from noninvasive cancers, because the histologic architecture of the lesion is preserved. However, core-needle biopsy can be technically difficult with small mobile masses and is most commonly used with mammographic (stereotactic) or ultrasound guidance to confirm accurate needle placement.

18. What is a stereotactic breast biopsy?

Interpreting free-hand needle biopsy results is problematic, because the operator cannot be certain that the needle has passed through the lesion of concern. Stereotactic biopsy uses a specialized table and computer system in conjunction with mammographic guidance to locate a breast lesion of concern for core-needle biopsy. The advantage of stereotactic biopsy over the free-hand approach is that one can document the tract of the needle. Ultrasound may be used in an analogous fashion to guide the biopsy needle to document accurate needle placement.

19. What is meant by needle localization biopsy?

Although the term may sound like a needle biopsy technique, needle localization biopsy is in fact a method of needle guidance to assist the surgeon in performing an excisional biopsy of a nonpalpable lesion. When an abnormality is seen only on mammography or ultrasound and cannot be felt, a fine needle or wire is inserted into the breast by mammographic or ultrasonic guidance to mark the abnormal area. The external tip of the needle is visible outside the skin and is used by the surgeon as a guidepost to locate the nonpalpable mammographic abnormality deep within the breast parenchyma at operation. A roentgenogram of the biopsy specimen, after it has been excised, confirms that the lesion has been removed as intended.

20. What is the approach to lumpy breasts, especially in young women?

Lumpy breasts are common, and there is no perfect answer. Normal breasts have normal lumps (see question 1). The role of the diagnostician is to determine whether a breast has a lump or region of lumps that seems different from the surrounding tissues, i.e., lacks uniformity or symmetry (see question 5). One should use all available modalities to examine the breast. Whether to biopsy or observe may come down to the judgment and experience of the physician.

21. Is cystic disease of the breast a premalignant condition?

Some clinicians use the terms "fibrocystic changes" or "fibrocystic disease" to refer to breast tissue that they find lumpy and difficult to evaluate. Both terms are imprecise and meaningless, because there is no commonly accepted definition. On the other hand, some premenopausal women have a clinically defined syndrome in which they form multiple gross cysts (≥ 3 mm diameter) within the breast parenchyma. Although it is often a diagnostic challenge to differentiate such cysts from solid masses, no clear evidence suggests that women who form macroscopic breast cysts are at increased risk for breast cancer. Microscopic findings of florid or severe intraductal hyperplasia or atypia may be associated with an increased incidence of carcinoma. Such microscopic findings have no relationship to the development of cysts in the breast.

22. Does prophylactic mastectomy have a role in the prevention of breast cancer?

Cancer prophylaxis is a complex issue that requires definitive indications of high risk. Family history alone is not an indication for prophylactic mastectomy, because no improvement in mortality rate has been shown compared with careful surveillance by mammography and physical examination. In occasional women with extreme family histories, surveillance appears unwise because of dense or cystic breasts; prophylactic mastectomy may be offered as one, **but not the only**, option in guarding against breast cancer. The role of prophylactic mastectomy among women who carry BrCa1 gene mutations remains to be determined.

23. What sort of anesthesia should be used in conjunction with a biopsy procedure?

Either a local or general, depending on the patient's wishes and, to some extent, the nature of the nodule. Almost all biopsies can be performed on an outpatient basis using local anesthesia, particularly if supplemented with intravenous sedation.

24. If a breast biopsy is positive for malignancy, should one proceed with a more definitive procedure at the same time?

Unless a specific condition of the patient dictates otherwise or unless the patient specifically requests this course of action, the definitive procedure is probably better done at a later time in a two-step procedure. This method permits the assessment of surgical margins. Currently, if the breast is preserved for irradiation, the surgical margins must be clear of cancer to ensure that no cancer from the primary tumor remains within the breast. The minor delay in definitive surgery does not change the prognosis. Psychologically, it may be distressing for a woman to undergo anesthesia with the uncertain prospect of losing a breast. When cancer is suspected on clinical grounds, a preoperative needle biopsy may be helpful by confirming the diagnosis of malignancy and allowing the definitive operative procedure to be performed under a single anesthesia, if this approach is preferred.

25. Do males develop breast cancer?
Yes—1% of breast cancers occur in males. Masses in the male breast should not be ignored on the basis of gender.

BIBLIOGRAPHY

 1. Borgen PI, Wong GY, Ylamis V, et al: Current management of male breast cancer. A review of 104 cases. Ann Surg 215:451–459, 1992.
 2. Claus EB, Risch N, Thompson WD: Autosomal dominant inheritance or early-onset breast cancer. Implications for risk prediction. Cancer 73:643–651, 1994.
 3. Hamed H, Coady A, Chaudary MA, Fentiman IS: Follow-up of patients with aspirated breast cysts is necessary. Arch Surg 124:253–255, 1989.
 4. Kaelin CM, Smith TJ, Homer MJ, et al: Safety, accuracy, and diagnostic yield of needle localization biopsy of the breast performed using local anesthesia. J Am Coll Surg 179:267–272, 1994.
 5. Lagios MD, Westdahl PR, et al: Paget's disease of the nipple: Alternative management in cases without or with minimal extent of underlying breast carcinoma. Cancer 54:545–551, 1984.
 6. Layfield LJ, Chrischilles EA, Cohen MB, Bottles K: The palpable breast nodule. A cost-effectiveness analysis of alternate diagnostic approaches. Cancer 72:1642–1651, 1993.
 7. Mikhail RA, Nathan RC, Weiss M, et al: Stereotactic core needle biopsy of mammographic breast lesions as a viable alternative to surgical biopsy. Ann Surg Oncol 1:363–367, 1994.
 8. Rosen PP: Proliferative breast "disease." An unresolved diagnostic dilemma. Cancer 71:3798–3807, 1993.

57. PRIMARY THERAPY FOR BREAST CANCER

Benjamin O. Anderson, M.D.

1. How is breast cancer diagnosed?
A diagnosis of cancer requires tissue confirmation. A diagnosis of breast cancer is usually made by **excisional biopsy** (removal of the entire mass) performed under local anesthesia. Needle biopsies are helpful in selected patients, as long as the limitations of sampling techniques are understood. **Fine-needle aspiration** (FNA) is useful for verifying a clinical impression of malignancy but requires formal histologic (as opposed to cytologic) confirmation at some point, because false-positive cytologies occasionally occur. **Core-needle biopsy**, if positive for cancer, may be considered a definitive diagnosis of cancer (see question 17 of chapter 56). However, a negative core-needle biopsy may represent sampling error and therefore is difficult to interpret. Core-needle biopsies can distinguish invasive from noninvasive (in situ) cancers (see question 4), whereas FNA cytology cannot.

2. What is the role of mammography after biopsy of a cancer?
Mammography after diagnosis is most valuable for identifying additional cancers in the same breast or opposite breast. Mammography also may be useful in counseling patients who must choose between breast conservation (lumpectomy and radiation) and mastectomy (see question 8). Women with highly dense or cystic breasts often have mammograms that defy accurate interpretation.

Such women may consider mastectomy instead of breast conservation, because local cancer recurrence in the conserved breast is difficult to detect promptly.

3. Does a delay between biopsy and definitive treatment adversely affect cure?
Probably not—if the delay is only a few days or weeks. Delays of more than 3–4 weeks should be avoided. A possible exception is the pregnant patient, in whom tumor growth may be quite rapid; prompt treatment appears to be particularly important.

4. What is the difference between noninvasive (in situ) and invasive breast cancers?
Noninvasive (in situ) cancers are malignant cells that remain confined to the duct or lobule in which they originated. In situ cancers have essentially no chance of spreading to nodes or distant sites, because they have contacted neither lymphatic nor vascular channels through which they metastasize. Invasive cancers have traversed the basement membrane of their originating duct or lobule and, therefore, have metastatic potential. With no chance for spread, in situ cancers without invasion do not warrant lymph node dissection as part of definitive surgery.

5. How is breast cancer staged?

	HISTOLOGY	TUMOR SIZE	NODAL METASTASES	DISTANT METASTASES
Stage 0	Noninvasive	Any	—	—
Stage I	Invasive	< 2 cm	No	No
Stage II	Invasive	2–5 cm	No	No
		< 5 cm	Yes	
		> 5 cm	No	
Stage III	Invasive	> 5cm	Yes	No
		Any size	Fixed nodes	
		Skin or chest wall invasion	Yes or no	
Stage IV	Invasive	Any size	Yes or no	Yes

6. Why is staging of breast cancer important?
Cancer staging is important because (1) it defines a common descriptive vocabulary and (2) the stages correlate with likelihood of relapse and fatality. The TNM (tumor, node, metastasis) staging summarizes data about tumor size, axillary node metastases, and distant metastases. In general, stage I breast cancers are small cancers without nodal metastases; stage II cancers are intermediate-sized cancers with or without axillary nodal metastases; stage III cancers are locally advanced cancers, usually with axillary nodal metastases; and stage IV cancers have already metastasized to distant sites.

7. Where does breast cancer spread (other than to lymph nodes)? Which diagnostic tests are useful for identifying such metastases?
Breast cancers most commonly metastasize to bone, lung, liver, and brain. Screening for bone metastases begins with whole-body radionuclide bone scanning. Bone scans are quite sensitive but less specific for metastases. Lesions seen on bone scan are further studied by standard radiographic techniques to distinguish metastases from benign inflammatory conditions. Lung metastases are identified by chest radiograph or CT scan. Liver function tests (LFTs) are commonly used to screen for liver metastases. Unfortunately, LFTs are neither specific nor sensitive for this purpose. LFTs are most commonly elevated because of benign hepatic pathology rather than metastases, and 25% of breast cancer patients with known liver metastases have normal LFTs. Liver imaging tests (ultrasound or abdominal CT), although more expensive, are more reliable for the diagnosis of liver metastases. Brain metastases are generally imaged by CT or MRI scanning.

8. Which preoperative studies should be done before mastectomy or lumpectomy to identify metastases?

Identifying stage IV (metastatic) cancers at first presentation is infrequent, because they represent 5% or fewer of all initially diagnosed breast cancers. Metastatic studies, therefore, should be used selectively at first diagnosis. All patients with symptoms suggesting metastatic disease (bone pain, pulmonary symptoms, jaundice, seizures) should be evaluated by appropriate preoperative testing once invasive breast cancer has been diagnosed. The asymptomatic patient, by comparison, warrants a limited evaluation. The standard minimal preoperative work-up for invasive cancer consists of a chest radiograph and liver function tests (LFTs). In reality, the utility of these tests among early-stage cancers is quite low. Routine chest radiography identifies unsuspected lung metastases in fewer than 1% of patients. Chest radiography is often justified for other reasons and is useful as a baseline test for future comparison. LFTs, on the other hand, may become eliminated from the standard preoperative breast cancer work-up because of their limited sensitivity and specificity for metastatic disease (see question 7).

9. What are the alternatives for primary treatment of invasive breast cancer?

1. **Modified radical mastectomy.** Removal of the breast, including the nipple-areolar complex, and removal (dissection) of axillary lymph nodes have survival benefit equivalent to radical mastectomy, which also removes the pectoralis major muscle. The true radical mastectomy is rarely performed today. The pectoralis minor muscle may be removed, with minimal morbidity, in a modified radical mastectomy to facilitate dissection of the highest (level III) lymph nodes.

2. **Partial mastectomy (lumpectomy or quadrantectomy).** Breast conservation therapy includes resection limited to removal of the breast tumor with a margin of normal breast tissue (negative margins), axillary dissection, and postoperative adjuvant breast irradiation. Breast conservation therapy has been shown in retrospective and prospective randomized studies to have survival rates equivalent to those for modified radical mastectomy among defined patient subgroups (see question 13). Although some surgeons have reserved breast-conserving therapy for patients without axillary node metastases, this restriction is no longer thought to be correct. Treatment of the breast tumor and treatment of axillary nodes appear to be independent issues, according to current data.

3. **Primary irradiation to the breast.** Primary breast irradiation without surgery—not to be confused with postoperative adjuvant irradiation—is under evaluation in European cancer centers. Primary breast irradiation is not accepted currently as standard treatment in the United States, because it has not been shown to have curative potential equivalent to that of surgically based approaches with proved efficacy.

10. What is the overall survival rate after definitive treatment?

    Stage I: 70–90% 10-year survival rate
    Stage II: 50–70% 10-year survival rate
    Stage III: 20–50% 10-year survival rate

11. What is the National Surgical Adjuvant Breast Project B-06 (NSABP B-06)? What is its significance?

The NSABP B-06 is a multicenter study that randomized nearly 2,000 women with stages I and II tumors (< 4 cm) to three treatment modalities: segmental mastectomy (SM) alone, segmental mastectomy with radiation, and total mastectomy (TM). All patients underwent axillary dissection, and patients with positive nodes received adjuvant chemotherapy. At least two significant conclusions were reached. Patients who underwent SM without radiation therapy had lower rates of disease-free survival than patients who underwent SM with radiation therapy. There was **no difference in overall survival rates** between the two groups, but radiation therapy was of benefit in control of local tumor. In patients who underwent SM (with or without radiation), there was **no difference in disease-free survival or overall survival rates**, indicating that breast-conserving surgery is an effective treatment in the appropriate setting.

12. What is a quadrantectomy (as opposed to lumpectomy or segmental mastectomy)?
A quadrantectomy is resection of the tumor along with the involved quadrant of the breast, including the skin. Quadrantectomy, lumpectomy, and segmental mastectomy are clinically the same procedure, differing primarily in the amount of breast tissue that is removed.

13. Are some patients poor candidates for breast conservation therapy?
Patients should be counseled against lumpectomy and irradiation in certain circumstances. Contraindications (relative or absolute) to breast conservation include (1) cancers that cannot be excised with negative margins without mastectomy, (2) cancers that are too large relative to the breast to obtain acceptable cosmetic results, (3) multicentric cancers (i.e., multiple cancers in the same breast), (4) breasts in which cancer recurrence would be difficult to identify by mammographic follow-up (see question 2), and (5) patients who do not desire or who have a specific contraindication to adjuvant radiation therapy (e.g., pregnancy). Knowledge and recommendations continue to evolve as additional well-controlled clinical data unfold.

14. Which patients who have undergone modified radical mastectomy may undergo immediate breast reconstruction (i.e., at the same operation)?
Controversy surrounds patient selection for immediate reconstruction. Most agree that patients with noninvasive (in situ) or early invasive (stage I and selected stage II) breast cancers may be offered immediate reconstruction with either a myocutaneous flap or a breast implant. It is disadvantageous to perform immediate reconstruction in patients with locally advanced (stage III) breast cancer because (1) the patient may require chest wall irradiation and (2) a subsequent chest wall recurrence, which is more likely with more advanced cancers, becomes difficult to detect with an overlying flap of tissue.

15. Which studies should be obtained after definitive surgery to screen for metastases and as baseline studies for future comparison?
The utility of metastatic screening tests correlates with the locoregional tumor and nodal (TN) staging determined at surgery. Patients with locally advanced (stage III and some stage II) cancers are at high risk for developing cancer recurrence with metastases. Bone scan and liver imaging (CT or ultrasound) are generally helpful as baseline studies. These tests occasionally reveal previously unappreciated metastatic disease. Conversely, such baseline studies are best avoided in asymptomatic patients with stage I (small, node-negative) cancers, because the chance of cure is high and the likelihood of finding metastases is remote. With stage I breast cancer, for example, the likelihood of a false-positive result on bone scan exceeds the likelihood of a true positive result by 250%. Brain imaging (CT or MRI), because of low yield in asymptomatic patients, is usually reserved for patients with neurologic symptoms.

16. What is the treatment of ductal carcinoma in situ (DCIS)?
In the past DCIS—also known as intraductal carcinoma—was thought to be a multicentric disease demanding mastectomy. This belief led to the paradoxical conclusion that a noninvasive cancer (DCIS) without the potential for metastatic spread required a more aggressive surgical approach than an invasive cancer of similar dimensions. As widespread screening mammography resulted in the detection of more cases of smaller, nonpalpable DCIS, this approach was reevaluated. Data from the NSABP B-17 trial (randomized excision vs. excision with radiation therapy) suggest that DCIS can be safely treated by breast conservation therapy (lumpectomy plus adjuvant radiation), provided that it can be excised with negative margins and that the remainder of the breast can be adequately evaluated and followed for development of subsequent malignancy.

17. Can some cases of DCIS be treated by lumpectomy without radiotherapy?
Lagios studied 79 patients with mammographically detected DCIS treated with lumpectomy without radiation and identified a subset of patients who were unlikely to develop local recurrence. On the basis of Lagios' report, a number of cancer centers no longer recommend the use of

radiation after lumpectomy for cases of DCIS that are (1) nonpalpable (mammographically detected); (2) smaller than 2.5 cm; (3) detected with negative margins; and (4) without comedo-type necrosis on histologic examination. However, forgoing radiation treatment after lumpectomy for low-grade DCIS remains controversial. Recent reports suggest that late local recurrence rates (15–25 years) without radiation may exceed 25%.

18. What should be the treatment of lobular carcinoma in situ (LCIS)?

LCIS behaves differently from its ductal counterpart. LCIS may not invariably degenerate into invasive cancer, but women with proven LCIS have a 20–25% chance of developing breast cancer during their lifetime. Unfortunately, the cancer may be ductal or lobular in origin and may develop with equal likelihood in the ipsilateral or contralateral breast. Most authorities interpret the histologic finding of LCIS to be a significant marker for high risk of breast cancer and suggest careful surveillance with serial mammography and physical examination. Bilateral mastectomy, the only logical surgical procedure for this condition, is extreme and has not been shown to improve overall survival rates. Chemoprevention of breast cancer with tamoxifen is under evaluation in a prospective randomized trial, but is not standard therapy at this time. Tamoxifen, although an effective treatment for some breast cancers, may increase the incidence of uterine cancers.

19. What is inoperable breast cancer?

Inoperable breast cancer has advanced beyond the boundaries of surgical resection. The spread may be regional (internal mammary lymph nodes, stage IIIB) or distant (distant metastases, stage IV). Supraclavicular lymph node metastases, which are beyond the margins of surgical resection, convey the same unfortunate prognosis as metastases to distant solid organs and are staged as such. Primary therapy with such advanced cancers is systemic treatment (chemotherapy or hormonal therapy) rather than surgery. Surgery combined with radiation therapy becomes an adjuvant therapy for local control of disease after a good response to systemic treatment.

20. What is neoadjuvant therapy for breast cancer?

Locally advanced but operable (stage IIIA and some stage II) cancers have a high likelihood of recurrence after surgery. Neoadjuvant therapy is induction chemotherapy before surgery to decrease the local tumor burden and to begin treatment of micrometastatic disease at the earliest possible time. It is not yet known whether the timing of chemotherapy relative to surgery influences survival time from diagnosis. The role of neoadjuvant therapy is under evaluation in prospective randomized trials. If a cancer is so locally advanced that negative margins are likely to be unobtainable even by mastectomy, neoadjuvant chemotherapy should be considered. In addition, preliminary data suggest that neoadjuvant therapy may convert some cancers that would otherwise require mastectomy into potential candidates for breast conservation surgery, although the safety of this approach warrants careful scrutiny.

BIBLIOGRAPHY

1. Anderson BO, Petrek JA, Byrd DR, et al: Pregnancy influences breast cancer stage at diagnosis in women 30 years of age and younger. Ann Surg Oncol 3(2): 1996.
2. Ciatto S, Pacini P, Azzini V, et al: Preoperative staging of primary breast cancer. A multicentric study. Cancer 61:1038–1040, 1988.
3. Fisher B, Redmond C, Fisher ER, et al: Ten-year results of a randomized clinical trial comparing radical mastectomy and total mastectomy with or without radiation. N Engl J Med 312:674–681, 1985.
4. Fisher R, Redmond C, Poisson R, et al: Eight-year results of a randomized clinical trial comparing total mastectomy and lumpectomy with or without irradiation in the treatment of breast cancer. N Engl J Med 320:822–828, 1989.
5. Harris JR, Recht A, Schnitt S, et al: Current status of conservation surgery and radiotherapy as primary local treatment for early carcinoma of the breast. Breast Cancer Res Treat 5:245–255, 1985.
6. Lagios MD, Margolin FR, Westdahl PR, Rose MR: Mammographically detected duct carcinoma in situ. Frequency of local recurrence following tylectomy and prognostic effect of nuclear grade on local recurrence. Cancer 63:618–624, 1989.

7. Osborne MP, Hoda SA: Current management of lobular carcinoma in situ of the breast. Oncology 8:45–49, 1994.
8. Page DL, Dupont WD, Rogers LW, et al: Continued local recurrence of carcinoma 15–25 years after a diagnosis of low-grade ductal carcinoma in situ of the breast treated only by biopsy. Cancer 76:1197–1200, 1995.
9. Singletary SE, McNeese MD, Hortobagyi GN: Feasibility of breast-conservation surgery after induction chemotherapy for locally advanced breast cancer. Cancer 69:2849–2852, 1992.
10. Solin LJ, Yeh I, Kurtz J, et al: Ductal carcinoma in situ (intraductal carcinoma) of the breast treated with breast-conserving surgery and definitive irradiation. Correlation of pathologic parameters with outcome of treatment. Cancer 71:2532–2542, 1993.
11. Wilson LD, Beinfield M, McKhann CF, Haffty BG: Conservative surgery and radiation in the treatment of synchronous ispsilateral breast cancers. Cancer 72:137–142, 1993.

VI. Other Cancer

58. MELANOMA

William R. Nelson, M.D.

1. What are the different types of moles or nevi?
Intradermal, junctional, compound, and Spitz nevi and nevi of the dysplastic nevus syndrome.

2. What is a Spitz nevus?
Formerly known as juvenile melanoma, the Spitz nevus has a characteristic cellular appearance and may mimic early melanoma. It is completely benign.

3. What characteristics typify the patient with melanoma?
The great majority of patients have auburn or reddish brown hair and fair, poorly tanning skin.

4. Is melanoma hereditary?
The inherited familial atypical mole and melanoma syndrome (FAM-M) has been defined as the occurrence of melanoma in one or more first- or second-degree relatives, and the presence of many moles (over 50) of variable size, some of which are atypical histologically. The risk of melanoma in this syndrome runs as high as 100% in the individual's life time. With only the positive family history, the risk of melanoma is still high but not nearly as great as in the FAM-M syndrome.

5. Do some people have a specific gene that leads to melanoma development, as in the FAM-M syndrome?
Genetic studies have revealed a specific gene (p16) in many people with the FAM-M syndrome.

6. Does sunlight have any effect on production of melanoma?
The great majority of melanomas occur in sun-exposed areas in sun-sensitive people. A small number of melanomas develop on the soles of the feet and on the genitalia.

7. Do blacks get melanomas?
The numbers are small, but blacks can develop melanoma. If they do, the lesions are often on unexposed and lightly pigmented areas, such as the soles of the feet and the palms of the hands.

8. In which part of the world is melanoma most common?
Melanoma is most common in Australia, especially the northern part of the continent, where light-skinned descendants of the original settlers are exposed to the tropical sun.

9. Which moles should be removed?
Growing and darkening nevi should be considered for removal, especially in sun-sensitive patients. Itching is a sign of early malignant change; ulceration is a very late sign. Melanoma may be familial in origin, and children of patients with melanomas should be carefully screened for very dark nevi.

10. Should nevi be biopsied, or should all nevi be totally excised?
It was once believed that incisional biopsy was contraindicated in all lesions suspected of being melanomas. Currently wedge biopsy is believed to be safe for any large lesion requiring complex repair. The best method, however, is total excision of the lesion with a narrow margin of normal skin plus primary repair. Thorough pathologic study is essential.

11. What are the types of melanoma? Is the term malignant melanoma a redundancy?
The term malignant melanoma is truly a redundancy, because melanoma is a malignant lesion. Nevertheless, the term persists in the literature. Types of melanoma are superficial spreading, nodular, lentigo maligna, and acral-lentiginous (usually on the palms and soles). Site-specific melanomas include those arising in giant hairy nevi, mucosal (oral and anorectal), conjunctival, ocular, and genital melanoma. Unknown primary or disappearing primary lesions may result in metastasis. The outlook for such patients is poor, even though the primary tumor may have regressed.

12. What is the importance of the Clark and Breslow classifications of melanoma invasion?

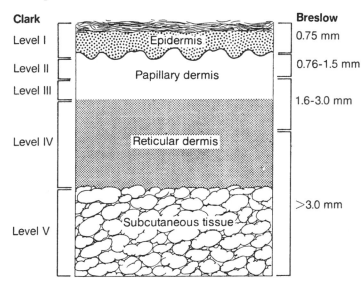

(From Young OM, Mathes ST: In Schwartz SI (ed): Principles of Surgery, 6th ed. New York, McGraw-Hill, 1994.)

Clark selected five levels of melanoma thickness in the skin:
Level I: an intradermal melanoma that does not metastasize; may be better termed "atypical melanotic hyperplasia," a benign lesion.
Level II: a melanoma that penetrates the basement membrane into the papillary dermis.
Level III: a melanoma that fills the papillary dermis and encroaches on the reticular dermis in a pushing fashion.
Level IV: a melanoma that invades the reticular dermis.
Level V: a melanoma that works its way into the subcutaneous fat.
The Breslow method requires an optical micrometer fitted to the ocular position of standard microscopes. This technique is generally thought to be a more exact determination of tumor invasion. Lesions are classified as follows: < 0.75 mm, 0.76–1.5 mm, 1.51–3.99 mm, > 4.0 mm. Lesions less than 1 mm include melanoma in situ and thin invasive tumors. The cure rate is over 99% with excision. Tumors of 1.0–4.0 mm are called intermediate but involve risk of metastases and death. Lesions over 4.0 mm are high-risk lesions with a relatively poor cure rate.

Thin melanomas should be checked by both methods, because some tumors may show a low Breslow measurement with a deeper Clark level, indicating a great risk of recurrence and spread.

13. What are the chances of metastases to nodes and systemic spread with the different degrees of melanoma invasion of the skin?

In melanoma < 0.76 mm in depth, regional node metastases occur in about 2 or 3%; the distant spread is almost 0%. Nodes are positive in 25% of tumors 0.76–1.5 mm and distant spread is 8%. In tumors of 1.5–4.0 mm thickness, node metastases occur in 57% and distant spread is 15%. In tumors over 4.0 mm, node metastases occur in up to 62% and distant spread is about 72%.

14. Does elective node dissection improve survival rates?

Data by Balch from American and Australian studies indicate that elective node dissections significantly increase actuarial survival rates for patients with primary melanomas of depths between 1.50 and 3.99 mm (intermediate tumors in the level III range). However, a recent report from the Sydney Australia Unit demonstrates no benefit with elective lymph node dissection in truncal and limb melanomas over 1.5 mm in depth. Thus, the subject continues to be controversial. A prospective, randomized trial is underway. For clinically positive nodes without evidence of systemic spread, lymph node dissection is definitely indicated.

15. Can lymph node spread be present without microscopic evidence?

Recent work from the University of South Florida indicates that the presence of tyrosinase messenger RNA (m RNA) indicates metastatic melanoma even without positive microscopic findings. This high-tech method may be useful in the future for determining the need for node dissection or other therapy in patients without apparent melanoma spread.

16. In some truncal primaries, how does a surgeon determine which node-bearing region to dissect? Is there a better method to determine preoperatively if node dissection is indicated?

Lymphoscintography (the injection and scanning of a radioactive material, technetium 99) is used to identify the routes of potential spread of melanoma. The tracer is injected into the skin at the site of the melanoma and lymph node spread is detected by scanning. A blue dye also has been used to determine the spread. The surgeon must search for a sentinel node indicated by blue dye collection in a lymph node nearest the primary tumor. This technique is at times difficult and may be replaced in the future by a hand-held probe (Krag), with which the surgeon locates the sentinel node with minimal invasive surgery. A small incision is made over the hot spot, and the node is removed for histologic study. This method requires special training and equipment and is not yet a routine maneuver.

17. How important is anatomic site in the prognosis of melanoma patients?

Patients with melanoma of the trunk have a poorer prognosis than patients with lesions of the extremities. Melanomas arising in the skin of the upper part of the back, back of the arms, neck, and scalp (once characterized as the ominous BANS [back, arm, neck, scalp] region) have somewhat similar prognoses as lesions in other parts of the body. Stage II lesions with positive regional nodes have a poorer prognosis in the BANS region than in other areas.

18. Do women with melanoma have a better prognosis than men?

For unexplained reasons, survival rates are definitely higher in female patients. This factor has been substantiated in series controlled for variables of age, site, Clark's level, histology, and Breslow's thickness.

19. Does ulceration of a melanoma make a difference in the aggressiveness of the tumor?

According to the Alabama and Sydney data, patients with ulcerated stages I and II melanomas have a 10-year survival rate of 50%, whereas patients with nonulcerated lesions of the same stages have a 10-year survival rate of 78%. Tumor thickness and ulceration are the two most dominant features of aggressive primary melanomas.

20. What is the characteristic of toenail or subungual melanomas?
Most patients with subungual melanomas present quite late; in general, they are also older than patients with other forms of cutaneous melanoma. The lesions are most often on the great toe. Frequently, the observer thinks first of an inflammatory process. Amputation at or proximal to the metatarsophalangeal joint and regional lymph node dissection are advised by most authors. The primary lesions are usually deeply invasive, and lymph nodes are positive in the great major-ity of the cases, either at the time of the original diagnosis or at subsequent follow-up.

21. In the attempt to cure, regional lymph node removal may be indicated. What type of node dissection should be done?
In elective cases (without obvious spread of melanoma) most authors agree that a so-called func-tional dissection should be done, with preservation of vital nerves and vessels. In the neck, this means preservation of the sternocleidomastoid muscle, internal jugular vein, and spinal acces-sory nerve. If obvious metastases are present with vein, nerve, or muscle attachment, sacrifice of these structures may be necessary.

22. Should a primary melanoma of intermediate depth be removed in continuity with the lymph nodes? When is deep groin dissection indicated along with superficial removal of the nodes?
In-continuity removal of primary nodes is carried out if the primary lesion is near a lymph node area. For example, a melanoma of the mid thigh can be excised in continuity with the nodes, whereas a lesion below the knee cannot logically be treated in this fashion. A deep groin dissec-tion is often done if the nodes in the area of the femoral canal are tested by frozen section and found to contain melanoma. This procedure is controversial.

23. How widely should the primary melanoma site be resected? When is a skin graft indi-cated?
Melanoma in situ can be cured with an excisional margin of 0.5 mm, whereas a thin melanoma of < 0.75 mm in depth can be excised with a 1.0-cm margin of normal skin and underlying subcuta-neous tissue (down to the fascia). For thicker lesions, a 2–3-cm margin is required. With evidence of satellite spread around the primary tumor, a much wider excision is usually advised. Skin grafting is used only if the wound edges cannot be approximated. In facial lesions, some compro-mise may be necessary to prevent serious deformity.

24. Does pregnancy affect the outcome of melanoma?
In the past it was believed that pregnancy decreased survival rates in melanoma patients, but more recent studies have indicated no significant alterations in rates of cure. However, in preg-nancy the disease-free interval between treatment of the primary tumor and the first sign of spread is shorter.

25. Is chemotherapy or radiation helpful in the treatment of melanoma?
In the past chemotherapy has been disappointing in patients with disseminated melanoma, al-though short-term responses of 15–25% were seen with the older regimens. More recently, com-binations of Dacarbazine, vinblastine, and tamoxifen have been used with high-dose interleukin-2, This regimen is toxic, but objective response rates have been as high as 56%. In clinical trials biologic agents such as systemic interleukin-2 plus lymphokine-activated killer cells give responses as high as 25%, primarily in skin, nodal disease, and lung metastases. Clinical trials to determine which agents—and in which combinations—provide the most effec-tive therapy are ongoing.

Isolation perfusion is often used in the treatment of local spread of melanoma in an extrem-ity ("in transit" spread). Chemotherapy drugs or biologic preparations (such as interferon or tumor necrosis factor) are circulated through an isolated extremity. This method is highly effective in many cases, although recurrence remains a possibility.

Radiotherapy, once believed to be ineffective in melanoma, has been shown recently to be quite helpful in various clinical settings. The most frequent indication for radiotherapy is palliative treatment of metastatic disease. In recent years, radiotherapy has been reevaluated for curative treatment, either as an adjunct to surgery or as a substitute for surgery in regional approaches. Clinical trials are ongoing. At this time, radiotherapy is seldom used for curative treatment, unless the patient is inoperable for medical reasons.

26. Is amputation ever indicated in the treatment of melanoma?
In selected cases, amputation of locally advanced lesions may be palliative. This guideline applies to huge, fungating masses or masses of satellites that are confined to an extremity and did not respond to isolation perfusion chemotherapy. Occasional cures have been reported.

27. Is it possible to cure a patient with metastatic melanoma in nodes of unknown primary origin?
If metastases are confined to one node-bearing region (after careful ruling out of other metastatic foci), radical dissection should be done. Cures rates as high as 15–20% have been reported.

28. Can serious edema of the lower extremity be prevented after radical groin dissection?
Edema of the lower extremity can be kept to a minimum with the use of tailor-made support stockings immediately after surgery. Some swelling occurs in most patients who undergo radical groin dissection. Care must be taken to prevent infection in the limb, a common complication.

29. How can wound complications be prevented after lymph node dissection?
Healing in the groin area often is delayed after such surgery. It is imperative to institute proper wound drainage. Fluid collections are common. Careful handling of skin flaps is essential to prevent skin slough and delayed healing.

30. After surgery for curable melanoma, what follow-up procedures are indicated?
Besides frequent physical examinations, chest radiographs and liver function tests are important. In patients with poor prognoses, gallium scans may detect isolated metastases in soft tissue and brain before symptoms develop. If metastases are suspected for any reason or if deep nodes have been positive, MRI scans may be used to detect otherwise hidden metastases.

31. Is it possible to cure a patient with a single, isolated distant spread of melanoma?
In a series reported by Overett and Shiu, a survival rate of 33% was achieved in a large series of patients with a single, isolated distant metastasis. Such patients, of course, must be carefully studied to rule out other evidence of spread.

BIBLIOGRAPHY

1. Balch CM: The role of elective lymph node dissection in melanoma: Rationale, results, and controversies. J Clin Oncol 6:163–172, 1988.
2. Balch CM, et al: A comparison of prognostic factors and surgical results in 1,786 patients with localized (stage I) melanoma treated in Alabama, USA and New South Wales, Australia. Ann Surg 196:677–684, 1982.
3. Balch CM, et al: Efficacy of 2.0 cm margins for intermediate thickness melanoma (1–4 mm). Results of multi-institutional randomized surgical trial. Ann Surg 218:202–207, 1993.
4. Coates AS, et al: Elective lymph node dissection in patients with primary melanoma of the trunk and limbs treated at the Sydney Melanoma unit from 1960 to 1991. J Am Coll Surg 180:402–409, 1995.
5. Day CL, et al: Malignant melanoma patients with positive nodes and relatively good prognosis: Microstaging retains prognostic significance in clinical stage I melanoma patients with metastases to regional nodes. Cancer 47:955–962, 1981.
6. Ebskov LD, et al: Major amputation for malignant melanoma: An epidemiological study. J Surg Oncol 52:89–91, 1993.

7. Hayes IM, Thompson JF, Quinn MJ: Malignant melanoma of the toenail apparatus. J Am Coll Surg 180:583–588, 1995.
8. Hilaris BS, Raben M, Calabrese AS, Phillips RF: The value of radiation therapy for distant metastases from malignant melanoma. Cancer 16:765, 1963.
9. Hussussian CF, et al: Germline p16 mutations in familial melanoma. Natl Genetics 8:15–21, 1994.
10. Keilholz U: Chemoimmunotherapy of melanoma. Cancer 75:905–907, 1995.
11. Krag, et al: Minimal-access surgery for staging of malignant melanoma. Arch Surg 130:654–660, 1995.
12. Morton DL, et al: Active specific immunotherapy in malignant melanoma. Semin Surg Oncol 5:420–425, 1989.
13. Overett TK, Shiu MH: Surgical treatment of distant metastatic melanoma. Cancer 56:1222–1230, 1985.
14. Pontikes LA, Temple WJ, et al: Influence of level and depth on recurrence rate in thin melanomas. Am J Surg 165:225–228, 1993.
15. Urin RF: Lymphoscintigraphy in high risk melanoma of the trunk—predicting drainage node groups, defining lymphatic channels and localizing the sentinel node. J Nucl Med 34:1435–1440, 1993.

59. PAROTID TUMORS

William R. Nelson, M.D.

1. How is a parotid tumor diagnosed?
A well-defined mass in the parotid gland as determined by physical examination is a parotid tumor until proved otherwise. Mumps, suppurative parotitis, stone in the parotid duct, and bilateral diffuse parotid enlargement should be excluded.

2. What is the most common location of a parotid tumor?
In the superficial lobe just beneath the lobe of the ear.

3. What is the most common cause of a mass high in the parotid gland in front of the tragus of the ear?
An enlarged parotid lymph node. In older patients, especially those with a history of skin cancer, such a mass must be considered as a site of metastatic cancer until proved otherwise.

4. What is the ratio of malignant to benign tumors of the parotid?
At least 60% of tumors of the parotid are benign.

5. Name the types of benign tumors of the parotid.
Mixed tumor (the term "benign mixed tumor" has been dropped, because such lesions recur locally and may be considered as local types of cancer)
Warthin's tumors
Oxyphilic adenoma
Oncocytoma
Benign lymphoepithelial lesion

6. Name the types of malignant tumors in order of frequency.
Mucoepidermoid carcinoma
Malignant mixed tumor
Acinic cell carcinoma
Adenocarcinoma
Adenoid cystic carcinoma
Epidermoid carcinoma

7. Should parotid tumors be biopsied before surgery?

In the past preoperative biopsy was believed to be rarely indicated. Many surgeons did needle aspiration of tumors that seemed malignant (rapid growth, nerve paralysis, extremely hard masses). In general, moveable, benign-appearing tumors are not biopsied preoperatively. A parotid lobectomy is normally carried out with dissection and preservation of the facial nerve, followed by frozen section of the tumor. If a tumor is found to be malignant preoperatively by needle aspiration biopsy, a complete lobectomy can be performed without violation of the tumor surface (as with wedge biopsy). Lobectomy may be followed with removal of adjacent upper neck nodes. Heller and others have recently advised fine-needle aspiration biopsy in all parotid tumors; in their series, 35% of patients underwent a change in clinical approach after the biopsy report. This procedure must be carried out with great care to prevent facial nerve injury.

8. Do tumors occur in the deep lobe of the parotid? If so, how are they treated?

Deep-lobe tumors are uncommon, because this portion is only about one-fifth of the total parotid substance and lies beneath the nerve. Superficial parotid lobectomy is first performed with dissection and preservation of the nerve, followed by removal of the tumor in the deep-lobe area along with any remaining deep-lobe tissue.

9. Is MR imaging helpful in diagnosing such lesions or in any parotid mass?

MR imaging easily diagnoses parotid lesions, some of which protrude into the oropharynx or oral cavity. It is possible to show infiltration or lack of sharpness in the margins of malignant parotid tumors with MRI. It is not possible otherwise to differentiate between benign and malignant lesions. Deep-lobe tumors, unsuspected preoperatively, are easily diagnosed with MRI. Routine MR imaging is not necessary in the usual moveable, apparently superficial parotid tumor.

10. What is the significance of partial or complete nerve paralysis in the presence of a parotid tumor?

If the onset of paralysis is gradual (as opposed to the rapidly developing Bell's palsy) in patients with a parotid tumor, the diagnosis is cancer until proved otherwise. In rare instances, benign tumors have been known to cause nerve weakness.

11. Is it possible to cure patients that present with nerve paralysis from cancer of the parotid?

The outlook is poor, but with radical parotidectomy (including nerve resection) and postoperative radiotherapy cures have been obtained.

12. Do parotid tumors occur in children?

Parotid tumors are uncommon in children, but the types of tumors are quite similar to those seen in adults.

13. Has radiation been known to cause parotid tumors?

Major and minor gland neoplasms have developed in patients previously treated for benign conditions of the face and neck. There is no proof that inflammatory disease of the parotid or stones in the parotid duct have produced tumors. One recent report indicates that smoking may play a part in the production of Warthin's tumors.

14. Should all apparently benign tumors of the parotid be removed?

The only exceptions to removal are longstanding parotid lesions of apparently benign type in aged or infirm patients. Aspiration biopsies should be performed to confirm the diagnosis of mixed tumors in situations in which surgery would be life-threatening.

15. In HIV-positive patients, what is the significance of a recent parotid enlargement or mass?

In HIV-positive patients the most likely diagnosis is a benign lymphoepithelial lesion. If needle biopsy confirms this diagnosis, surgery is not indicated because of the benign nature of this process in the face of eventual AIDS development. If a cyst is present, fluid aspiration decreases or temporarily eliminates the swelling.

16. If cancer is found in the parotid lobectomy specimen, what is the next step in treatment?
In high-grade cancers, adjacent nodes of the upper neck are removed along with the total parotid gland, but the entire nerve is not removed unless there is obvious tumor involvement.

17. When is nerve grafting used in the treatment of parotid cancer?
If a branch or the entire nerve is involved, resection must be performed, and frozen sections should be obtained from the nerve ends. A nerve graft of the greater auricular nerve from the opposite side of the neck is usually preferred. The graft is normally sutured in place with magnification.

18. Is it possible to remove a parotid tumor without dissecting the facial nerve?
Nerve dissection should be carried out in nearly all cases. For a known Warthin's tumor (which usually develops in the lower part of the parotid), careful local excision has been advocated by some authors; local recurrence is uncommon. Mixed tumors arising in rare anterior locations are commonly excised locally. Recurrence and/or peripheral nerve injury is possible.

19. What is the most common type of nerve injury in parotidectomy?
The most commonly injured nerve is the ramus marginalis mandibularis, the lowest branch of the nerve that innervates the depressor muscles of the lower lip. This nerve must be carefully preserved during the operation, and, if it is not injured, weakness of the lower lip (a common complication even of careful surgery) resolves within 4–6 weeks.

20. Is bone resection indicated in the treatment of malignant parotid tumors?
Bone resection is rarely necessary and should be carried out only in the presence of deep recurrence of cancer or in patients in whom cancer has invaded the mandible.

21. Is it possible to reduce the incidence of temporary postparotidectomy facial nerve palsy when the nerve has been preserved?
If great care is taken with nerve dissection, postoperative palsy should be minimal. Coagulation of bleeding vessels near the nerve, careless suctioning around the nerve itself, and unnecessary pulling and stretching of the nerve may result in several weeks of distressing palsy.

22. Is it possible to prevent anesthesia of the ear lobe after parotid surgery?
The greater auricular nerve can be preserved in small benign tumors if the branches are uninvolved and not adherent to the tumor itself.

23. When is radiation therapy indicated after treatment of a parotid cancer?
In all except the very low-grade cancers, many authors state that radiation therapy should be used after total parotidectomy and removal of adjacent upper neck nodes. A radical neck dissection is not done unless there is evidence of nodal involvement. At the M.D. Anderson Hospital, aggressive surgery in the treatment of parotid cancer, including upper neck node removal followed by radiotherapy, has been shown to improve cure rates.

24. What is the cure rate in cancer of the parotid gland?
In low-grade cancers, the cure rate may approach 80–90%, but in one overall series of cancers, the 5-, 10-, and 15-year cure rates were approximately 62%, 54%, and 47%, respectively.

25. Which is more important in adenoid cystic carcinoma—stage of the tumor or histologic grade?
Spiro and Huvos have shown that stage of the tumor is more important than the grade. Early-stage tumors, even in the face of high-grade histology, were found to have a relatively good prognosis.

26. Does salivary fistula occur after superficial parotid lobectomy?
If all except a few fragments of the superficial lobe are removed cleanly, fistulas should not occur. The deep lobe itself is rarely, if ever, the source of salivary leak after removal of the superficial lobe.

27. What is Frey's syndrome?
Also called gustatory sweating, Frey's syndrome occurs with eating in 30% or more of patients who have had parotidectomy. Regeneration of parasympathetic fibers within the auriculotemporal nerve is thought to result in stimulation of the sweat glands.

28. Is chemotherapy beneficial in patients who have had radical removal of cancers of the parotid plus radiotherapy?
Chemotherapy has not had a great impact on the cure rate. Studies from the M.D. Anderson Hospital have shown some definite chemotherapeutic effect but generally it is of short duration. Pulmonary lesions regressed and occasionally the response was complete. Combination chemotherapy with multidrug regimes has shown temporary responses.

29. Do mixed tumors turn into true cancers?
Most authors believe that truly malignant mixed tumors can develop from the benign type after many years, but this phenomenon is certainly not common. Many advanced mixed tumors are benign, even though they may have achieved incredible growth. On the other hand, the incidence of malignant mixed tumors is quite a bit higher in older patients than in patients under 60. This observation, along with studies in the pathology laboratory, give credence to the theory that carcinomatous transformation occurs in unusual settings. Beahrs of the Mayo Clinic has documented this phenomenon.

30. Can facial function return spontaneously after removal of the facial nerve?
Although rare, spontaneous return of facial function has been well recorded in isolated cases. The exact mechanism has not been determined, but a takeover by fifth-nerve fibers and regrowth of facial nerve fibers are possibilities. Martin and Helsper, who discuss this phenomenon in great detail, believe that fifth-nerve takeover is the most likely mechanism. One patient with spontaneous return underwent injection of the fifth nerve for neuralgia. Temporary, rapid loss of facial function resulted.

31. Is a tumor suppressor gene involved with parotid gland carcinoma?
One of the best known tumor suppressor genes is p53. Parotid cancers showing a moderate or high degree of expression of p53 are usually more advanced and larger than those with no expression. Tumors with moderate or high expression of p53 were more often involved with regional and distant metastases.

BIBLIOGRAPHY

1. Beahrs OH, Woolner LB, Kirklin JW, Devine KD: Carcinomatous transformation of mixed tumors of the parotid gland. Arch Surg 75:605, 1957.
2. Blevins NH, Jackler RK, Kaplan MJ, Oles R: Facial paralysis due to benign parotid tumors. Arch Otol/Head Neck Surg 118:427–430, 1992.
3. Brown JS, Ord RA: Preserving the greater auricular nerve in parotid surgery. Br J Oral Maxillofac Surg 27:459–466, 1989.
4. Frankenthaler RA, Byers RM, Luna MA, et al: Predicting occult lymph node metastasis in parotid cancer. Arch Otol/Head Neck Surg 119:517–520, 1993.
5. Freiling NJ: Malignant parotid tumors: Clinical use of MR imaging and histologic correlation. Radiology 185:691–696, 1992.
6. Gallo O, et al: p53 Oncoprotein expression in parotid gland carcinoma is associated with clinical outcome. Cancer 75:2037–2044, 1995.
7. Guillamondegui OM, Byers RM, Luna MA, et al: Aggressive surgery in treatment for parotid cancer: The role of adjunctive postoperative radiotherapy. Am J Roentgenol Radiat Ther Nucl Med 123:49–54, 1975.

8. Hanna DC, Gaisford JC, Richardson GS, Bindra RN: Tumors of the deep lobe of the parotid gland. Am J Surg 116:524–527, 1968.
9. Heller KS, Dubner S, Chess Q, Attie JN: Value of fine needle aspiration biopsy of salivary gland masses in clinical decision-making. Am J Surg 164:667–670, 1992.
10. Kotwall CA: Smoking as an etiological factor in the development of Warthin's tumor of the parotid gland. Am J Surg 164:646–647, 1992.
11. Martin H, Helsper JT: Supplementary report on spontaneous return of function following surgical section or excision of the seventh cranial nerve in the surgery of parotid tumors. Ann Surg 151:538–541, 1960.
12. Shaha AR, et al: Benign lymphoepithelial lesions of the parotid. Am J Surg 166:403–406, 1993.
13. Skibba JL, Hurley JD, Ravelo P: Complete response of a metastatic adenoid cystic carcinoma of the parotid to chemotherapy. Cancer 47:2543–2548, 1981.
14. Spiro IJ, Wang CC, Montgomery WW: Cancer of the parotid gland, analysis of treatment results and patterns of failure after combined surgery and radiation therapy. Cancer 71:2699–2705, 1993.
15. Spiro RH, Huvos AG: Stage means more than grade in adenoid cystic carcinoma. Am J Surg 164:623–628, 1992.

60. DEBULKING (CYTOREDUCTIVE) SURGERY

John A. Ridge, M.D., Ph.D.

1. What is debulking surgery?
Debulking is performed to enhance survival or to improve quality of life through incomplete surgical removal of cancer, even though the surgeon recognizes that tumor is left behind.

2. Is debulking to achieve cure contrary to Halsted's principles?
Yes. But Halsted lived in different times.

3. Does it make sense to put a patient through a major operation if all of the tumor cannot be removed?
Certainly. Operations are often performed to alleviate the mechanical symptoms of cancer (such as bleeding or obstruction), thus improving quality of life (palliation), even if the cancer is incurable. In addition, some patients live longer after debulking (or cytoreductive) surgery.

4. Does debulking surgery have a role in managing most types of cancer?
No. However, in special cases it has considerable benefit.

5. What is cytoreductive surgery?
Cytoreductive procedures are designed to decrease tumor burden so that the planned addition of radiation therapy, chemotherapy, or biologic modifiers will prolong survival.

6. Is cytoreductive surgery just a fancy way of saying debulking?
Yes.

7. Do some patients benefit from debulking surgery alone?
Patients with advanced functioning endocrine tumors (whose hormone secretion makes them ill) benefit from reduction in tumor mass alone. This principle makes sense, because smaller amounts of tumor should secrete less hormone and the patient feels better. Such cancers are uncommon, but patients may enjoy dramatic benefits. Debulking benefits selected patients with insulinoma, vasoactive intestinal polypeptide-secreting tumor, glucagonoma, somatostatinoma, carcinoid tumor, adrenal cancer, pheochromocytoma, and medullary thyroid cancer. Although not commonly considered in such terms, operations for parathyroid hyperplasia represent debulking surgery.

8. Which patients may be expected to benefit from cytoreductive surgery?
The better the chemotherapy and radiation therapy, the greater the role of cytoreductive surgery. If the surgeon can reduce the total tumor mass to a manageable size, oncologists can clean up the remaining metastases of some types of cancer. Fancy specialists call this approach **multimodality therapy of neoplastic disease**.

9. Why do chemotherapy and radiation therapy not work alone?
Experiments suggest that the proportion of rapidly proliferating cells is increased by cytoreduction. Rapidly dividing cells are most sensitive to radiation and current chemotherapeutic agents. As the tumor volume increases, growth slows. Hence, reduction in tumor burden should lead to enhanced sensitivity to treatment. In addition, cytotoxic chemotherapy seems to kill a constant proportion of tumor cells with each course. Because treatment side effects and mutations leading to drug resistance limit the use of chemotherapeutic drugs, treating smaller initial numbers of cancer cells should increase the chance of cure.

10. So if nonsurgical treatments improve, cytoreductive surgery may not be needed?
Exactly. In the past Burkitt's lymphoma and pediatric tumors were often treated with cytoreductive surgery. This approach does not seem to be necessary with current chemotherapy and radiation treatment.

11. How is cytoreductive surgery most commonly used today?
Cytoreductive surgery is standard care in the management of ovarian cancer and glioblastoma. Operations in patients with advanced ovarian cancer are followed by cytotoxic chemotherapy. With current chemotherapy, patients whose unresectable tumor masses are reduced to < 2 cm in diameter live longer than patients whose tumor bulk cannot be reduced to this extent. Surgical removal of residual metastatic disease after chemotherapy treatment of nonseminomatous testis tumors cures a gratifying percentage of patients.

12. What is second-look surgery for ovarian cancer?
Second-look operations are procedures that follow chemotherapy or radiation treatments to evaluate response and to remove any residual tumor. Although often performed for ovarian cancer in the past, the benefit has been uncertain. A recent well-designed, randomized clinical trial demonstrated a survival advantage for patients who underwent second-look surgical cytoreduction after three courses of chemotherapy followed by three additional chemotherapy courses. Such patients lived longer than women who received six courses of chemotherapy without second-look surgery.

13. When chemotherapy improves, cytoreductive surgery may become unnecessary. Could improvements in surgery or other treatments increase the role for cytoreductive surgery?
Probably. **Peritoneal carcinomatosis** from colorectal cancer was once thought to be incurable, and most patients died within weeks. It is still a serious problem, but some patients have derived significant benefit and long-term survival after cytoreductive surgery and intraperitoneal chemotherapy. **Anaplastic thyroid cancer** can seldom be cured, and most patients succumb to local tracheal invasion and suffocation. The combination of chemotherapy, radiation treatment, and subsequent debulking surgery may improve local control and survival.

14. Are there other forms of debulking surgery for cancer?
Patients with metastatic thyroid cancer offer a cytoreductive opportunity. The use of radioactive iodine to treat distant disease is frustrated by the presence of the normal thyroid gland, which steals essentially all of the radioactive iodine from the metastasis. Removal of the normal thyroid gland thus facilitates treatment of the cancer by reducing the burden of iodine-avid tissue and allowing higher doses to reach the cancer. Similarly, resectable metastatic thyroid cancer is often removed before radioactive iodine treatment.

CONTROVERSIES

15. Do patients with ovarian cancer whose postoperative tumor bulk is small live longer because most of their tumor has been removed or because they have less aggressive cancers? If a surgeon leaves "some" cancer behind, does it make any difference how much?
No prospective trials have been performed to compare cytoreductive surgery followed by chemotherapy with chemotherapy alone for patients with advanced ovarian cancer. Patients with only a small amount of postoperative tumor clearly live longer than patients with bulky residual neoplastic disease. This may be due to individual tumor biology, because patients whose residual tumor is initially 1 cm in diameter live longer than patients whose remaining cancer is reduced to 1 cm by surgery. Perhaps the prolonged survival with low tumor burden reflects some diminished virulence of ovarian cancer that does not produce bulky unresectable metastases. However, the debulking operation must play a role in survival, because patients whose initial exploration is conducted by a trained oncologist live longer than those treated by generalist gynecologists.

BIBLIOGRAPHY

1. Grant CS: Surgical management of malignant islet cell tumors. World J Surg 17:498–503, 1993.
2. Hoskins WJ: Epithelial ovarian carcinoma: Principles of primary surgery. Gynecol Oncol 55:S91–S96, 1994.
3. Kulkarni RP, Reynolds KW, Newlands ES, et al: Cytoreductive surgery in disseminated nonseminomatous germ cell tumours of testis. Br J Surg 78:226–229, 1991.
4. Ozols RF: Treatment of ovarian cancer: Current status. Semin Oncol 21(Suppl 2):1–9, 1994.
5. Sugarbaker PH, Jablonski KA: Prognostic features of 51 colorectal and 130 appendiceal cancer patients with peritoneal carcinomatosis treated by cytoreductive surgery and intraperitoneal chemotherapy. Ann Surg 221:124–132, 1995.
6. Tennvall J, Lundell G, Hallquist A, et al: Combined doxorubicin, hyperfractionated radiotherapy, and surgery in anaplastic thyroid carcinoma. Cancer 74:1348–1354, 1994.
7. Van der Burg MEL, van Lent M, Buyse M, et al: The effect of debulking surgery after induction chemotherapy on the prognosis in advanced epithelial cancer. N Engl J Med 332:629–634, 1995.
8. Wong RJ, DeCosse JJ: Cytoreductive surgery. Surg Gynecol Obstet 170:276–281, 1990.
9. Zogakis TG, Norton JA: Palliative operations for patients with unresectable endocrine neoplasia. Surg Clin North Am 75:525–538, 1995.

61. HODGKIN'S DISEASE AND THE MALIGNANT LYMPHOMAS

Christina A. Finlayson, M.D.

1. What is the differential diagnosis of lymphadenopathy?
It is common for cervical, axillary, or inguinal lymphadenopathy to be identified during physical examination. The significance of this finding depends on the character of the lymph nodes and associated symptoms. Infection, autoimmune disease, and malignancy should be considered in the differential diagnosis.

2. What historical information helps to direct the diagnostic evaluation of lymphadenopathy?
A focused evaluation with a comprehensive history. It is unusual for a patient over the age of 40 to have nonspecific lymphadenopathy; in fact, over 70% of enlarged cervical lymph nodes in this age group are malignant. Patients under 40 are more likely to have a nonspecific or infectious etiology, although the mean age of onset of Hodgkin's lymphoma is 32 years.

Duration of symptoms can provide an indication of the cause of the adenopathy. Recent awareness of an enlarged lymph node is more suggestive of infection; however, an enlarging lymph node may undergo internal hemorrhage with rapid increase in size. Travel and occupation history, exposure to pets, geographic area of residence, and sexual history can provide clues to infectious agents. A history of smoking is associated with lung, upper gastrointestinal, and head and neck malignancy.

Systemic symptoms, including fever, weight loss, night sweats and pruritus, are present in approximately 30% of patients with Hodgkin's and 10% of patients with non-Hodgkin's lymphoma. Unfortunately, such symptoms are associated with a wide variety of diseases and, therefore, are neither sensitive nor specific.

3. A 25-year-old man presents for evaluation of a 1-cm, soft inguinal lymph node that has been present for 1 month. How should the diagnostic evaluation proceed?

A comprehensive history provides direction for further diagnostic maneuvers. The physical examination must draw particular attention to all draining lymph node basins: cervical, submandibular, auricular, occipital, supraclavicular, axillary, epitrochlear, inguinal, and popliteal. Supraclavicular adenopathy is virtually always associated with malignant or granulomatous disease. Peripheral adenopathy in the groin and axilla often is a response to trauma, frequently occult. The limb should be thoroughly examined.

The size and consistency of an enlarged lymph node helps to discriminate malignant or granulomatous lymphadenopathy from other causes. A lymph node less than 1 cm in size is usually from a nonspecific and nonsignificant cause. Nodes greater than 2 cm are often malignant or granulomatous. Soft lymph nodes do not indicate a particular diagnosis; however, hard nodes are typical of metastatic malignancy.

In this patient, if historical or physical findings do not lead to a specific diagnosis, a period of observation is appropriate. Follow-up examination in 1 month is required, and, if regression has not occurred, biopsy is indicated.

4. A 48-year-old woman presents with a 3-cm, firm lymph node in the left supraclavicular area. How may her evaluation differ from that of the previous patient?

The age of the patient and the size, consistency, and location of the lymph node virtually exclude the possibility that the node can be safely ignored. If historical or physical findings do not indicate an infectious etiology, malignancy must be ruled out. Both Hodgkin's and non-Hodgkin's lymphomas as well as metastatic disease from a primary tumor of the abdomen, genitals, lung, or breast may initially present with supraclavicular adenopathy. Primary tumors of the head and neck rarely metastasize to this location but tend to spread first to cervical lymph nodes. A period of observation is not appropriate; an early diagnosis with fine-needle aspiration or open biopsy is indicated.

5. Should antibiotics be used during a watch-and-wait period when a specific site of infection has not been identified?

Lymphadenopathy is a common response to infection. Rarely, however, are lymph nodes themselves the target of invading organisms. When infected nodes are present, other signs of inflammation, including warmth, erythema, and pain, accompany the swelling. A careful search for infection should be conducted during the history and physical examination. If a potential bacterial infection is identified, cultures should be taken and appropriate antibiotics instituted. If such a process is not identified, the empiric use of shot-in-the-dark antibiotics is without therapeutic or diagnostic benefit.

6. Can fine-needle aspiration be used if lymphoma is in the differential diagnosis?

Fine needle-aspiration (FNA) is an established diagnostic tool in several clinical situations, including the evaluation of breast, thyroid, and metastatic disease. It is easy to do, and benefits include minimal patient invasion, rapid diagnosis, and low expense. The overall reliability in any given institution depends on the interest and experience of the pathologist; however, many reports indicate an accuracy greater than 90%. Definitive diagnosis of lymphoma by cellular aspirate is much less reliable. The pathologist looks for malignant cells in a background of normal lymphocytes and often requires intact lymph node architecture to reach a diagnosis. The immunohistochemistry involved in typing lymphoma requires a relatively large quantity of tissue that cannot be retrieved by aspiration alone. However, when a mass is being evaluated and the differential is broad, as in the example given above, an FNA often establishes the diagnosis. If a positive identification is not made or if the cytology is suspicious for lymphoma but tissue is inadequate for typing, the patient must proceed to open biopsy.

7. What particular considerations must a surgeon keep in mind when performing a lymph node biopsy for suspected lymphoma?
The primary role of the surgeon in most cases of lymphoma is to diagnose and stage the disease. The cervical lymph nodes are usually the site of involvement (65–80%), followed by axillary (10–15%), and inguinal (6–12%) lymph nodes. A primary node involved with tumor is often accompanied by smaller reactive lymph nodes. Therefore, it is important to select the largest, most suspicious lymph node for biopsy. Because the architecture of the lymph node is important for the pathologist, it should be removed in one piece. Care should be taken during the dissection to avoid crushing, clamping, or cauterizing the tissue. The specimen must go to the laboratory fresh, preferably wrapped in saline-soaked gauze. The cellular architecture should not be distorted by placing the node in water or formalin. Careful communication between the surgeon and the pathologist before and during the procedure can avert most misadventures. A frozen section can determine if an adequate tissue sample has been obtained.

8. What are the clinical differences between Hodgkin's and non-Hodgkin's lymphoma?
    Hodgkin's lymphoma usually presents with either a neck mass or a mediastinal mass. It most commonly arises in lymph nodes and rarely involves extranodal sites initially. It tends to spread contiguously to adjacent nodal stations rather than skipping to more distant sites. Most patients present with early stage I or II disease. It is unusual to have epitrochlear, popliteal, or mesenteric nodal involvement. The age distribution is bimodal with an early peak in the 20s and a later peak in the 60s.
    Non-Hodgkin's lymphomas originate predominantly from lymphocytes and are also referred to as lymphocytic lymphomas. The incidence of these tumors has increased significantly over the past 20 years. Some of the increase has been attributed to association with AIDS, but this association does not account for all of the observed increase. In contrast to Hodgkin's lymphoma, the non-Hodgkin's lymphomas are often extranodal and spread noncontiguously. They rarely present as localized disease; bone marrow and liver involvement are common. It is more common for non-Hodgkin's lymphoma to involve the epitrochlear, popliteal, and mesenteric lymph nodes as well as Waldeyer's ring. It accounts for almost all gastrointestinal lymphomas. Most patients present with advanced-stage disease.

9. What is Waldeyer's ring?
The mucosa of the posterior oropharynx covers a bed of lymphatic tissue and nodules, some of which aggregate to form the palatine, lingual, pharyngeal, and tubal tonsils. When viewed from the posterior aspect, they form a ring around the pharyngeal wall—hence the name Waldeyer's lymphatic ring. It may be the site of both primary or metastatic tumor.

10. How is lymphoma staged?
A careful history and physical examination elicit systemic symptoms and identify involved lymph node stations. Laboratory evaluation includes complete blood count, creatinine, liver function tests, erythrocyte sedimentation rate, lactate dehydrogenase, and alkaline phosphatase. If a chest radiograph is abnormal, a CT scan of the chest is required. A CT scan of the abdomen and pelvis and bilateral bone marrow aspiration and biopsy are required in all cases. The use of lymphangiography and staging laparotomy is controversial and should be limited to select situations.

11. Why are tumors staged?

The foundation of communication is a standard nomenclature that has consistent meaning to all participants. Tumors are staged on the basis of extent of disease at the time of clinical presentation. Under the TNM method of staging, the size of the tumor, the presence of nodal metastasis, and the presence of distant metastasis are used to quantify tumor burden. This system allowed patients with a similar tumor burden to be evaluated together to determine the natural history of cancer progression. Staging allowed clinicians to predict prognosis for groups of patients with similar disease.

Once the natural history of cancer was defined, the outcome of therapeutic trials could be evaluated. Because patients with a lower tumor burden are expected to do better than patients with advanced disease, it is important not to place them in the same category when evaluating response to therapy. The staging system allows researchers to communicate results with standard nomenclature.

It is unusual for all stages of a given tumor to be treated the same way. Therefore, staging an individual patient directs a clinician to the appropriate therapy.

For a staging system to have value, therefore, it must be designed to predict prognosis for a group of patients with similar tumor burden, to facilitate communication between researchers and clinicians, and to assist in the selection of the appropriate treatment plan for individual patients with cancer.

12. What staging system is used for lymphoma?

Because lymphoma is a malignancy of the lymph nodes and the initial site of disease is rarely identifiable, the TNM staging system does not apply. Staging, therefore, is based on the distribution of the disease and systemic symptoms. Both Hodgkin's and low-grade non-Hodgkin's lymphoma use the same staging system (Ann Arbor Staging Classification):

Stage I   Involvement of a single lymph node region or localized involvement of a single extralymphatic organ or site.

Stage II   Involvement of two or more lymph node regions on the same side of the diaphragm.
Localized involvement of a single extralymphatic organ or site and its regional lymph nodes.

Stage III   Involvement of lymph node regions on both sides of the diaphragm, including localized involvement of an associated extralymphatic organ or site, involvement of the spleen, or both.

Stage IV   Disseminated involvement of one or more extralymphatic organs (including bone marrow) with or without associated lymph node involvement.
Isolated extralymphatic organ involvement with distant nodal involvement.

The subscript $_E$ is used to denote extralymphatic organ involvement, and the subscript $_S$ is used to denote splenic involvement in stage III or IV disease. They may be combined with involvement of both an extralymphatic site and the spleen.

Each stage is subdivided into either A or B, depending on the presentation of associated systemic symptoms. A patient who presents without systemic symptoms is classified as A. A patient who presents with unexplained weight loss of more than 10% in the 6 months preceding diagnosis, unexplained fever with temperatures above 38°C, or drenching night sweats is classified as B; these are referred to as B-symptoms. Pruritus is often included in the description of B-symptoms but does not qualify for B classification when it is the only presenting symptom.

For example, a 24-year-old man who presents with an asymptomatic mass in the neck, no systemic symptoms, and no other sites of disease on staging work-up is classified as stage IA. A 70-year-old woman who presents with a localized small bowel lymphoma (low grade) that involves the mesenteric (regional) lymph nodes and has had a temperature of 38.5°C nightly over the past 6 weeks would be classified as stage II_EB.

Intermediate- and high-grade non-Hodgkin's lymphomas are staged according to the National Cancer Institute Modified Staging System:

Stage I   Localized nodal or extranodal disease.

Stage II   Two or more nodal sites of disease or one localized extranodal site plus draining lymph nodes with no poor prognostic features.

Stage III   Stage II plus one or more poor prognostic features.

Poor prognostic features include (1) performance status < Karnofsky 70%, (2) B-symptoms, (3) any mass > 10 cm in diameter, (4) serum lactate dehydrogenase > 500, or (5) three or more extranodal sites of disease.

13. What is the difference between clinical and pathologic staging?

An initial diagnosis of lymphoma cannot rely solely on history, physical examination, or radiographs; it requires a biopsy that confirms pathologically the presence of tumor cells. Staging, however, can be done clinically or pathologically. Clinical staging is based on history, physical examination, and radiographic evaluation. Abnormal lymph nodes identified by abdominal CT scan or lymphangiography imply clinical subdiaphragmatic disease. Pathologic staging requires the histologic evaluation of all potentially involved tissues. To stage pathologically abnormal lymph nodes identified by abdominal CT scan or lymphangiography, a staging laparotomy with biopsies is required. To identify the method of staging, a lower-case c for clinical staging or lower-case p for pathologic staging precedes the staging nomenclature. For example, cIII indicates a tumor staged clinically with abnormal lymph nodes identified by abdominal CT scan or lymphangiography. If a staging laparotomy was performed and involved lymph nodes were identified by biopsy and pathologic confirmation, the tumor is classified as stage pIII.

14. What are the indications for staging laparotomy?

A laparotomy for Hodgkin's lymphoma was developed to define the presence and extent of tumor in the abdomen for accurate staging and subsequent coordination of therapy. It should be performed only when the results may change the clinical stage and when a change in stage will alter the planned treatment. Pathologic staging of surgically removed tissue is more accurate than clinical staging. In the Stanford experience, 43% of patients had a change in stage after laparotomy. Of patients in clinical stage (CS) I and II, approximately 30% are upstaged to pathologic stage III or IV disease after surgery. Conversely, 10–20% of patients with clinical stage III or IV disease are downstaged. In some subgroups of patients, however, the risk of subdiaphragmatic disease is so low (< 10%) that staging laparotomy rarely adds information and is not indicated. Examples include all CS IA patients with a high neck presentation, lymphocyte-predominant histology, or disease confined to the mediastinum.

Whether or not a change in stage results in a change in therapy depends on the treatment philosophy of the attending medical oncologist. At one institution, 22% of CS IIIB–IVB patients were downstaged by staging laparotomy, but nearly 100% received chemotherapy as part of the initial treatment. Therefore, treatment proceeded regardless of the surgical results.

Further obscuring the role of staging laparotomy in treating Hodgkin's disease is its demonstrated lack of effect on survival because of the highly effective salvage chemotherapy for patients who relapse. Evidence suggests, however, that patients staged surgically have a lower incidence of recurrence and, therefore, are less likely to require a second course of treatment. Thus, it is important that the surgeon have a close working relationship with the medical oncologist so that laparotomy can be used appropriately.

Staging laparotomy is not performed for non-Hodgkin's lymphoma.

15. What is a staging laparotomy?

A midline incision is used to enter and explore the abdomen, with particular attention to lymph node-bearing areas. Abnormal lymph nodes are sampled. Splenectomy is performed first, followed by wedge and core biopsies of each lobe of the liver. Lymph nodes are obtained from the celiac, mesenteric, portal, paraaortic, and paracaval areas. In premenopausal women, an oophoropexy is performed. This procedure secures the ovaries behind the uterus and preserves fertility in approximately one-half of women who require pelvic radiation. When the abdomen is closed, repeat bone marrow biopsies are done bilaterally.

16. How is Hodgkin's lymphoma treated?
Early stage disease (stage I, II and IIIA) may be treated with radiation alone whereas more advanced disease (stage IIIB and IV) may be treated with combined chemotherapy with different regimens using from four to eight different agents. The most popular combinations include four or more of the following: nitrogen mustard, vincristine, procarbazine, prednisone (MOPP), doxorubicin, bleomycin, vinblastine, and dacarbazine (ABVD). Some centers are utilizing combined modality treatment with radiation and chemotherapy.

17. What is the Working Formulation for non-Hodgkin's lymphoma?
Non-Hodgkin's lymphoma is a broad category encompassing any lymphoma that is not Hodgkin's lymphoma. It includes many diverse histologic patterns, each with its own natural history and prognosis. Early attempts to classify these subtypes resulted in six separate classification schemes. The Working Formulation was created to standardize the nomenclature for non-Hodgkin's lymphomas. It categorizes each cytologic description into three general categories: low-grade, intermediate-grade, and high-grade. Lymphomas in the same category have a similar natural history, treatment plan, and prognosis.

18. How does the natural history for each category of non-Hodgkin's lymphoma differ?
Histologic classification is the primary determinant for the natural history and, therefore, the treatment of patient's with non-Hodgkin's lymphoma. Low-grade lymphomas tend to be indolent and slow-growing, often waxing and waning in symptoms over a long period. Aggressive lymphomas, which include the intermediate- and high-grade lymphomas, progress rapidly and may be fatal in a short period. Ironically, chemotherapy has had the most success in the intermediate and aggressive subtype. Whereas the rare patient with a localized low-grade lymphoma may be cured with radiotherapy, more extensive disease is rarely eradicated with chemotherapy, although the median survival is still measured in years because of the indolent nature of the disease. Intermediate-grade lymphomas often respond to standard combination chemotherapy. Aggressive lymphoma, when treated promptly and aggressively with combination chemotherapy, has a 70–80% complete response rate and an approximately 50% chance of long-term survival.

19. Does surgery have a role in the treatment of lymphoma?
Localized non-Hodgkin's lymphoma of the gastrointestinal tract most commonly arises from the stomach. It originates in the lymphoid tissue of the submucosa. Surgery has been the mainstay of treatment, and complete resection of early stage disease is considered curative. More advanced disease may benefit from adjuvant radiation and chemotherapy.

Lymphoma at other locations within the gastrointestinal tract often presents as a surgical emergency. The diagnosis is often made at the time of the operation, and attention is focused on dealing with the situation at hand, whether it be perforation, obstruction, or hemorrhage. The primary tumor should be resected if the disease is localized and can be removed safely.

BIBLIOGRAPHY
1. DeVita V Jr, Hellman S, Rosenberg S: Cancer: Principles and Practice of Oncology, 4th ed. Philadelphia. J.B. Lippincott, 1993, pp 1819–1927.
2. Fleming I (ed): The surgeon and malignant lymphoma. Surg Oncol Clin North Am 2:1993.
3. Mauch P, Larson D, Osteen R, et al: Prognostic factors for positive surgical staging in patients with Hodgkin's disease. J Clin Oncol 8:257–265, 1990.
4. Pangalis G, Vassilakopoulos T, Boussiotis V, Fessas P: Clinical approach to lymphadenopathy. Semin Oncol 20:570–582, 1993.
5. Pilotti S, Di Palma S, Alasio L, et al: Diagnostic assessment of enlarged superficial lymph nodes by fine needle aspiration. Acta Cytol 37:853–866, 1993.
6. Suhrland M, Wieczorek R: Fine needle aspiration biopsy in the diagnosis of lymphoma. Cancer Invest 91:61–68, 1991.
7. Taylor M, Kaplan H, Nelsen T: Staging laparotomy with splenectomy for Hodgkin's disease: The Stanford experience. World J Surg 9:449–460, 1985.

62. NECK MASSES

Nathan Pearlman, M.D.

1. A 21-year-old woman presents with a 3–4 cm mass below the angle of the mandible and slightly anterior to the sternomastoid muscle. What is a reasonable differential diagnosis?

Tuberculosis

Infectious mononucleosis

Lymphoma

Metastatic carcinoma

Tumor of the submaxillary or parotid gland

Carotid body tumor

Branchial cleft cyst

Reactive lymphadenopathy

2. Metastatic neck cancer in a 21 year old?
Yes. Thyroid cancer, tongue cancer, and nasopharyngeal cancer are infrequent but far from rare in young patients.

3. The differential diagnosis is a long list. Is there any way to narrow it?
Inflammatory nodes, most of which are involved with mononucleosis, tend to be soft, less than 3 cm in diameter, bilateral, and tender. There is also usually a history or signs of systemic illness. Metastatic or lymphomatous neck nodes, in contrast, tend to be greater than 3–4 cm, unilateral, and nontender; in many patients, they are the only sign of disease. Nodes involved by lymphoma are generally soft, with the consistency of the submaxillary gland, whereas nodes harboring carcinoma are relatively hard, with a consistency more like that of the thyroid. Parotid tumors may be soft or hard but tend to have an indistinct upper border merging with the body of the parotid gland. Tumors of the submaxillary gland generally occupy the same position as that of the contralateral gland and are often rubbery in consistency. Carotid body tumors are also rubbery but usually tender and cannot be separated from the carotid pulse. Unfortunately, tuberculous nodes share many of these characteristics and may be difficult to distinguish from a neoplasm in early-stage disease. Branchial cleft cysts, on the other hand, rarely present in patients older than 21 years of age, have often been present for long periods of time, and transilluminate.

4. Beyond a detailed history and examination of the neck mass, what else should be done at this time?
In 90% of cases, digital and visual evaluation of the face, contralateral neck, scalp, thyroid and parotid glands, oral cavity, pharynx, and larynx reveals the primary tumor or narrows the list of possibilities and obviates the need for an expensive, shotgun approach to diagnosis.

5. Most physicians acknowledge the eventual need for such an examination but feel awkward trying to use a mirror to examine the pharynx or larynx. Few have a flexible endoscope. Instead, they immediately carry out an open biopsy of the node/mass. What is wrong with this approach?
Open biopsy of a mass or enlarged neck node, as the initial diagnostic maneuver, unduly complicates further management if a malignancy is found. If lymphoma is present but not suspected, the node may be mishandled when sent to pathology, and chances for an accurate diagnosis are lost. The inflammation and fibrosis surrounding the biopsy site may be difficult to distinguish from tumor on CT or MRI scan; on occasion, the result is inaccurate staging and inappropriate treatment. The scar tissue also may resemble cancer at subsequent surgery (tumor removal, neck dissection), leading to a larger operation and more complications. A much better choice for histologic diagnosis at this stage is fine-needle aspiration (FNA) of the mass. This procedure is 85–95% accurate and avoids the problems inherent in open biopsy.

6. A complete head and neck examination reveals nothing. What next?
An examination under anesthesia of the neck, mouth, pharynx, larynx, esophagus, and tracheo-bronchial tree allows more detailed evaluation. If nothing is found, blind biopsies of the naso-pharynx, tonsils, and tonsillar beds, base of tongue, and pyriform sinuses are carried out.

7. Why esophagoscopy and bronchoscopy?
A second primary lesion is found in the aerodigestive tract of 10–20% of patients with squamous cancer.

8. Why blind biopsies of the sites listed above?
In about 10–15% of cases in which nothing is seen grossly, the primary tumor is found by blind biopsy.

9. Why not proceed to examination under anesthesia at the outset and skip the mirror and/or flexible endoscope examination?
The two procedures are complementary, not competitive. Examination while the patient is awake provides information about tongue and laryngeal function that cannot be obtained when the patient is asleep, and treatment planning often depends on such knowledge. In addition, examination of the patient under anesthesia may be something of a blind search, because of collapse of the tongue and pharyngeal walls, unless directed by findings on awake examination.

10. The patient undergoes direct and mirror examination, while awake and asleep, as well as blind biopsies of the aforementioned areas. Nothing is found. What about MRI or CT scan?
MRI is increasingly used to stage head and neck tumors and in fact is quite accurate—more accurate than CT scan. Thus, it may be of use in identifying an otherwise occult primary lesion.

11. MRI provides no new information. FNA of the neck mass reveals only lymphocytes. What should the patient be told?
The presence of lymphocytes most likely represents inflammation or lymphoma, but, given the location of the mass, it may also be a salivary gland (Warthin's) tumor. An operation is still necessary to rule out lymphoma and/or to remove the tumor, but a neck dissection is unlikely.

12. What if FNA or needle biopsy shows only fat or muscle?
The needle probably missed the node or mass. An open biopsy is indicated and, if metastatic squamous carcinoma is found, a neck dissection.

13. A radical neck dissection?
Most of the distaste for neck dissection is historical—a product of the time when the **standard radical dissection** was used for all forms of neck disease. This procedure sacrificed the jugular vein, sternomastoid muscle, and spinal accessory nerve and often resulted in significant cosmetic and functional deformities. Although a standard radical dissection may still be needed to remove bulky or fixed nodes, it has been supplanted in recent years by **functional, or modified radical dissection** for lesser disease—as in the patient under discussion. These procedures preserve jugular vein, sternomastoid muscle, and spinal accessory nerve and have a better cosmetic/functional outcome than a standard dissection; in appropriate patients, however, they provide the same degree of tumor control.

The best time for any neck dissection is when normal tissue planes exist. This time comes only once—when the neck is entered for biopsy. Reasons have already been discussed. Thus, the proper time to carry out an open biopsy is when the surgeon is ready to proceed with a neck dissection, radical or functional, if carcinoma is found.

14. If the mass or node is in the posterior triangle of the neck, is the same work-up still necessary?
Yes. Although most oral or pharyngeal tumors spread first to nodes in the angle between the mandible and sternomastoid muscle, it is not uncommon for nasopharyngeal, posterior hypopharyngeal, and thyroid tumors to present initially as metastases in the posterior triangle.

15. What if the FNA or open biopsy shows adenocarcinoma?

Although most malignant lymph nodes high in the ipsilateral neck are metastatic squamous or thyroid cancer or lymphoma, on occasion one encounters metastatic adenocarcinoma. At this point, the chances are about equal that the patient has an occult lung cancer, a renal, prostatic, or gastrointestinal primary tumor, or a salivary gland tumor. In this case, it makes sense to stop and try to locate the primary tumor before proceeding to a neck dissection.

16. How about undifferentiated carcinoma?

Proceed to neck dissection. The patient has either metastatic melanoma or metastatic squamous cancer and a primary tumor that has either spontaneously regressed or is too small to be found.

17. Thyroid cancer?

Neck dissection, exploration of the thyroid gland, and, at a minimum, ipsilateral lobectomy and isthmusectomy.

18. Should other therapy be offered after surgery?

If the problem is metastatic squamous or undifferentiated carcinoma, postoperative irradiation should be considered. Experience suggests that cancer in the neck recurs in 10–25% of patients with surgery alone (depending on amount of disease) and 5–10% with surgery plus irradiation. If the problem is metastatic thyroid cancer, the patient needs lifetime thyroid suppression with T3, T4, or dessicated thyroid, and consideration of ablation of residual thyroid tissue with radioactive iodine (I-131).

19. What if a primary tumor is not found? Does this influence prognosis?

No. Prognosis is determined primarily by the presence of metastatic neck disease, not by whether the primary tumor is found.

20. What is the role of adjuvant chemotherapy in such patients?

Chemotherapy before surgery reduces the tumor significantly (> 50%) in 80–90% of patients with bulky squamous head and neck tumors. On occasion, such reduction makes an inoperable tumor resectable or allows less extensive resection than originally planned. Unfortunately, it has yet to be shown that the ability to shrink tumors before surgery improves survival. This is also the case for postoperative chemotherapy. Thus, in the absence of metastatic disease, the role for chemotherapy in the treatment of head and neck cancer remains to be determined.

21. Lumps in the neck are common, and relatively few patients have cancer. Does *everyone* with a neck mass require this work-up?

True midline lesions, if situated cephalad to the thyroid isthmus, are unlikely to be anything other than a thyroglossal duct cyst, and true branchial cleft cysts transilluminate. Thus, when such findings are present, one can proceed directly to removal. On the other hand, the noncompulsive physician will be surprised by unsuspected cancer 3–4 times more often than he or she will encounter true branchial cysts in adults. The message is clear: branchial cleft and thyroglossal cysts are uncommon in adults; cancer is not.

BIBLIOGRAPHY

1. Attie JN, Setzin M, Klein I: Thyroid cancer presenting as an enlarged cervical lymph node. Am J Surg 166:428–430, 1993.
2. Erwin BC, Brynes RK, Chan WC, et al: Percutaneous needle biopsy in the diagnosis and classification of lymphoma. Cancer 57:1074–1078, 1986.
3. Frankenthaler RA, Sellin RV, Cangir A, Goepfert H: Lymph node metastasis from papillary-follicular thyroid carcinoma in young patients. Am J Surg 160:341–343, 1990.
4. Harwick RD: Cervical metastases from an occult primary site. Semin Surg Oncol 7:2–8, 1991.
5. Lee NK, Byers RM, Abbruzzese JL, Wolfe P: Metastatic adenocarcinoma to the neck from an unknown primary source. Am J Surg 162:306–309, 1991.

6. Lefebvre JL, Coche-Dequeant B, Ton Van J, et al: Cervical lymph nodes from an unknown primary tumor in 190 patients. Am J Surg 160:459–462, 1990.
7. Lufkin RB, Hanafee W: Magnetic resonance imaging of head and neck tumors. Cancer Metastasis Rev 7:19–38, 1988.
8. Kline TS, Kannan V, Kline IK: Lymphadenopathy and aspiration biopsy cytology. Review of 376 superficial nodes. Cancer 54:107–108, 1984.
9. Shah JP, Kraus DH, Dubner S, Sarkar S: Patterns of regional lymph node metastases from cutaneous melanomas of the head and neck. Am J Surg 162:320–323, 1991.
10. Shah JP: Patterns of cervical lymph node metastasis from squamous carcinomas of the upper aerodigestive tract. Am J Surg 160:405–409, 1990.

VII. Vascular Surgery

63. ARTERIAL INSUFFICIENCY

Thomas F. Rehring, M.D., and Robert B. Rutherford, M.D.

1. Atherosclerotic occlusive disease involving the lower extremities, also known as arteriosclerosis obliterans, progresses in severity through three distinct stages. What are they?

1. Claudication
2. Ischemic rest pain
3. Ischemic tissue necrosis

The French surgeon Fontaine originally described the three clinical stages. Since his time, a zero (asymptomatic) stage has been added to allow for categorization of pulse deficits in sedentary patients who do not exercise enough to experience claudication. The final stage of ischemic tissue loss is commonly subdivided into two subtypes—nonhealing ulcers and gangrene. The ulcers may result from focal ischemic infarcts or, at least initially, from other factors (pressure neuropathy, venous insufficiency, trauma); **ulcers do not heal** because of diffuse pedal ischemia due to arteriosclerosis obliterans. Similarly, one may have **focal gangrene without diffuse pedal ischemia**, as in atheromicroembolism (commonly referred to as "the blue toe syndrome") or digital artery thrombosis. It is important to distinguish patients with focal gangrene alone, who are capable of local healing, from patients with ulcers or gangrene and diffuse pedal ischemia, who will not heal unless circulation is improved by therapeutic intervention.

2. Describe claudication and the clinical features that distinguish it from other forms of extremity pain.

Claudication is defined by extremity pain (typically of the calf muscle) regularly produced by the same degree of exercise and relieved promptly by rest.

In order of frequency, claudication occurs in the calf, buttock, hip/thigh, or foot. Calf claudication is typically a cramping pain, but buttock, hip, or thigh claudication may not be very painful (it is often described as an aching discomfort). The rare foot claudication is typically a severe metatarsalgia associated with a wooden numbness. In general, the more proximal the location of the symptoms, the more proximal the distribution of the responsible arterial occlusive lesion.

3. What other disease entities should be considered in the differential diagnosis of claudication? How are they distinguished?

Sporadic calf cramps
Osteoarthritis
Neurogenic pseudoclaudication (sciatica)

Sporadic calf cramps may occur at rest, after exercise and, particularly in elderly patients, at night when they stretch during periods of arousal from sleep. Buttock, hip, or thigh discomfort, aggravated by exercise, may occur with **osteoarthritis of the hip**, but the presence of pain at rest and the lack of relationship with duration and degree of exercise distinguish it from claudication. **Narrowing of the neurospinal canal** by osteoarthritic hypertrophic changes in the lumbar spine causes compression of the cauda equina and an aching numbness of the hips and thighs. Such patients may regularly experience weakness and discomfort when they get up and walk; however, stopping does not relieve their distress. Other forms of metatarsalgia do not have the clear-cut relationship to duration of exercise and prompt relief by rest that is observed in patients with foot claudication due to severe infrapopliteal occlusive disease.

4. What percentage of patients presenting with claudication progress to eventual limb loss without intervention?

The 5-year rate of limb loss with expectant therapy is only 5–10%.

Several major studies have shown that 75% of claudicators remain relatively stable over a 5-year period. Of the 25% who require therapeutic intervention, 8% lose the limb because of acute progression of disease before limb salvage surgery. The remaining 17% elect surgical intervention for increasing symptoms. Of importance, during the same 5-year period, nearly 40% suffer a significant new systemic complication of arteriosclerosis (myocardial infarction, cerebrovascular accident, mesenteric ischemia, ruptured aneurysm) with an overall mortality rate of almost 25%. Patients who present with rest pain, ulcerations, or gangrene have a completely different prognosis. They initially present with a "threatened limb" (i.e., they will lose the extremity without intervention).

5. What is the ankle-brachial index (ABI)? How is it measured?

The ABI is an integral part of the physical examination of patients with peripheral arterial disease. With a blood pressure cuff at the mid-calf, a systolic pressure is recorded at the dorsalis pedis and posterior tibial arteries with Doppler. A brachial artery systolic pressure is also taken with the Doppler, and the ratio is computed. The ABI in normal patients should be 1.0. In claudicators, the index is typically 0.6–0.9. In patients with rest pain or ulcerations, the ABI drops to < 0.5. Diabetics may have falsely elevated ABIs as a result of calcified tibial vessels.

6. What therapeutic interventions should be initiated to improve the functional capacity of claudicators in whom surgery is not yet required?

   Cessation of smoking
   Progressive exercise programs
   Pharmacologic agents (possibly)

Cessation of smoking cannot be overemphasized. Smokers are nine times more likely to develop claudication and compose the overwhelming majority of patients requiring lower extremity amputation for ischemia. Abstinence from smoking improves symptoms, graft patency, and prognosis for prevention of limb loss. Other factors that promote the progression of peripheral arterial disease include diabetes, hypertension, and hyperlipidemia. Aggressive measures to control these factors may slow the progression of disease but will not relieve the symptoms of intermittent claudication. Benefits of **progressive exercise programs** have been known since 1966. Several prospective, randomized trials have now confirmed improvement in pain-free walking time (averaging 134%) and peak walking time (averaging 96%) in response to an exercise program. Vasodilators and antiplatelet and anticoagulant agents have not proved to be of benefit to patients with claudication. **Pentoxyphylline**, a hemorrheologic agent, remains the only drug approved by the Food and Drug Administration for intermittent claudication. In patients with moderately severe disease, pentoxyphylline exhibited a 50–100% improvement in treadmill walking ability.

7. What is the Leriche syndrome?

The syndrome represents the symptoms resulting from the gradual occlusion of the terminal aorta, which were initially described by Leriche in 1940. The symptoms include (1) impotence, (2) claudication, (3) lower extremity muscular atrophy, (4) trophic changes of the feet, and (5) pallor of the legs.

8. What are the indications for surgery in patients with chronic ischemia of the lower extremity?

   Disabling claudication (with significant life-style limitation)
   Rest pain
   Gangrene or ulceration
   Leriche syndrome

As with any other surgery, the indications for arterial reconstruction must be justified by a risk-to-benefit analysis. The risk of loss of life or limb weighs heavily in such deliberation. When the benefit is only increased walking distance, the risk of surgery must be small and an extended benefit must be anticipated (i.e., durable procedure with prolonged patency and expected longevity of the patient).

9. How does the coexistence of diabetes affect the distribution, natural history, and surgical indications for peripheral arterial disease?

Arteriosclerosis in diabetics more commonly affects **arteries of supply** (the infrapopliteal branches, profunda femoris, and hypogastric arteries) than **arteries of conduction** (such as the superficial femoral). Diabetics have approximately 5 times the risk of limb loss as nondiabetics (34% vs. 8% in 5 years), although much of this difference is also due to neuropathy and local sepsis. Once arterial occlusive disease becomes apparent, life expectancy is greatly shortened (38% in 10 years vs. 10% in nondiabetics), primarily because of the greater visceral artery involvement with atherosclerosis (e.g., coronary, carotid, renal, mesenteric disease). Diabetics also have a lower operability rate (because of infrapopliteal disease) and patency rate (because of poor run-off) than nondiabetics. In one report, the 5-year survival after amputation in diabetics was 39% (vs. 75% for nondiabetics), and the risk of losing the other leg approached 50%. For these reasons, arterial reconstruction should be limited to limb salvage in diabetics; surgery rarely is justified for claudication alone.

10. What are the invasive options for the treatment of aortoiliac occlusive disease? What patency rates can be expected with each option?

    Aortobifemoral bypass   Axillobifemoral bypass
    Femoral-femoral bypass   Percutaneous transluminal angioplasty

    Aortobifemoral bypass has almost completely replaced aortoiliac bypass or endarterectomy as the direct reconstructive approach to aortoiliac occlusive disease. It carries an approximately 3% mortality rate, a 2% risk of amputation, and a 5-year patency of 85–95%. In patients with unilateral iliac occlusion, **femoral-femoral** bypass may be an excellent option. It has a slightly lower mortality rate, patency rates of 80–85% at 5 years, and may be performed under local anesthesia. The **axillobifemoral graft** (subcutaneous axillary to femoral artery bypass with a suprapubic femoral-femoral artery crossover graft) carries a lower risk, but because it is reserved for high-risk patients, its operative mortality is paradoxically higher than for aortobifemoral bypass. With the aid of secondary thrombectomy, 5-year patency rates approach 75%, but the actual primary patency rate is 33–50%. This operation should be reserved for categorically high-risk patients and patients with hostile intraabdominal pathology (multiple adhesions, malignancy, ostomies, radiation damage, inflammatory bowel disease). **Transluminal angioplasty** gives 2-year patencies that are equivalent to the 5-year patency rates for femoral-femoral bypass if applied to favorable lesions (discrete, focal lesion, common iliac location, good run-off). Its major advantages are negligible mortality and minimal morbidity. Complete occlusion, extensive disease, or multiple lesions (especially involving the external iliac artery) respond much more poorly to angioplasty (50–60% success) and should be treated by surgical bypass grafting.

11. Infrainguinal bypasses fare less well than proximal bypasses, with a direct correlation between patency and length of graft (i.e., the more distal the anastomosis, the worse the patency rate). The type of graft is also correlated with patency. Identify and rank the graft options for infrainguinal bypass. What patency and limb salvage rates can be expected with each option?

    1. In situ saphenous vein
    2. Reversed saphenous vein
    3. Other autologous grafts (e.g., lesser saphenous or cephalic venous conduits)
    4. Expanded polytetrafluoroethylene (PTFE)
    5. Umbilical vein
    6. Dacron

Saphenous vein carefully harvested from the same leg and reversed to avoid valvular obstruction to flow has been the gold standard in femoropopliteal bypass with a 5-year patency of 75%. Unfortunately, it is also the ideal graft for coronary arterial bypass, which many patients also require. Furthermore, the vein may be unsuitable or unavailable in 10–20% of patients. **In situ bypass** describes a procedure in which the vein is left in place, the valves are rendered incompetent with valvulotomies, and the major branches are ligated to avoid arteriovenous fistulas. Advantages to this technique may include improved vein utilization, improved anastomotic compliance matches, and maintenance of inherent nutrient supply beds to the vein. In patients requiring distal bypasses to the peroneal or tibial arteries, significantly improved patency rates can be attained (+10%) with the in situ technique. Results with **PTFE** are clearly inferior to saphenous vein (-10% at the above-knee popliteal level, -20% at the below-knee popliteal level, and -30% at the peroneal/tibial level). **Umbilical vein** grafts attain similar rates of patency as PTFE but may deteriorate and dilate after 5 years. **Dacron** grafts, in general, suffer at least 10% worse patency than PTFE.

12. Why do grafts occlude? What is the relationship between time and cause of graft failure?
Grafts fail because of poor inflow, poor outflow (run-off), or structural changes at the anastomosis or graft itself.
1. **Less than 30 days:** technical errors, surface thrombogenicity with low flow
2. **Less than 18 months:** myointimal hyperplasia
3. **More than 18 months:** venous graft structural changes (e.g., valve site stenosis, segmental fibrosis), aneurysm, or new atheromatous change
4. **Greater than 36 months:** dilation or aneurysmal change in umbilical vein, PTFE, or Dacron graft. Risk factor modulation may affect long-term patency (see question 6).

13. What are the roles of noninvasive vascular testing and arteriography in the evaluation of patients with arteriosclerosis obliterans?
Noninvasive testing detects, localizes, and gauges the functional severity of arteriosclerotic occlusive lesions and is ideal for screening and follow-up monitoring. Arteriography yields two-dimensional, anatomic detail (i.e., morphologic, not physiologic, information), which is needed only in patients who are already probable candidates for therapeutic intervention (i.e., arterial reconstruction or transluminal angioplasty).

Segmental limb pressures and plethysmography detect and localize lesions with a 97% accuracy. Arteriography is like an up-to-date road map—the clinician needs it only if he or she is about to make a trip (operate).

14. What is the most common arteriosclerotic occlusive lesion in the lower extremity? Why is it now bypassed less frequently than other sites?
The most common site (50–60% of all claudicators) of occlusion for patients with peripheral arterial disease is in the superficial femoral artery at the adductor canal (Hunter's canal). As an isolated, well-collateralized lesion, it causes at worst only two-block claudication and therefore is not very disabling. More disabled patients (half-block claudicators and patients with rest pain) invariably have multilevel disease. If the additional block is **proximal** (e.g., iliac stenosis), it may be bypassed or dilated alone, with enough improvement that the superficial femoral artery lesion is no longer symptomatic. Similarly, if the additional block is **parallel** (e.g., in the profunda femoris) profundoplasty or dilation may suffice. Only when the additional occlusive lesions are in the distal vessels is femoropopliteal or tibial bypass indicated. Because of the additional incidence of isolated aortoiliac disease and its common association with superficial femoral occlusion, proximal iliac bypass (direct or extraanatomic) or balloon dilation is twice as common as infrainguinal bypass.

15. What are the classic signs and symptoms of acute arterial insufficiency?
The five Ps: pain, pulselessness, pallor, paralysis, and paresthesias.

Admittedly a bit contrived and by no means universally present, this pentad provides a useful reminder in evaluating patients presenting with acute extremity symptoms. Sudden, shooting **pain** down the extremity is common at the moment of embolism and is often associated with rapidly diminishing numbness and weakness. Thrombosis tends to be silent at the outset. However, if severe ischemia persists, typical ischemic rest pain, as described above, soon develops. **Pulses** are absent beyond the level of occlusion and should be compared with the opposite extremity. **Pallor** is common at the outset but after a few hours may convert to a mottled cyanosis. Temperature changes may be more marked than color change, but, alas, coolness does not begin with a p. **Paralysis** develops in time if severe ischemia persists, beginning in the distribution of the peroneal nerve, with weakness on dorsiflexion of the toe or foot. Loss of motor function is a grave sign, often correlating with permanent loss of function and necessity of an amputation. Considerable motion of the toes and ankle may persist because the origins of the responsible muscles are far proximal and may not suffer from much ischemia. **Paresthesias** and a sensation of increasing numbness portend serious consequences. Sensory loss may be subtle at first. Loss of appreciation of light touch, vibration, and sense of position should be assessed rather than perception of pain, pressure, or two-point discrimination. Depending on the presence and degree of sensory and motor changes, acutely ischemic limbs may be categorized as (1) viable, (2) threatened but salvageable, or (3) major irreversible ischemic changes.

16. How can the clinician determine whether an acute occlusion of the extremity was provoked by an embolus or thrombosis? How does this knowledge affect therapy?
Prompt surgical embolectomy is the preferred treatment for patients with acute arterial emboli. However, an attempted thrombectomy for acute thrombosis may worsen the ischemic insult. Better results may be obtained with angiography and lytic therapy of a thrombosed vessel and subsequent bypass or endarterectomy in patients whose collateral flow can sustain the limb for the 24–72 hours necessary for clot lysis. Despite the cause, once acute arterial occlusion is recognized, heparin should be administered **immediately** (before angiography, embolectomy, or acute reconstruction) to prevent clot propagation.

In general, patients with an embolic occlusion have a historical source for embolus, typically a history of atrial fibrillation. They have no prior history of claudication or any physical stigmata of peripheral arterial disease. In contrast, patients presenting with thrombosis of a diseased vessel have no historical predisposition to embolic phenomenon but may have a history of claudication and morphologic changes characteristic of chronic ischemia of the lower extremity. Angiography also may yield some clues as to the cause of the occlusion (normal vs. diseased vessels, collateralization, location), but in cases of clear-cut embolism angiography provides little benefit and only prolongs the ischemic insult to the limb.

17. What is the most likely source for an embolus causing an acute arterial occlusion?
Of all emboli, 80–90% have a cardiac origin. Atrial fibrillation is an associated finding in 65–75% of patients with peripheral vascular embolic disease. Other, less common, cardiac causes of emboli include mural thrombus after myocardial infarction, prosthetic valves, rheumatic heart disease, and intracardiac tumors. Noncardiac sources, which account for only 5–10% of emboli, generally occur secondary to diseased proximal large vessels (aneurysm, atherosclerotic plaque). In the remaining 5–10% the source of emboli remains undetermined, even at autopsy.

18. In what location is an embolus from a cardiac source most likely to lodge?
The common femoral artery bifurcation is the most frequent site of embolic occlusion (35–50% of all patients). The axial limb vessels are involved in 70–80% of embolic episodes in most series. In general, the lower extremities are involved 5 times as frequently as the upper extremities. Because vessel diameters change most abruptly at branching points, emboli are most likely to lodge at bifurcations of major vessels. In decreasing order of incidence, embolic occlusions occur at common femoral bifurcation (36%), aortic or common iliac bifurcation (22%), popliteal artery (15%), upper extremity (14%), visceral arteries (7%), and other (6%).

BIBLIOGRAPHY

1. Boyd A: Natural course of arteriosclerosis of lower extremities. Proc R Soc Med 53:591, 1962.
2. Brewster DC: Acute peripheral arterial occlusion. Cardiol Clin 9:497, 1991.
3. Couch N: On the arterial consequences of smoking. J Vasc Surg 3:807, 1985.
4. Gordon T, Kannel W: Predisposition to atherosclerosis in the head, heart and legs: The Framingham Study. JAMA 221:661, 1972.
5. Hiatt W, Regensteiner J, Hargarten M, et al: Benefit of exercise conditioning for patients with peripheral arterial disease. Circulation 81:602, 1990.
6. Imparato A, Kim G, Davidson T, et al: Intermittent claudication: Its natural course. Surgery 78:795, 1975.
7. Lundgren F, Dahllof A, Lundholm K, et al: Intermittent claudication—surgical reconstruction or physical training? A prospective randomized trial of treatment efficiency. Ann Surg 209:346, 1989.
8. Rutherford RB: The vascular consultation. In Rutherford RB (ed): Vascular Surgery, 4th ed. Philadelphia, W.B. Saunders, 1995.

64. CAROTID DISEASE

David J. Minion, M.D., and B. Timothy Baxter, M.D.

1. What diseases affect the carotid arteries?
Atherosclerosis is by far the most common. It can be accelerated by radiation treatment. The carotid may also be affected by fibromuscular dysplasia and arteritis (e.g., giant cell or Takayasu's arteritis).

2. What does a carotid bruit signify?
A carotid bruit is a generalized marker for atherosclerosis; it is more predictive of a cardiac event than a neurologic event. Although a carotid bruit indicates increased risk of neurologic events, they are as likely to occur on the contralateral side as on the side of the bruit.

3. Describe a bruit produced by internal carotid artery stenosis.
Cervical bruit begins in systole and extends into diastole; it is unaffected by superficial temporal artery occlusion.

4. Will a severe internal carotid artery stenosis produce a bruit?
No. With progression of stenosis the bruit may disappear as flow decreases.

5. What test should be ordered to evaluate a cervical bruit?
Duplex scanning.

6. What are some of the symptoms of carotid artery disease?
Transient ischemic attack   Cerebrovascular accident
Reversible ischemic neurologic deficit   Amaurosis fugax

7. Define transient ischemic attack, reversible ischemic neurologic deficit, and cerebrovascular accident.
These clinical terms describe a spectrum of cerebral ischemic syndromes. **Transient ischemic attack** (TIA) is a neurologic deficit that lasts less than 24 hours. **Reversible ischemic neurologic deficit** (RIND) is a neurologic event that lasts longer than 24 hours and completely resolves within days. **Cerebrovascular accident** (CVA), or acute stroke, is a stable neurologic deficit that may show gradual improvement over a long period of time. These definitions are clinical and may not represent actual pathology. CT may show evidence of ischemic stroke in some asymptomatic patients or in patients with TIA.

8. Define crescendo TIA and stroke in evolution.
Crescendo TIA: repeated neurologic events without interval neurologic deterioration.
Stroke in evolution: repeated neurologic event in which neurologic function does not return to baseline between events.

9. Define amaurosis fugax.
Amaurosis fugax is an episode of transient (minutes to hours) monocular blindness, often likened to a window shade pulled across the eye, due to temporary ischemia.

10. What are Hollenhorst plaques?
Hollenhorst plaques are bright yellow plaques of cholesterol in the retinal vessels that have embolized from the carotid bifurcation. Clinically, this finding indicates that the atheromatous plaque in the carotid is quite friable; other microemboli may occur spontaneously with manipulation at surgery.

11. What mechanisms produce neurologic deficits?
  1. Artery-to-artery embolus
  2. Low perfusion, especially with multivessel occlusive disease
  3. Occlusive disease with thrombosis
  4. Intracranial hemorrhage

12. When posterior cerebral circulation is impaired, what symptoms occur? What extracranial arteries may be diseased?
Ischemia to the brainstem produces near-syncope, bilateral visual disturbances, and bilateral motor paralysis. Extracranial arterial lesions that may produce vertebrobasilar insufficiency include subclavian artery stenosis, vertebral artery stenosis, or carotid artery stenosis in combination with vertebral artery stenosis. Basilar artery disease and small-vessel disease also may cause posterior circulation ischemia.

13. What is the natural history of a TIA?
The natural history of a TIA is defined by the pathology of the ipsilateral carotid artery. In patients with significant stenosis (> 70%), the risk of ipsilateral stroke within 24 months is 26%. The risk appears to increase in direct proportion to the degree of carotid stenosis. For patients with minimal (< 30%) stenosis the risk of ipsilateral stroke is 1% at 3 years.

14. What is the effect of aspirin on TIAs?
Acetylsalicylic acid is a cyclooxygenase inhibitor that affects platelets and decreases the incidence of both TIAs and stroke.

15. When is surgery indicated for symptomatic carotid artery disease?
Surgery is strongly indicated for symptomatic carotid artery disease associated with > 70% stenosis. The absolute risk reduction of stroke is 17% at 2 years. Indications for surgery in patients with a symptomatic stenosis of 30–70% are not well defined. Aspirin alone is recommended for symptomatic stenoses of < 30%.

16. Should a patient with an asymptomatic stenosis undergo surgery?
In asymptomatic patients with > 60% stenosis, as confirmed by angiography, there is an absolute reduction in the risk of stroke of 6% over a 5-year period in patients who undergo carotid endarterectomy with aspirin compared with those who are treated with aspirin alone (5.1% vs. 11%). Thus, carotid endarterectomy should be performed for asymptomatic carotid artery disease when the following criteria are met: (1) the patient is expected to live at least 3 years; and (2) the carotid endarterectomy can be performed with a combined stroke and mortality rate of < 3%.

17. What surgical procedure should be performed on a totally occluded carotid artery?
None or an extracranial-intracranial (ECIC) bypass operation. In patients with chronic total occlusion, surgery is rarely helpful. When the occlusion is acute, the associated severe neurologic deficits and risk of creating a hemorrhagic infarct are contraindications to surgery. ECIC bypass may be indicated in the rare situation of complete occlusion of the internal carotid artery with evidence of persistent hemispheric ischemia without CVA.

18. When the internal carotid artery is occluded, what branches of the external carotid artery form collaterals and reestablish circulation in the circle of Willis?
Periorbital branches of the external carotid artery form communications with the ophthalmic artery, a branch of the internal carotid.

19. How many branches of the internal carotid artery are located in the neck?
None.

20. What is the landmark of the carotid artery bifurcation?
Facial vein.

21. What are the functions of the carotid sinus and the carotid body?
Both are located at the carotid bifurcation and are innervated by the glossopharyngeal and vagus nerves, respectively. The function of the carotid sinus is regulation of blood pressure. Hypertension stimulates efferent impulses to the vasomotor center in the medulla, inhibiting sympathetic tone and increasing vagal tone. The carotid body regulates respiratory drive and acid/base status via chemoreceptors. It also induces bradycardia when manipulated.

22. What is a shunt?
A shunt is a plastic conduit that diverts blood flow around the surgically opened carotid artery while endarterectomy is performed. Several varieties are available. The use of shunts is discussed in the section on controversies.

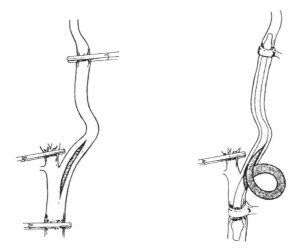

Intraluminal shunt for carotid artery surgery.

23. What is stump pressure?
Stump pressure is the back pressure of the internal carotid artery after clamping; it indicates adequacy of cerebral perfusion. The safe pressure for cross-clamping varies according to author; the mean is 25–50 mmHg.

24. When do neurologic events occur during carotid endarterectomies?
1. Dissection: dislodgement of arterial wall diseases
2. Carotid artery clamping: ischemic infarct
3. Postoperatively: intimal flap, reperfusion, and external carotid artery clot

25. What are the complications of carotid endarterectomy?
Intraoperative complications include neurologic deficits and cerebral ischemia. New deficits or exacerbations of old deficits may occur by embolization of debris during vessel manipulation or by poor flushing technique after arteriotomy closure. Cerebral ischemia may occur because of hypotension or poor protection during cross-clamping. There may be no clinical symptoms, or the ischemia may be manifested as TIA or acute stroke. The overall incidence of neurologic deficits during endarterectomy is about 2–3%.

26. Which cranial nerves may be injured during carotid endarterectomy? What are the clinical signs of nerve injury?
   Hypoglossal (XII): deviation of the tongue to the operated side; difficulty with speech and mastication.
   Vagus (X): minor swallowing difficulty, recurrent laryngeal cord paralysis with hoarseness.
   Glossopharyngeal (IX): difficulty in swallowing with ipsilateral Horner's syndrome.
   Facial (VII): droop of the ipsilateral corner of the lip and decreased ability to smile.
   Superior laryngeal: easy fatigability of the voice.

27. What is the danger of wound hematoma after carotid surgery?
The main danger is airway compromise. The risk of wound hematoma can be reduced by careful attention to hemostasis. Sudden airway compromise may require emergent decompression by opening the wound.

28. What are the possible causes of postoperative hypertension?
   Denervation of the carotid sinus
   Cerebral renin production
   Preexisting hypertension
   Central neurologic deficit

29. When was the association between carotid artery disease and neurologic deficit first reported and by whom?
In 1857 by Savory.

30. When was the first carotid endarterectomy performed and by whom?
In 1954 by Eastcott.

31. In what layer of the artery is the endarterectomy performed?
Tunica media.

CONTROVERSIES

32. Cerebral protection.
Adequate cerebral protection is essential to avoid intraoperative ischemia. Some surgeons believe that temporary clamping under local anesthesia is an adequate test of the effectiveness of the collateral circulation. Others use the stump pressure to assess the collateral circulation. Alternatives include the use of intraoperative electroencephalography or transcranial Doppler. Because none of these methods is 100% accurate, many surgeons routinely use an intraoperative shunt, whereas others use it selectively or rarely, if at all.

33. Intraoperative shunts.

For: Ensures adequate cerebral protection in all patients.

Against: Prolongs time of operation, results in increased manipulation of friable vessel, and usually is not necessary.

BIBLIOGRAPHY

1. CASANOVA Study Group: Carotid surgery versus medical therapy in asymptomatic carotid stenosis. Stroke 22:1229–1235, 1991.
2. Endarterectomy for asymptomatic carotid artery stenosis. JAMA 273:1421–1428, 1995.
3. European Carotid Surgery Trialists' Collaborative Group: European Carotid Surgery Trial: Interim results for symptomatic patients with severe (70–99%) or with mild (0–29%) carotid stenosis. Lancet 337:1235–1243, 1991.
4. Hobson RW II, Weiss DG, Fields WS, et al: For Veterans Affairs Cooperative Study Group: Efficacy of carotid endarterectomy for asymptomatic carotid stenosis. N Engl J Med 328:221–227, 1993.
5. Mayo Asymptomatic Carotid Endarterectomy Study Group: Results of a randomized controlled trial of carotid endarterectomy for asymptomatic carotid stenosis. Mayo Clin Proc 67:513–518, 1992.
6. North American Symptomatic Carotid Endarterectomy Trial Collaborators. Beneficial effect of carotid endarterectomy in symptomatic patients with high-grade stenosis. N Engl J Med 325:445–452, 1991.

65. ACUTE ARTERIAL OCCLUSION

Glenn L. Kelly, M.D.

1. What are the causes of acute arterial occlusion?

The most common causes are an embolus (of cardiac origin [30%], from a proximal aneurysm [2%], or of undetermined origin [30%]) or thrombosis (of an arteriosclerotic stenosis [30%] or aneurysm [2%]). Other infrequent causes are venous thrombosis, vasospasm, extrinsic compression, or paradoxical embolism through a cardiac defect. Emboli of cardiac origin are usually associated with atrial fibrillation or recent myocardial infarction.

2. What are the symptoms and findings?

There is usually sudden coolness followed by ischemic pain. When tissue hypoxia is extreme, numbness and paralysis result. Patients with emboli may have a history of antecedent cardiac symptoms. Arterial thrombosis often is preceded by symptoms of claudication or rest pain due to antecedent arteriosclerotic stenosis. On examination the proximal pulse is absent; positive findings include pallor and reduced capillary and venous refill. Diagnosis may be confirmed when Doppler flow is absent or Doppler pressure is markedly reduced.

3. Is it important to distinguish between embolism and thrombosis?

It may be. Emboli can be expeditiously removed by surgery with a high expectation of circulatory recovery. Because emboli contain old, organized fibrin, they are less successfully dissolved by lytic enzymes. Conversely, thrombi usually are associated with underlying occlusive or aneurysmal disease, which requires repair or bypass during or after thrombectomy. Thrombi are usually less well organized, making them more responsive to enzymatic lysis.

4. What is the treatment?

After prompt evaluation and stabilization, full-dose intravenous heparin helps to prevent clot propagation prior to definitive treatment. Patients with suspected embolization, whose clot is usually well organized and localized, are more expeditiously and less expensively treated by surgical embolectomy. This approach is also indicated in patients with severe limb-threatening ischemia. With the patient under local or general anesthesia, the clot is extracted by using a

Fogarty balloon catheter. Emboli to the upper extremity should be treated in the same manner as those in the leg. Care must be taken not to overdistend the balloon, which may produce local arterial injury. Completion arteriography identifies unsuspected residual clots, which may be retrieved by further passages of the balloon catheter or lysed with intraoperative urokinase. Postoperative heparin therapy should prevent recurrent embolism. If underlying arterial stenosis or aneurysm has caused the thrombosis, concomitant or staged reconstruction is necessary. Occasionally patients with mild ischemic symptoms present several weeks after thromboembolic occlusion. Although chances of successful thromboembolectomy or lysis are diminished, it is usually worthwhile to attempt treatment, usually with lytic therapy even up to 3–6 months, especially if the radiologist can pass a guidewire through the occlusion.

Patients with suspected thrombosis of an arterial stenosis or aneurysm, especially those with mild ischemic symptoms, are best treated in the radiology suite with thrombolytic therapy. Urokinase is safer than streptokinase and somewhat less expensive than tissue plasminogen activator. Urokinase is delivered through a catheter fluoroscopically placed within the clot. Once lysis has occurred, baseline blood flow is restored, and abnormal vessel architecture can be evaluated for balloon angioplasty or future reconstruction. Lytic therapy is 75–80% effective in restoring flow. Complications, including distal embolization and bleeding, occur in 10% of patients but are usually incidental.

5. What is urokinase? How does it work? Why is it safer than streptokinase?
Urokinase (UK) is a serine protease isolated from urine or kidney cell cultures. UK directly converts the proenzyme plasminogen to the active fibrinolytic enzyme plasmin. Bleeding is the most common complication (7–15% of patients). UK is safer than streptokinase, which causes allergic or febrile reactions in up to 30% of patients.

6. What are the complications of thromboembolectomy?
Because of coexisting serious (typically cardiopulmonary) diseases, the mortality rate is 10–30% in patients with thrombosis. Revascularization, especially when ischemia is severe and surgery is delayed, may lead to four other problems:

  1. **Reperfusion shock** is due to systemic acidosis and hyperkalemia. It may be prevented by slow release of the vascular clamps and systemic administration of bicarbonate solution, glucose, and insulin.

  2. **Compartment syndrome** from muscle edema and subsequent neurovascular compression is treated by prompt fasciotomy of the involved muscle compartment.

  3. **Acute tubular necrosis** is due to release of myoglobin from damaged muscle tissue. Alkalinization of urine and diuretics are the recommended therapy.

  4. **Local tissue necrosis or neuropathy** due to prolonged preoperative ischemia may ensue.

7. What is a Fogarty catheter?
The Fogarty catheter is a flexible plastic catheter with a syringe at the proximal end and a soft, inflatable latex balloon at the distal end. It is passed through the clot, then gently inflated and withdrawn to remove the clot. It was invented in 1963 by Thomas Fogarty, a cardiovascular surgeon who also invented the friction clutch for the motor scooter.

8. How does heparin work?
Heparin complexes with and enhances the activity of circulating antithrombin III. Thus it inhibits the action of thrombin on fibrinogen but also interferes with activation of factors VIII, IX, and X and the effect of thrombin on platelet aggregation.

CONTROVERSIES

9. Is preoperative arteriography necessary?
Not always, especially when associated atrial fibrillation or recent myocardial infarction suggests embolism. Presumptive embolic arterial occlusion is often treated by rapid embolectomy without

the nephrotoxic risk, delay, and expense of arteriography. When a history of chronic ischemic symptoms or physical findings suggests thrombosis of an intrinsic arterial lesion, arteriography is useful in planning a concomitant or subsequent reconstructive procedure.

10. Is heparin alone an effective therapy?
A few authors have advocated heparin therapy over surgery, using 2000–4000 U of heparin/hour. Although the mortality rate is reduced slightly, the amputation rate is increased; thus, this modality is not used extensively in most centers.

BIBLIOGRAPHY

1. Abbott WM, Maloney RD, McCabe CC, et al: Arterial embolism: A 44-year perspective. Am J Surg 143:460, 1982.
2. Baxter-Smith D, Aston F, Slaney G, et al: Peripheral arterial embolism. A 20 year review. J Cardiovasc Surg 29:453:1988.
3. Blaisdell FW, Steele M, Allen RD: Management of acute lower extremity arterial ischemia due to embolism and thrombosis. Surgery 84:822, 1978.
4. Brewster DC: Acute peripheral arterial occlusion. Cardiol Clin 9:497, 1991.
5. Camerota AJ, White JV: Intraoperative, intra-arterial thrombolytic therapy as an adjunct to revascularization in patients with residual and distal arterial thrombus. Semin Vasc Surg 52110, 1992.
6. DeMaioribus CA, Mons JL, Fujitani RM, et al: A reevaluation of intraarterial thrombolytic therapy for acute lower extremity ischemia. J Vasc Surg 17:888, 1993.
7. Fogarty TJ, Cranley JJ, Krause RJ, et al: A method for extraction of arterial emboli and thrombi. Surg Gynecol Obstet 116:241, 1963.
8. Fogarty TJ, Hermann GD: New techniques for clot extraction and managing acute thromboembolic limb ischemia. In Vieth FJ (ed): Current Critical Problems in Vascular Surgery. St. Louis, Quality Medical Publishing, 3:197, 1991.
9. McNamara TO: Thrombolysis of peripheral arterial and graft occlusions: Improved results using high-dose urokinase. Am J Radiol 144:769, 1985.
10. Quriel K, Shortell CK, DeWeese JA, et al: A comparison of thrombolytic therapy with operative revascularization in the initial treatment of acute peripheral arterial ischemia. J Vasc Surg 19:1021, 1994.
11. Patman RD: Fasciotomy: Indications and techniques. In Rutherford RB (ed): Vascular Surgery, 3rd ed. Philadelphia, W.B. Saunders, 1989.
12. Quinones-Baldrich WJ: Principles of thrombolytic therapy. In Rutherford RB (ed): Vascular Surgery, 4th ed. Philadelphia, W.B. Saunders, 1995, p 334.
13. Tawes RL, Beare JP, Scribner RG, et al: Value of postoperative heparin therapy in peripheral arterial thromboembolism. Am J Surg 146:213, 1983.

66. VASCULAR INJURIES

William H. Pearce, M.D., and Sandra C. Carr, M.D.

1. By what mechanisms can arterial trauma occur?
Blunt trauma   Iatrogenic trauma
Penetrating trauma   Orthopedic injuries

2. What is the kinetic energy of a bullet? Why is it important?
The kinetic energy (K) of a bullet is determined by the following equation:

$$K = \frac{1}{2}MV^2$$

where M = mass and V = velocity. The tissue energy is related to the square of the velocity. A high-velocity bullet causes more damage and requires more extensive debridement than a bullet of smaller mass and lower velocity.

3. In what four ways can an arterial injury manifest?

Hemorrhage   Pseudoaneurysm
Thrombosis (with or without ischemia)   Arteriovenous fistula

4. Can a patient with an arterial injury present with palpable distal pulses in the affected extremity?

Yes. Depending on the location and nature of the injury, 15–20% of patients with significant arterial injuries present with distal palpable pulses.

5. Does the presence of Doppler signals over an artery rule out an arterial injury?

No. Nor does it indicate adequate perfusion.

6. What test can one do in the emergency room to assess the adequacy of perfusion to an extremity in a patient with suspected arterial injury?

Segmental blood pressures using a hand-held Doppler device is a good test. The ankle/brachial index should be greater than 1:1 in a healthy young person.

7. What are the symptoms of complete acute arterial occlusion?

The six Ps: pain, pallor, pulse deficit, paresthesia, paralysis, and poikilothermia (coldness).

8. What are the hard signs of arterial injury?

Massive external bleeding   Expanding hematoma
Palpable thrill and continuous murmur   The six Ps

9. What is the appropriate management of a patient with hard signs of arterial injury?

The patient should undergo prompt operative exploration and appropriate repair. Arteriogram is usually not necessary and only delays appropriate treatment.

10. What are the soft signs of arterial injury?

History of significant prehospital hemorrhage   Peripheral nerve deficit
Wound in proximity to a major artery   Small nonpulsatile hematoma
Diminished pulse   Fracture dislocation of the knee or elbow

Arteriography is usually indicated in patients with soft signs of arterial injury.

11. Which two fractures are associated with a significant risk of arterial injury?

Supracondylar humeral fracture (brachial artery)
Posterior dislocation of the knee (popliteal artery)

12. What important arterial injury is seen with deceleration injury, as in a high-speed motor vehicle accident or a fall from a significant height?

Blunt injury to the thoracic aorta, which occurs most commonly at the insertion of the ligamentum arteriosum distal to the origin of the left subclavian artery.

13. What is the mortality rate from blunt injury to the thoracic aorta?

Eighty-five percent of patients do not survive the initial impact; 50% of patients who reach the hospital rupture and die within 24–48 hours of admission.

14. What are the signs and symptoms associated with blunt injury to the thoracic aorta?

Patients may be asymptomatic, have severe chest or back pain, or may have asymmetry of blood pressures or pulse characteristics in the upper and lower extremities.

15. What findings on chest radiograph are associated with injury to the thoracic aorta?

Widened mediastinum (> 8 cm at the aortic knob in adults)
Obliteration of the aortopulmonary window

Indistinct aortic knob
Deviation of the trachea, nasogastric tube, or endotracheal tube to the right
Depression of the left mainstem bronchus more than 140°
Elevation of the right mainstem bronchus
Pleural apical cap of blood
Fractures of the first and second ribs
Scapula fracture

16. Which arterial injury bleeds more—a complete transection or an incomplete transection? Why?
The incomplete transection bleeds more because it does not have the ability to undergo retraction, vasoconstriction, and thrombosis as the complete transection often does.

17. What are the three layers of an artery?
Tunica intima, tunica media, and tunica adventitia

18. What is the difference between a true aneurysm and a false aneurysm?
A true aneurysm is a localized dilation of an artery covered by all three layers of the vessel. A false aneurysm (pseudoaneurysm), usually caused by trauma, is a disruption of all three vessel layers that results in a pulsating hematoma covered by fibrous tissue.

19. What is the mechanism of arterial injury from blunt trauma?
As the arterial wall is stretched, the elastic adventitial and muscular layers remain intact while the intima fractures. Blood dissects beneath the fractured intima, resulting in an intimal flap that occludes the lumen.

20. What are the three zones in the neck? Why are they important in preoperative evaluation?
Zone I is below the cricoid cartilage, zone II is from the cricoid cartilage to the angle of the mandible, and zone III is above the angle of the mandible. Because these areas are difficult to access surgically, patients with zone I and III injuries require aortography with selective injection of the carotid and vertebral arteries. Patients with zone II injuries may undergo surgical exploration or evaluation with arteriography (also esophagogram, esophagoscopy, and sometimes bronchoscopy) to exclude injury.

21. What is the best way to control external bleeding acutely?
External pressure is best. Blind clamping should be avoided to prevent injury to adjacent nerves.

22. Why should tourniquets be avoided if possible?
The tourniquet occludes collaterals, making distal ischemia worse. If applied improperly, it may allow arterial inflow and occlude venous outflow, making the bleeding worse.

23. What is the initial step in the surgical management of vascular injuries?
Obtain proximal and distal control of the injured vessel.

24. What are the steps involved in arterial repair?
Debridement, removal of distal thrombi, arterial reconstruction, and soft-tissue coverage.

25. What is the first choice of conduit for repairing an extensive arterial injury that cannot be closed primarily?
Reversed saphenous vein from an uninjured lower extremity.

26. If the nerve, artery, vein, and bone are injured, what is the order of repair?
    With a short period of ischemia: bone, artery, vein, nerve.
    With a longer period of ischemia: artery, vein, bone, nerve.

27. What intraabdominal vessel is most often injured?
The inferior vena cava is injured in 10–20% of intraabdominal vessel injuries and 30–50% of abdominal venous injuries.

28. Should venous injuries below the inguinal ligament be repaired? Why?
Yes. Although the long-term patency for venous repair is not excellent, short-term patency is beneficial. It allows the development of collateral venous and lymphatic drainage, increased arterial inflow during the acute postoperative period, and reduction in peripheral edema.

29. What is the most important complication after successful repair of an injury to the thoracic aorta? Why?
Paraplegia, because the anterior spinal artery originates from branches of the thoracic intercostal arteries.

30. What are the four compartments in the lower leg? Why are they important in arterial injuries to the leg?
Anterior, lateral, superficial posterior, and deep posterior. With a significant injury to the leg, edema may occur in the compartments secondary to ischemia or massive soft tissue trauma, leading to a compartment syndrome.

31. What are the local and systemic consequences of a compartment syndrome?
Locally, the increased pressure decreases capillary blood flow and leads to tissue necrosis. Neurologic injury occurs first, because the nerves are most sensitive to ischemia, and may result in a foot drop syndrome from peroneal nerve injury and paresthesias of the foot. Systemic manifestations are hyperkalemia, myoglobinuria, and sepsis.

32. What is the treatment for a suspected compartment syndrome?
Prompt fasciotomy.

33. What is the most sensitive sign of a compartment syndrome?
Pain on passive stretch of the involved muscle. Signs such as foot drop and loss of pulses are late signs and usually indicate permanent damage from ischemia.

34. What factors suggest the need for a fasciotomy?

Prolonged period (6 hours or more) between injury and restoration of perfusion

Associated crush injury

Preoperative calf swelling

Combined arterial and venous ligation

Postoperative signs of disproportionate muscle pain, pain on passive stretch, or tender and firm muscles

Elevated compartment pressures

35. In an extremity with a neurovascular injury, what injury results in major disability?
Whereas injury to the vessels may be repaired, frequently with good results, injury to the nerve may be impossible to repair, leading to significant disability.

36. If an arterial injury is ligated but not repaired, what is the chance of amputation?
It depends on which artery is ligated:

Femoral	81%	Subclavian	29%
Popliteal	72%	Axillary	43%
Tibial	69%	Brachial	56%

37. Significant swelling in the early postoperative period is suggestive of what complication? How should it be evaluated?
Venous thrombosis, which should be evaluated by a duplex scan.

38. Who performed the first venous interposition for arterial injury?
Goyanes in 1906.

40. Who performed the first end-to-end repair?
John Murphy in 1896.

BIBLIOGRAPHY

1. Cameron JL (ed): Current Surgical Therapy, 4th ed. St. Louis, Mosby, 1992, pp 865–873.
2. Ernst CB, Stanley JC (eds): Current Therapy in Vascular Surgery, 2nd ed. Philadelphia, B.C. Decker, 1991, pp 609–690.
3. Greenfield LJ (ed): Surgery: Scientific Principles and Practice. Philadelphia, J.B. Lippincott, 1993, pp 247–331.

67. ABDOMINAL AORTIC ANEURYSM

William C. Krupski, M.D.

1. What is an abdominal aortic aneurysm?
The term aneurysm refers to a permanent, focal dilatation of a blood vessel with respect to the original or adjacent artery. Although a uniform definition of abdominal aortic aneurysm (AAA) does not exist, most authorities agree that a localized enlargement of the aorta greater than or equal to twice the size of normal diameter is aneurysmal. CT measurements of the infrarenal aorta in adult men average 2.3 cm, whereas the corresponding diameter in women is 1.9 cm. Thus, aneurysms begin at about 4 cm. In referring to the size of the aneurysms, it is customary to use the maximal external transverse diameter of the aorta, regardless of how the measurement was obtained (ultrasound, CT, MRI, or direct operative assessment).

2. Who gets AAAs?
Aneurysm of the abdominal aorta is mostly a disease of elderly men; men outnumber women by approximately 4 to 1. Estimates of prevalence range from 2–5% in men over the age of 60. The incidence of AAA appears to be increasing. Two reports from the Mayo Clinic indicate a three-fold increase in prevalence from 12.2 per 100,000 to 36.2 per 100,000 during the period 1951 through 1980. The increasing age of the population plays a role in the increasing incidence.

3. Are screening programs for AAAs worthwhile?
Screening the general population for AAAs is not cost effective. Most aneurysms detected by screening are small. In contrast, selective screening may be cost effective. Patients who have peripheral vascular disease, who are heavy cigarette smokers, and who have a family history of aneurysm disease have a particularly high incidence.

4. What causes AAAs?
Because the aortic wall of most patients with aneurysms shows atherosclerosis, in the past AAAs have been called atherosclerotic aneurysms, and atherosclerosis was assumed to cause aneurysmal degeneration. Patients with AAAs have risk factors associated with occlusive vascular disease, particularly smoking and hypertension. However, concurrent occlusive disease in the aortoiliac distribution is uncommon in patients with AAAs. Therefore, atherosclerotic aneurysms are more appropriately described as **degenerative** or **nonspecific aortic aneurysms**.

5. Can one inherit AAAs?
A high incidence of AAAs in members of several large families suggests that genetic factors are sometimes involved in the pathogenesis. An abnormality in the long arm of chromosome 16 has

been implicated in some familial aneurysms. Rare hereditary defects of type III collagen, a primary structural component of the arterial wall, are found in Ehlers-Danlos syndrome, which is associated with aneurysms of many arteries. In Marfan's syndrome, which is associated with arterial dilations and dissections of the entire aorta, mutations of the fibrillin-1 gene on chromosome 15 have been implicated. During the 1980s, several studies showed a familial clustering of AAAs; at least 18% of patients with AAAs have a first-degree relative also affected.

6. What are the other causes of AAAs?

Degenerative aneurysms account for more than 90% of all infrarenal aortic aneurysms. Additional causes include cystic medial necrosis, arteritis, trauma, genetic connective tissue disorders, and anastomotic disruption. Infection also may be present in AAAs. Infected aneurysms result from localized infections of the arterial wall. Most infected aneurysms develop from bacteremias associated at distal sites (e.g., endocarditis). Infected aneurysm is the most common type of aortic aneurysm in children.

7. How do AAAs present clinically?

In clinical practice, about three-fourths of all patients with AAAs are asymptomatic at the time of initial diagnosis. Aneurysms are commonly diagnosed during routine physical examination when an otherwise asymptomatic pulsatile epigastric mass is discovered. Patients often find such masses and seek medical attention. Radiographic examinations performed for other reasons also frequently detect aneurysms. The widespread use of abdominal ultrasonography and CT scanning has increased detection of smaller AAAs.

8. Do any patients develop symptoms from AAAs?

Vague abdominal pain is the most common complaint described by patients with symptoms from AAAs. Rapid expansion may cause more intense pain, probably from stretching of the overlying peritoneum. Pain is typically constant or throbbing and located in the epigastrium. Encroachment by an aneurysm on adjacent structures may produce various symptoms. Vertebral body erosion is usually associated with large aneurysms causing severe back pain. Gastrointestinal symptoms, including early satiety, nausea, and weight loss, may indicate intestinal compression. Hydronephrosis may occur from ureteral compression. Ureteral obstruction may produce flank pain that radiates into the groin and is occasionally associated with pyelonephritis. Mural thrombus within the aneurysm may embolize and produce acute lower extremity ischemia. Rare presentations include thrombosis with profound lower extremity ischemia and aortocaval fistulas producing acute congestive heart failure. Another unusual manifestation is primary aortoenteric fistula, which results from erosion of an aneurysm into the third portion of the duodenum.

9. Why operate on AAAs?

Rupture of an abdominal aortic aneurysm is the most feared complication. Most patients have no premonitory symptoms. Aneurysms often go undetected until sudden rupture prompts discovery because of dramatic symptoms and signs (see chapter 68). Patients with ruptured aneurysm often present in extremis; despite rapid operative intervention, the mortality rate exceeds 50%.

10. When should AAAs be repaired?

The decision to operate on a patient with an AAA requires that the risk of death from the aneurysm exceeds the risk of surgery. According to the law of Laplace, wall tension is proportional to the diameter of the vessel. Thus, larger aneurysms rupture more frequently than smaller ones. Based on old natural history studies, small aneurysms do rupture, but rarely. Available data, subject to numerous limitations, suggest that aneurysms between 5 cm and 5.9 cm have a 5-year rupture rate of about 25%. For aneurysms of 6 cm, the 5-year rupture rate is approximately 35%; for aneurysms 7 cm or larger, the 5-year rupture rate exceeds 75%. There are insufficient data upon which to estimate accurately the risk of rupture in aneurysms less than 5 cm.

11. What is the risk of elective aneurysm surgery?
The risk of elective aneurysm surgery depends on the physiologic status of the patient. Surgical risk is increased significantly by the presence of cardiac disease, recent myocardial infarction, evidence of atherosclerotic disease elsewhere, hypertension, decreased renal function, and chronic obstructive pulmonary disease. Chronologic age is not as important as physiologic age in determining the risk of surgery. Octogenarians can safely undergo the operation. Recent series commonly report elective mortality rates of 2–5%.

12. Do all aneurysms eventually expand and rupture?
Numerous studies have reported mean expansion rates ranging from 0.2–0.8 cm/year, for an average rate of expansion of about 0.4 cm/year. Larger aneurysms generally expand more rapidly. Some aneurysms may remain stable for long periods, exhibiting little or no enlargement, whereas others undergo progressive expansion. The single factor that consistently correlates with aneurysm expansion and rupture is the size of the aneurysm. Additional factors that may favor expansion are hypertension, obstructive pulmonary disease, and renal insufficiency.

13. How is the diagnosis of AAA best established?
The accuracy of physical examination varies widely. In thin patients, aneurysms are more easily detectable. Ultrasonography is the preferred method for evaluating suspected AAAs. CT scans and MRI also effectively image aneurysms, but they are much more expensive. Arteriography notoriously underestimates or misses aneurysms because of laminated thrombus within the aneurysm walls.

14. What preoperative studies are required for AAAs?
Contrast-enhanced CT scans are best for preoperative assessment of AAAs; they provide both accurate measurements and important architectural information. Relationship of the AAA to surrounding structures is well-delineated by CT. Major venous and renal abnormalities are accurately defined preoperatively. Iliac aneurysms, which are present in at least 20% of cases, are also correctly identified. Aortography is used routinely by some surgeons, whereas others obtain aortograms for aneurysms only in specific circumstances.

15. What does surgery involve?
Temporary clamping of the abdominal aorta and replacement of the abdominal aorta and iliac arteries are required for interposition grafting with prosthetic material. Because 90% of AAAs are infrarenal, clamps are usually placed below the renal arteries. Prosthetic material may be woven or knitted Dacron graft or polytetrafluoroethylene (PTFE). Anatomic considerations dictate whether the distal anastomosis is made to the lower abdominal aorta, iliac arteries, or femoral arteries.

16. What complications occur after AAA repair?
Although the mortality rate associated with elective AAA repair has declined to less than 5%, major morbidity is still common. Complications include myocardial infarction, congestive heart failure, renal insufficiency, pulmonary insufficiency, ischemic colitis, limb ischemia, graft thrombosis, wound infection, stroke, and paraplegia.

17. What are the late complications of aortic aneurysm surgery?
Late complications, which occur in up to 10% of patients, include anastomotic aneurysm, aortoenteric fistula, graft limb occlusion, and infection.

18. What are the alternatives to operative management of AAAs in high-risk patients?
Before development of current operative techniques, nonresective operations, including aneurysm ligation and wrapping and attempts at inducing aneurysm thrombosis yielded uniformly dismal results. Smaller aneurysms in high-risk patients should be followed with ultrasound or CT scan. Alternatively, axillobifemoral grafting and inducement of thrombosis of aneurysms with either ligation of outflow or ligation of the neck of the aneurysm have been moderately successful.

19. What are the future therapeutic options for AAAs?

The concept of repairing AAAs with an endoprosthesis introduced into the aorta through the femoral or external iliac arteries has quickly progressed to early clinical trials. Currently, at least seven different delivery systems are under development. The basic principle of endoluminal repair involves expansion of a graft within an aneurysm through a femoral cutdown. An expandable metal stent is used to anchor the proximal end of the intraluminal graft in position in the infrarenal aorta. The distal end of the graft may or may not be stented. As yet, it is uncertain how durable such procedures will be.

BIBLIOGRAPHY

1. Adamson J, Powell JT, Greenhalgh RM: Selection for screening for familial aortic aneurysms. Br J Surg 79:897, 1992.
2. Brown PM, Pattenden R, Gutelius JR: The selective management of small abdominal aortic aneurysms: The Kingston study. J Vasc Surg 15:21, 1992.
3. Cronenwett JL, Sargent SK, Wall MH, et al: Variables that affect the expansion rate and outcome of small abdominal aortic aneurysms. J Vasc Surg 11:260, 1990.
4. Drott C, Arfvidsson B, Ortenwall P, et al: Age-standardized incidence of ruptured aortic aneurysm in a defined Swedish population between 1952 and 1988: Mortality rate and operative results. Br J Surg 79:175, 1992.
5. Ernst CB: Abdominal aortic aneurysm. N Engl J Med 328:1167, 1993.
6. Farkas J, Fichelle J, Laurian C, et al: Long-term followup of positive cultures in 500 abdominal aortic aneurysms. Arch Surg 128:284, 1993.
7. Hollier LH, Taylor LM, Ochsner J: Recommended indications for operative treatment of abdominal aortic aneurysms. J Vasc Surg 15:1046, 1992.
8. Katz DA, Littenberg B, Cronenwett JL: Management of small abdominal aortic aneurysms: Early surgery vs. watchful waiting. JAMA 268:2678, 1992.
9. Krupski WC: Abdominal aortic aneurysm: Defining the dilemma. Semin Vasc Surg 8:115, 1995.
10. Lazarus HM: Endovascular grafting for the treatment of abdominal aortic aneurysm. Surg Clin North Am 72:959, 1992.
11. Lee B, Godfrey M, Vitale E, et al: Linkage of Marfan syndrome and a phenotypically related disorder to two different fibrillin genes. Nature 352:330, 1991.
12. Mesh CL, Baxter BT, Pearce WH, et al: Collagen and elastin gene expression in aortic aneurysms. Surgery 112:256, 1992.
13. Mitchell MB, Rutherford RB, Krupski WC: Infrarenal aortic aneurysms. In Rutherford RB (ed): Vascular Surgery, 4th ed. Philadelphia, W.B. Saunders, 1995, p 1032.
14. Olscn PS, Schroeder T, Agerskov K, et al: Surgery for abdominal aortic aneurysms: A survey of 656 patients. J Cardiovasc Surg 32:636, 1991.
15. Ouriel K, Green JRM, Donayre C, et al: An evaluation of new methods of expressing aortic aneurysm size; relationship to rupture. J Vasc Surg 15:12, 1992.
16. Todd GJ, Nowygrod R, Benvenisty A, et al: The accuracy of CT scanning in the diagnosis of abdominal and thoracoabdominal aortic aneurysms. J Vasc Surg 13:302, 1991.

68. RUPTURED ABDOMINAL AORTIC ANEURYSM

William C. Krupski, M.D.

1. How often do abdominal aortic aneurysms (AAAs) rupture?

Ruptured AAAs are the fifteenth leading cause of death in the United States. The incidence of ruptured AAAs has increased in the last three decades. In England, ruptured AAAs caused death in 22 per 100,000 men aged 60–64 and 177 per 100,000 men aged 80–84.

2. What is the difference between ruptured aneurysm, leaking aneurysm, and dissecting aneurysm?

When the integrity of the arterial wall of a AAA is lost, blood extravasates first into the retroperiteum and later freely into the peritoneal cavity. The terms **leaking** and **ruptured** AAA are essentially synonymous. The term **dissecting** aneurysm is misleading. Spontaneous dissections occur when blood "takes a wrong turn" between the layers of the media of a blood vessel. It occurs most frequently in the thoracic aorta and gives rise to a multitude of symptoms, primarily severe pain associated with hypertension. Dissection can later lead to aneurysmal enlargement of the blood vessel near the same location. However, it is unusual for a dissection to occur in a preexistent aneurysm.

3. How does a ruptured AAA most commonly manifest?

The fundamental clinical triad of a ruptured AAA consists of (1) abdominal or back pain of sudden onset, (2) hypotension, and (3) a pulsatile abdominal mass. Unfortunately, the complete triad is present in only about one-half of patients.

4. What physical findings are associated with a ruptured AAA?

A pulsatile abdominal mass is a helpful clue to the diagnosis but is present in only one-half of patients with ruptured AAAs. In obese patients, the aneurysm may not be palpable. Abdominal distention is frequently present, caused by retroperitoneal or intraperitoneal hematoma, intraperitoneal bleeding, or secondary ileus. Lateral and distal extension of the retroperitoneal hematoma may result in ecchymoses and discoloration of the flank, groin, scrotum, or penis.

5. What diagnostic tests should be obtained?

The diagnosis of ruptured AAA should be based on clinical presentation. Diagnostic tests should be kept to a minimum. If the clinical signs and symptoms are not sufficient to confirm the diagnosis of ruptured AAA, a few studies are permissible if performed simultaneously with initial resuscitation.

6. What is the best emergency study in a stable patient?

Emergency B-mode ultrasound imaging confirms the presence of AAAs but rarely shows extravasated blood. If the diagnosis is uncertain and the patient has been hemodynamically stable, CT may be performed under vigilant supervision. **CT scan should be performed only in hemodynamically stable patients.**

7. Should the patient be resuscitated?

Resuscitation of hypotensive patients with ruptured AAA should be initiated during rapid prehospital transport by paramedics. During the initial physical examination after arrival at the emergency room, large-bore catheters are placed in peripheral veins, and blood is sent for cross-matching and routine tests. The ideal amount of intravenous fluids infused in hypotensive patients is controversial. Most authorities recommend elevating systemic blood pressure only to 80–100 mmHg, because additional increases in pressure may contribute to more blood loss through the ruptured aorta. An arterial line to monitor blood pressure and a urinary catheter to monitor urine output should be placed. A chest radiograph and electrocardiogram are performed if time allows.

8. What is the correct surgical technique for repair of ruptured AAAs?

The patient with a ruptured AAA should be transported from the emergency room to the operating room without delay. Anesthesia is not induced until the skin of the chest, abdomen, and groin is prepared and sterile drapes are applied. Control of the proximal aorta should be obtained by the most experienced vascular surgeon. The abdominal aorta can be isolated at the level of the diaphragm or at the infrarenal segment. Rapid control of the upper abdominal aorta below the diaphragm should be obtained if the patient is unstable, if there is free intraperitoneal bleeding, or if the retroperitoneal hematoma extends superiorly to the level of the left renal vein. Alternatively, some authorities recommend controlling the proximal aorta through a left thoracotomy or by intraluminal placement of a Fogarty balloon catheter introduced either through a direct cutdown of the brachial artery or through the ruptured aneurysm.

9. What is the most common technical misadventure in the repair of ruptured AAAs?
Use of excessive haste in obtaining proximal control of the aorta or imprudent dissection of the iliac arteries may result in associated injuries to the inferior vena cava or iliac veins. Venous injuries are much more difficult to control than arterial injuries and may result in massive bleeding with subsequent coagulopathy.

10. What is the best graft material for repair of ruptured AAAs?
Woven Dacron or polytetrafluoroethylene (PTFE) is best used to avoid bleeding through the graft. The use of heparin for repair of ruptured AAAs is controversial. There is no time to preclot a standard knitted graft, but a knitted graft impregnated with collagen or albumin is a good alternative to woven Dacron grafts.

11. What are the most common postoperative complications of ruptured AAAs?
In order of decreasing frequency, the most common complications are respiratory failure, renal failure, sepsis, cardiac failure, bleeding, stroke, ischemic colitis, and lower extremity ischemia. Paraplegia and paraparesis are extremely unusual.

12. Why has the mortality rate of ruptured AAAs remained high, even in modern series?
The persistently high mortality rate can be attributed to several factors, including improved prehospital care and rapid transport and advanced age of the population with multiple cardiovascular risk factors.

13. What clinical variables are associated with the increased mortality?
The available experience from collected series suggests that patients with preoperative cardiac arrest and profound hypotension on admission and immediately before operation have the poorest likelihood of survival. Patients over 80 years of age also have an excessive death rate.

BIBLIOGRAPHY

1. Durham SJ, Steed DL, Moosa HH, et al: Probability of rupture of an abdominal aortic aneurysm after an unrelated operative procedure: A prospective study. J Vasc Surg 13:248, 1991.
2. Gloviczki P, Pairolero PC, Mucha P, et al: Ruptured abdominal aortic aneurysms: Repair should not be denied. J Vasc Surg 15:851, 1991.
3. Gloviczki P: Ruptured abdominal aortic aneurysms. In Rutherford RB: Vascular Surgery, 4th ed. Philadelphia, W.B. Saunders, 1995, p 1060.
4. Harris LM, Faggioli GL, Fiedler R, et al: Ruptured abdominal aortic aneurysms: Factors affecting mortality rates. J Vasc Surg 14:812, 1991.
5. Johansen K, Kohler RT, Nicholls SC, et al: Ruptured abdominal aortic aneurysm: The Harborview experience. J Vasc Surg 13:240, 1991.
6. Marston WA, Ahlquist R, Johnson G, et al: Misdiagnosis of ruptured abdominal aortic aneurysm. J Vasc Surg 16:17, 1992.
7. Meissner MH, Johansen KH: Colon infarction after ruptured abdominal aortic aneurysm. Arch Surg 127:979, 1992.
8. Ouriel K, Geary K, Green RM, et al: Factors determining survival after ruptured aortic aneurysm: The hospital, the surgeon, and the patient. J Vasc Surg 11:493, 1990.

69. VENOUS DISEASE

Thomas A. Whitehill, M.D., and Robert B. Rutherford, M.D.

1. Where does deep venous thrombosis (DVT) originate?
Over 95% of DVTs develop in the veins of the lower extremities; the majority originate in the valve sinuses of the calf veins.

2. What is the source of pulmonary emboli?

Calf vein thrombosis may propagate proximally into the deep venous system to involve the popliteal, femoral, and/or iliac veins. These proximal DVTs are the source of over 90% of pulmonary emboli. Solitary calf vein thrombosis is rarely the source of symptomatic pulmonary emboli.

3. What is Virchow's triad?

Virchow's triad defines the three factors that are necessary for venous thrombosis and pulmonary embolism: hypercoagulability, disruption of an intact venous intimal lining, and stasis of venous blood flow. In the majority of patients with DVT, at least two of these three components are operative.

4. What risk factors are associated with hypercoagulability?

Malignancy (especially of the pancreas, genitourinary tract, stomach, lung, colon, and breast)
Age greater than 40
Female sex
Obesity
Previous history of venous thrombosis or pulmonary embolism
Operative procedures
Pregnancy
Oral contraceptive use in premenopausal women
Nephrotic syndrome
Blood group A
History of smoking
Diabetes

5. What are the common procoagulant syndromes that increase the risk of thrombosis?

Heparin-associated thrombocytopenia
Antithrombin III deficiency
Protein C deficiency
Protein S deficiency
Dysfibrinogenemia
Lupus anticoagulant
Antiphospholipid antibodies
Abnormalities of fibrinolysis

6. What causes venous intimal injury?

Venous intimal changes may be secondary to vein wall trauma, infection, inflammation, indwelling catheters, or surgery. Venodilation during anesthesia and surgery may produce microscopic intimal tears as well as stasis. The injured venous intima initiates the release of thromboplastic substances that activate the coagulation cascade. Such endothelial denudation also facilitates platelet adhesion to the exposed collagen and basement membrane components, thus forming a nidus for further thrombus formation.

7. What causes stasis of venous blood flow?

Venostasis is common in surgical patients; it occurs during anesthesia, after certain types of trauma, and with perioperative immobility.

8. What signs and symptoms are suggestive of DVT? How can DVT be accurately diagnosed?

DVT may cause tenderness, increased skin temperature, edema, superficial venous dilation, and calf or thigh pain. None of these symptoms is specific for DVT. Even the well-known Homan's sign (calf pain on dorsiflexion of the foot) is quite unreliable. The overall accuracy of clinical diagnosis is close to 50%. Two noninvasive vascular tests—Doppler ultrasound examination and impedance plethysmography (IPG)—detect DVT proximal to the calf veins with over 90% accuracy when used together; unfortunately, they are not sensitive in detecting calf vein DVT.

9. What measures should be used for DVT prophylaxis? In which surgical patients?
Extensive evidence supports the use of DVT prophylaxis in the subset of patients who are over 40 years of age and scheduled for major general or orthopedic procedures. Other conditions are less well studied, but prophylaxis should be applied liberally. The best prophylaxis for DVT includes preoperative activity and early postoperative ambulation. No current regimen provides total protection. Intermittent pneumatic compression stockings and/or low-dose heparin is commonly used.

10. What is low-dose heparin? How does heparin work?
Heparin binds to antithrombin III [AT III], rendering it more active. Low-dose heparin (5000 units administered subcutaneously every 8–12 hours until the patient is fully ambulatory) activates AT III, inhibits platelet aggregation, and decreases availability of thrombin. The use of low-dose heparin has been disappointing in hip, pelvic, and prostate surgery. High-risk patients who cannot receive anticoagulation (e.g., patients with history of abnormal bleeding, recent peptic ulcer or esophageal bleeding, or recent intraocular or intracranial bleeding) should be given intermittent pneumatic compression stockings and elastic compression stockings.

11. What does dextran do?
Dextran reduces thrombotic events by decreasing blood thrombogenicity (platelet-endothelium factor VIII interaction) and viscosity and improves venous flow by expanding plasma volume.

12. What are antiplatelet drugs?
Antiplatelet drugs—aspirin and dipyridamole—interfere with platelet deposition, which is the key to DVT formation. However, antiplatelet drugs are ineffective once thrombus formation has been initiated and, generally, are not of much clinical value unless combined with intermittent pneumatic compression stockings. Low-dose sodium warfarin (Coumadin) may confer protection equal to low-dose heparin; its use in nonorthopedic operations has not been extensively studied.

13. What are the characteristics of chronic venous insufficiency and the postphlebitic syndrome?
The primary consequence of DVT is venous valvular incompetence with resultant distal ambulatory venous hypertension. After DVT, involved venous segments eventually recanalize to some degree. However, their delicate valves remain scarred or trapped by residual organized thrombus. The result is a patent but valveless venous segment with a gravitational pressure equal to an open blood column extending from the heart to the ankles. In addition, the loss of valvular function disables the venomotor pump. The vein walls become thicker and less compliant, impeding proximal blood flow. These factors result in distal venous hypertension whenever the patient is not recumbent. Elevated deep venous pressure is transmitted to the superficial tissues of the calf through incompetent perforator veins. Therefore, the location of the perforating veins often determines the location of stasis ulceration. Protein-rich fluids, fibrin, and red blood cells are extravasated and deposited through large pores in the distended microcirculation during periods of venous hypertension. This leads to inflammation, scarring, fibrosis of the subcutaneous tissues, and discoloration by hemosiderin deposition. The resultant inflammatory reaction, scarring, and interstitial edema create a further barrier to capillary flow and diffusion of oxygen; adequate nutrition to the skin is inhibited. With restricted capillary inflow, shunts may open that bypass the skin, leading to further steal of nutrition. Such changes may lead to tissue atrophy and ulceration (venous stasis ulcer).

14. Do all patients with DVT develop the postphlebitic syndrome? What is the treatment of postphlebitic syndrome?
It was generally believed that one-half of patients with DVT develop stasis dermatitis in 5 years and the other half in 10 years. However, more recent epidemiologic studies suggest that the incidence of venous ulceration is much lower—closer to 5%. As many as 1 in 5 patients have no symptoms and maintain normal noninvasive vascular test data. The median time for the appearance of a first stasis ulcer is 2½ years.

With proper patient education and compliance, postphlebitic stasis sequelae may be controlled by nonoperative means in well over 90% of patients, particularly if no residual venous outflow obstruction complicates valvular incompetence. Nonoperative treatment consists of graded elastic support stockings to retard swelling and periodic leg elevation during the day. Patients must be instructed to elevate their legs above the heart (big toe above the nose) at regular intervals (e.g., 10–15 minutes every 2 hours) and be warned that elastic stockings alone retard rather than prevent swelling.

15. Distinguish between phlegmasia alba dolens and phlegmasia cerulea dolens.

The two terms apply to the two clinical extremes of the progression of the same condition—iliofemoral venous thrombosis. Iliofemoral thrombosis is characterized by unilateral pain and edema of an entire lower extremity, discoloration, and groin tenderness. Three-fourths of the cases of iliofemoral venous thrombosis occur on the left side, presumably because of compression of the left common iliac vein by the overlying right common iliac artery. In phlegmasia alba dolens (literally, painful white swelling), the leg becomes pale and white. Arterial pulses remain normal. Progressive thrombosis may occur, with resultant propagation proximally or distally and into neighboring tributaries that function as collaterals. This stage, at which the entire leg becomes both strikingly edematous and also mottled or cyanotic, is called phlegmasia cerulea dolens (literally, painful purple swelling). Phlegmasia cerulea dolens is seen in 5% of all patients with iliofemoral venous thrombosis and may ultimately lead to compartment syndrome and/or venous gangrene. When venous outflow is seriously impeded, arterial inflow may secondarily be reduced by as much as 30%. Arterial pulsations may be faint. Edema is marked. Limb loss is a serious concern; aggressive management (venous thrombectomy and/or catheter-directed lytic therapy) is necessary.

16. What is venous claudication?

When venous recanalization fails to occur after iliofemoral venous thrombosis, venous collaterals develop to bypass the obstruction to venous outflow. These collaterals usually suffice when the patient is at rest. However, any leg exercise induces increased arterial inflow, which may exceed the capacity of the venous collateral bed and result in progressive venous hypertension. The pressure build-up in the venous system results in calf pain commonly described as tight, heavy, and/or bursting—venous claudication. Relief is obtained with rest and elevation but is not as prompt as with arterial claudication.

17. How can one distinguish primary varicose veins, associated with a normal deep venous system, from secondary varicose veins that result from a diseased deep venous system (e.g., postphlebitic syndrome)?

Primary varicose veins result from uncomplicated saphenofemoral venous valvular incompetence and have a greater saphenous distribution, a positive tourniquet test, no stasis sequelae (dermatitis or ulceration), and no morning ankle edema (lymphedema). **Secondary varicose veins** usually result from deep and perforator venous incompetence secondary to postphlebitic syndrome. Primary varicose veins may lead ultimately to stasis sequelae, even ulceration, because of retrograde flow down the superficial system and back into the deep system via perforating veins. At this end stage, the appearance may be indistinguishable from the postphlebitic syndrome, but the history is quite different.

18. Why do people develop primary varicose veins?

The most common cause is congenital absence of venous valves proximal to the saphenofemoral junction. Normally there are no valves in the vena cava or common iliac veins and only an occasional valve in the external iliac veins. Thus the sentinel valve in the common femoral vein just above the saphenofemoral junction is of critical importance. However, anatomic studies reveal that the sentinel valve is absent on one or the other side in 30% of patients. This alone does not guarantee the development of varicose veins but makes the system susceptible to breakdown under conditions that increase venous back pressure (e.g., pregnancy). Prolonged proximal saphenous vein distention causes sequential distal valvular incompetence. When this process progresses into the thinner-walled tributaries, they become dilated and tortuous and result in varicose vein formation.

19. How, when, and in whom should varicose veins be treated?

Varicose veins that cause discomfort or serious cosmetic embarrassment require treatment. Better results are obtained with early treatment before continuous retrograde pressure and flow down the superficial system and into communicating perforating veins (whenever the patient is standing) cause secondary, irreversible perforator incompetence. High saphenous vein ligation at an early stage arrests progression of this gravitation process. The varicosities can then be managed by selective surgical stripping and/or sclerotherapy. Sclerotherapy is better suited for control of smaller tributary varicosities.

BIBLIOGRAPHY

1. Cordts PR, Hanrahan LM, Rodriguez AA, et al: A prospective randomized trial of Unna's boot versus Duoderm CGF hydroactive dressing plus compression in the management of venous leg ulcers. J Vasc Surg 15:480–486, 1992.
2. Cordts PR, Hartano C, LaMorte WW, et al: Physiologic similarities between extremities with varicose veins and with chronic venous insufficiency utilizing air plethysmography. Am J Surg 164:260–264, 1992.
3. Heijboer H, Brandjes DPM, Buller H, et al: Deficiencies of coagulation-inhibiting and fibrinolytic proteins in outpatients with deep vein thrombosis. N Engl J Med 323:1512–1516, 1990.
4. Hull R, Raskub G, Pineo G, et al: A comparison of subcutaneous low-molecular-weight heparin with warfarin sodium for prophylaxis against deep-venous thrombosis after hip or knee implantation. N Engl J Med 329:1370–1376, 1993.
5. Markel A, Manzo RA, Bergelin RO, et al: Valvular reflux after deep vein thrombosis: Incidence and time of occurrence. J Vasc Surg 15:377–384, 1992.
6. Raju S, Fredericks R: Venous obstruction: An analysis of 137 cases with hemodynamic, venographic and clinical correlations. J Vasc Surg 14:305–313, 1991.

70. NONINVASIVE VASCULAR DIAGNOSTIC LABORATORY

Darrell N. Jones, Ph.D.

1. What is the role of the vascular diagnostic laboratory in the assessment and treatment of patients with suspected vascular disease?

Although traditional evaluation by an experienced clinician remains the foundation of vascular diagnosis, clinical assessment has its limitations. For example, only one-third of cervical bruits are associated with significant carotid artery disease; conversely, as many as two-thirds of patients with severe carotid disease present without a cervical bruit. One-half of patients with extensive deep venous thrombosis of the lower extremity lack signs and symptoms referable to the lower extremities, whereas more than one-half of patients presenting with clinical signs of DVT are venographically normal. As many as 40% of diabetic patients with abnormal clinical diagnosis have no peripheral arterial occlusive disease.

The vascular diagnostic laboratory (VDL) provides objective and quantitative data to identify and assess the severity of extracranial cerebrovascular disease, peripheral arterial occlusive disease, and acute and chronic venous disease. The VDL provides quantitative assessment of the disease status and functional status of the patient both in disease progression and in response to medical and surgical therapy.

2. What differentiates the VDL from diagnostic radiology and ultrasound?
In addition to its obviously specialized focus, the VDL provides **functional information** rather than or in addition to the morphologic data provided by radiology tests and general ultrasound images. This information is particularly important for peripheral arterial occlusive disease, in which anatomic information about the site of stenosis or occlusion is of limited value without knowledge of the functional significance.

CEREBROVASCULAR DISEASE

3. Which noninvasive tests should be used to diagnose extracranial carotid artery disease?
Duplex ultrasound has a sensitivity of approximately 97–99% in detecting carotid artery disease and an accuracy of 90–95% in correctly classifying carotid stenoses with greater than 50% reduction in diameter. No other noninvasive test has comparable accuracy.

4. What is duplex ultrasound?
Duplex ultrasound uses both image and velocity data (hence the name duplex) in a nearly simultaneous presentation of ultrasound echo images (B-mode ultrasound) and blood velocity waveforms obtained by Doppler ultrasound. The Doppler signals in a duplex ultrasound presentation are obtained from a single small region of the blood vessel using pulsed Doppler. With the sacrifice of precision, velocities can be estimated for many such regions over a large area of the blood vessel at the same time. By assigning colors to the average velocity in each such small region and displaying the colors as part of the echo image, blood flow can be represented. Such a presentation, called colorflow duplex ultrasound, aids the duplex examination but cannot replace the information obtained from the Doppler velocity waveform.

5. Why is blood velocity important in assessing the degree of carotid artery stenosis?
It is often difficult to measure accurately the residual arterial lumen on a B-mode ultrasound image, because the acoustic properties (and hence the image) of noncalcified plaque, thrombus, and flowing blood may be similar. However, the hemodynamic changes produced by arterial narrowing can be used to characterize the degree of narrowing. Current practice classifies the degree of internal carotid stenosis into categorical ranges based entirely on the Doppler velocity data.

6. What are the velocity criteria and categorical ranges of the degree of carotid artery stenosis?
The criteria developed at the University of Washington are the most widely accepted:

0% stenosis	Peak systolic velocity < 125 cm/sec and no velocity disturbance
1–15%	Peak systolic velocity < 125 cm/sec with turbulence during systolic deceleration
16–49%	Peak systolic velocity < 125 cm/sec with turbulence in the entire cardiac cycle
50–79%	Peak systolic velocity > 125 cm/sec and diastolic velocity < 140 cm/sec
80–99%	Diastolic velocity > 140 cm/sec
100%	Absent flow velocity signal

The category greater than 80% has been termed critical stenosis because of the high rate of disease progression and high incidence of neurologic symptoms for patients in this category.

VENOUS DISEASE

7. What noninvasive test is used to diagnose acute deep venous thrombosis (DVT)?
Duplex ultrasound has replaced venous occlusion plethysmography as the accepted standard. Imaging ultrasound is sometimes used alone but has less accuracy. Colorflow duplex is useful because it helps to identify small veins from the muscle and fascial layers. The ultrasound assessment involves the following steps:

1. Examine the vein for echogenic thrombus.
2. Compress the vein, using pressure on the ultrasound probe, and look for complete collapse. Inability to compress the vein suggests thrombosis. Partial compression suggests partial thrombosis.
3. Obtain a Doppler signal from the vein. A signal that is phasic with respiration suggests no proximal occlusive thrombus. A signal that is spontaneously present but nonphasic suggests flow around an occlusion via small collateral veins. Absence of a Doppler signal in the vein suggests absence of flow, but smaller veins often have no spontaneous flow and distal compression is required to force the venous blood cephalad.

8. Does venous occlusion plethysmography still have a role in the assessment of DVT?
Yes. Venous occlusion plethysmography or impedance plethysmography (IPG) has high sensitivity and specificity for detection of occlusive thrombi above the knee and particularly for iliofemoral occlusive thrombi (95%). Because IPG provides functional information about deep venous outflow from the legs, it provides diagnosis of nonvisualized caval or iliac thrombosis, diagnosis of recurrent acute proximal thrombosis superimposed on chronic thrombosis, and functional evaluation of residual or chronic outflow obstruction.

9. What is IPG?
IPG is the most widely used modality of venous occlusion plethysmography. Changes in calf volume are measured first during tourniquet occlusion of the deep thigh veins and then with release of the tourniquet (pneumatic cuff). The volume change is estimated from electrical impedance changes secondary to vein filling. Other forms of plethysmography have used air cuffs or strain-gauges to measure the calf volume. Reduced filling or volume increase and delayed outflow are diagnostic of proximal venous obstruction.

10. What noninvasive tests are useful for evaluation of venous incompetence?
Doppler ultrasound is used to detect venous reflux in the deep veins of the legs and also in the greater and lesser saphenous veins. With experience, the test can be done using a simple Doppler (continuous wave vs. pulsed Doppler), but duplex ultrasound is often used to facilitate identification of the vein segments and valves and to position a pulsed Doppler sample reliably. Some laboratories measure the duration of reflux during controlled proximal compression as an indicator of severity of valve incompetence, but unless a valvuloplasty or valve transposition is planned for the identified incompetent valve, such specific measures appear to have little clinical utility. The functional evaluation of venous incompetence relies on plethysmographic measures of venous reflux to the lower leg, including photoplethysmography (PPG) and air plethysmography (APG).

11. How is PPG testing performed?
The PPG test of venous refilling time uses an infrared photoelectric cell to detect the presence of red blood cells in the cutaneous tissue of the lower medial calf (same physical principle as pulse oximetry). Venous emptying is achieved by repeated plantar- and dorsiflexion of the foot to contract the calf muscles, followed by relaxation during which cutaneous refilling normally occurs by arterial inflow over an interval of 25 seconds or more. Refilling at a faster rate occurs by venous reflux. The measurements of refilling time are repeated with tourniquets placed at the upper thigh, lower thigh, and upper calf to evaluate the contribution of perforator incompetence.

PERIPHERAL ARTERIAL OCCLUSIVE DISEASE

12. What is the primary test for diagnosis of lower extremity ischemia?
The primary test is the measurement of systolic ankle artery pressures and systolic brachial artery pressure. The ankle/brachial pressure ratio (ABI) should be greater than or equal to 1.0. Typically, Doppler ultrasound is used as the flow sensor distal to the pressure cuff, but plethysmographic instruments also may be used. Doppler signals are usually monitored at the posterior tibial artery or dorsalis pedis artery. The ABI is not only sensitive and specific for the diagnosis of peripheral arterial disease (PAD); it also accurately assesses the severity of disease.

13. What is gained by measuring pressures at limb levels other than the ankle?
Segmental limb pressure measurements (SLP), performed at the upper thigh, lower thigh, calf, and ankle, localize the arterial segment(s) involved in peripheral arterial occlusive disease.

14. What tests are used for assessing PAD in diabetic patients who may have incompressible arteries due to medial calcification?
Pulse volume recording (PVR) is a pneumoplethysmographic technique that tracks the changes in limb volume over the cardiac cycle. It measures the pressure changes in segmental pneumatic cuffs as a function of the limb volume changes. The relative PVR amplitudes identify the presence of PAD and localize the arterial segment involved. The PVR is unaffected by medial calcification.

Great toe pressure also may be used to diagnose and assess disease severity in diabetic patients, because medial calcification rarely affects the digital arteries.

15. How should patients with suspected intermittent claudication be evaluated?
The patient should first be evaluated by obtaining ankle pressure indices or segmental limb pressures at rest. The patient with ischemia at rest does not normally need further evaluation. The patient with mild arterial insufficiency at rest or even normal resting pressures should perform an exercise stress test (the standard is a treadmill test at 2 mph, 12% grade), followed by ankle pressure indices. The distance that the patient is able to walk allows assessment of the functional disability, and the postexercise reduction in ankle pressure (or lack thereof) allows assessment of whether the disability is due to arterial insufficiency rather than musculoskeletal or neurologic pain.

CONTROVERSIES

16. Can carotid endarterectomy be performed on the basis of duplex study alone?
The argument for elimination of arteriography in selected cases is persuasive, because the carotid arteriogram alone has a morbidity rate greater than 1%. This rate may represent 1/4 of the total morbidity usually associated with carotid endarterectomy. However, to realize the benefit of surgery based on duplex ultrasound, the duplex study must have a high positive predictive value. Fortunately, the PPV is high for severe lesions that meet suitably strict criteria (e.g., peak systolic velocities > 290 cm/sec and end-diastolic velocities > 80 cm/sec).

17. Does duplex ultrasound have a role in the diagnosis of PAD?
Its role is limited. Peripheral arterial disease must be assessed functionally, not anatomically. Duplex ultrasound can be used to localize disease that has already been assessed for its functional significance by SLPs and PVRs. Localization may be of importance if transluminal angioplasty is considered.

18. Does transcranial Doppler have a role in the noninvasive diagnosis of cerebrovascular disease?
No. Although the technique is widely touted, recent large studies show that the results of Doppler evaluation of intracranial arteries did not change the clinical management of any patient.

BIBLIOGRAPHY

1. Gerlock AJ, Giyanani VL, Krebs C: Applications of Noninvasive Vascular Techniques. Philadelphia, W.B. Saunders, 1988.
2. Journal of Vascular Technology. Vol 18(5), 1994 (Special Topics Issue).
3. Moneta GL, Edwards JM, Papanicolaou G, et al: Screening for asymptomatic internal carotid artery stenosis: Duplex criteria for discriminating 60% to 99% stenosis. J Vasc Surg 21:989–997, 1995.
4. Zierler RE: Arterial duplux scanning. In Rutherford RB (ed): Vascular Surgery, 4th ed. Philadelphia, W.B. Saunders, 1995, pp 120–130.
5. Zierler RE, Sumner DS: Physiologic assessment of peripheral arterial occlusive disease. In Rutherford RB (ed): Vascular Surgery, 4th ed. Philadelphia, W.B. Saunders, 1995, pp 65 117.

VIII. *Cardiothoracic Surgery*

71. CORONARY ARTERY DISEASE

Joseph C. Cleveland, Jr., M.D., and Alden H. Harken, M.D.

1. What causes angina?

Angina typically results from a reduction in coronary flow reserve to a portion of the myocardium. The fixed obstruction creates an imbalance in myocardial oxygen supply and demand, with demand exceeding supply.

The cause of angina is usually related to atherosclerotic coronary artery disease, which produces a relatively fixed obstruction to blood flow in a coronary artery. This fixed obstruction limits blood flow (oxygen supply) in the setting of increased oxygen demand. Thus, the classic patient experiences chest pain with physical exertion, after eating, or with increased sympathetic activity.

2. What are the determinants of myocardial oxygen demand?

Braunwald has identified nine independent determinants of myocardial oxygen demand in the laboratory. Clinically, heart rate, contractility, and wall tension (an enlarged heart requires extra oxygen as defined by the law of Laplace) are the major determinants of myocardial oxygen demand.

3. What are the treatment options for angina?

In general, angina can be treated medically or with an interventional procedure. The medical management of angina is based on the principle that most patients with coronary artery disease have a limitation in blood flow with a fixed oxygen supply. Therefore, medical treatment is directed toward reducing oxygen demand. Medical therapy includes **nitrates** (nitroglycerin, isosorbide), which may minimally dilate coronary arteries, but work predominantly through decreasing systemic afterload, thereby decreasing wall tension and contractility; **beta blockers**, which decrease heart rate and contractility; and **calcium channel antagonists**, which may decrease afterload and prevent coronary vasoconstriction.

If medical therapy is unsuccessful in alleviating angina, percutaneous transluminal coronary angioplasty (PTCA), atherectomy, or coronary artery bypass grafting (CABG) may be appropriate.

4. What are the indications for coronary artery bypass grafting (CABG)?

1. **Continued angina despite aggressive medical therapy**. When a patient has stable angina, with documented coronary artery disease that limits daily activities, CABG is indicated if operative risk is not prohibitive. Data from the Coronary Artery Surgery Study (CASS), which compared medical therapy with CABG for stable angina, show that patients treated with surgery have less chest pain, fewer activity limitations, and an objective increase in exercise tolerance compared with patients treated with medical therapy.

2. **Left main coronary stenosis.** A stenosis of greater than 50% involving the left main coronary artery is an independent predictor of poor outcome in medically treated patients. Because of the large portion of myocardium supplied by this artery, PTCA is too hazardous to treat this lesion. Even if the patient is asymptomatic, longevity is sufficiently improved by CABG to warrant intervention.

3. **Three-vessel coronary artery disease (CAD) with depressed left ventricular function.**
Left ventricular function has a dominant role in determining indications and prognosis for all
modes of therapy. Three-vessel coronary artery disease in combination with depressed ventricular function confers a much poorer long-term outlook in medically treated patients. Thus, in patients with depressed left ventricular function and three-vessel CAD, CABG has a favorable
effect on survival. A caveat, however, is that the operative risk increases markedly at ejection
fractions less than 0.30; therefore, operative intervention mandates careful consideration of the
risks and benefits of surgery.

4. **Complications of PTCA.** If an unsuccessful PTCA has resulted in hemodynamic instability or was performed because of unstable angina or ongoing myocardial infarction with hemodynamic instability, emergency CABG is indicated.

5. Does CABG improve myocardial function?

Yes. Segments of myocardium that are akinetic, hypokinetic, or dyskinetic (indicating dysfunction) before myocardial revascularization with CABG may have improved postoperative function
associated with increased regional perfusion. Investigations describing global systolic function
after CABG also suggest that CABG improves both systolic and diastolic function. Both observations lend credence to the concept of hibernating myocardium.

6. Is CABG useful in patients with congestive heart failure?

CABG is likely to improve congestive heart failure related to ischemic myocardial dysfunction.
However, if heart failure is the longstanding result of irreversibly nonviable myocardium, CABG
should not prove beneficial. The trick is determining whether the nonfunctional myocardium is
still alive (hibernating).

7. What is stunned myocardium? Are myocardial stunning and hibernation the same?

Stunning describes postischemic, reversible contractile dysfunction of myocardium that responds to inotropic agents. Although stunning originally was believed to be relevant only in laboratory animals, clinical situations such as thrombolytic therapy for myocardial infarction and
CABG have emphasized its importance in humans. The definition of stunning requires that the
contractile abnormality is completely reversible and that the dysfunctional myocardium has
normal or near-normal blood flow. Experimental observations point toward two mechanisms that
may account for stunning: (1) the generation of oxygen-derived free radicals, with subsequent
oxidative injury (the oxyradical hypothesis), and (2) impaired calcium homeostasis, which results in increased intracellular calcium and leads to excitation-contraction uncoupling or decreased myofilament response to calcium (the calcium hypothesis).

It is important to differentiate stunning from hibernation. **Hibernation**, as originally described by Braunwald, refers to myocardial contractile dysfunction associated with a decrease in
coronary flow but preserved myocardial viability. The mechanisms of hibernation are less well
explored than the mechanisms of stunning, but hibernation is thought to be a teleologic mechanism that affords myocardial viability in the setting of reduced flow.

8. What is reperfusion injury?

Reperfusion injury constitutes a spectrum of events, including reperfusion arrhythmias, vascular
damage, myocardial stunning, acceleration of necrosis in cells nonlethally injured by ischemia,
and acceleration of necrosis in cells already irreversibly injured by ischemia. The pathogenesis
of reperfusion injury relates to the metabolic changes initiated during myocardial ischemia. A
hypothesis derived from several laboratory investigations links reperfusion injury to calcium
overload. Essentially, ischemia shifts the myocardium to anaerobic metabolism, which, in turn,
generates lactic acid. To deal with a progressive intracellular acidosis, a complex series of ionic
compensations occur. The myocyte pumps out hydrogen ions (acid) in exchange for sodium
ions. The sodium ions accumulate and, with the initiation of reperfusion, are exchanged for calcium. This calcium overload triggers alterations in mitochondrial energy utilization, sticks the

actin and myosin filaments together in contracture, and may generate oxygen free radicals through activation of membrane proteases. Thus, the initial reperfusion process can be highly destructive.

9. Is CABG valuable in preventing ventricular arrhythmias?
No. Most ventricular arrhythmias in patients with CAD derive from the borderline of irritable myocardium between well-perfused muscle and nonviable scar. Intuitively, CABG should restore flow and suppress arrhythmias. To everyone's disappointment, it does not seem to work that way.

10. Are PTCA and CABG equivalent?
Three of the five randomized clinical trials comparing PTCA with CABG—the Emory Angioplasty vs. Surgery Trial (EAST), the German Angioplasty Bypass Surgery Investigation (GABI), and the Randomized Intervention Treatment of Angina (RITA)—have reported interim results. Fewer than 8% of potential patients were randomized in any of these trials; most patients were excluded because they were not deemed candidates for PTCA by the cardiologists (due to total coronary occlusion or extensive coronary artery disease).

Nevertheless, the results illustrate important differences between two therapies. The procedure related mortality of patients with multivessel disease undergoing CABG and PTCA was equivalent (roughly 1% in both groups). CABG patients had a slightly higher rate of procedure-related myocardial infarction—8% vs. 2% in the PTCA group. Not surprisingly, CABG patients had a longer hospital stay than PTCA patients. However, the most striking findings pertain to the number of repeat interventions required in the PTCA group. Data from the EAST study show that at 3 years, over one-half (54%) of the PTCA patients required another intervention— either repeat PTCA or CABG. Conversely, 87% of the CABG group are free from repeat procedures at 3 years. Furthermore, the RITA trial indicates that at 2-year follow-up 66% of CABG patients were not taking antianginal medications compared with only 39% of PTCA patients. Lastly, surgery improves survival in the subset of patients with multivessel CAD and involvement of the left anterior descending artery or depressed ventricular function. Although PTCA may have a similar effect, its influence on survival in this group of patients still remains untested.

The unavoidable conclusion in directing therapy for patients is that the recommendation of PTCA or CABG must be individualized to each patient. Patients should be informed that CABG results in slightly higher initial morbidity than PTCA, but that CABG results in more effective and durable relief of angina with freedom from repeated procedures over a 2–3 year period in comparison with PTCA.

*Comparison of PTCA with CABG**

GROUP	SURVIVAL (%)	REPEAT PROCEDURES (%)	ANTIANGINAL MEDICATIONS (%)	PATENT VESSELS (%)	ANGINA (%)
PTCA	94	54	61	59	31
CABG	94	11	34	88	21

* Data presented in RITA and EAST investigations. Survival indicates percent of original number of patients surviving at 2 yrs; repeat procedures indicates percent of patients in each group that required either PTCA or CABG by 3 yrs; antianginal medications depicts percent of patients in each group still requiring at least 1 antianginal medication at 2 yrs: patent vessels refers to the percent of treated vessels remaining open at 3 yrs; and angina indicates the percent of patients still having angina at 2-yrs follow-up.

11. Is there a rule of thumb for vessel patency?
- Internal mammary (thoracic) bypass graft   90% patency at 10 years
- Saphenous vein bypass graft   70% patency at 10 years
- PTCA of stenotic vessel   60% patency at 6 months
- PTCA of totally occluded vessel   40% patency at 6 months

12. Does every patient with an acute myocardial infarction need a CABG procedure?

No. Although an acute myocardial infarction invariably indicates that coronary artery disease is present, CABG or PTCA is not absolutely indicated after a myocardial infarction. In fact, not everyone who has sustained a myocardial infarction undergoes cardiac catheterization. Either an exercise stress test or dipyridamole thallium test before hospital discharge can identify patients who have viable myocardium at risk. If tests are positive, cardiac catheterization appropriately sorts out potential therapy.

13. What is done in a CABG procedure?

CABG is an arterial bypass grafting procedure. A median sternotomy is performed with simultaneous removal of the greater saphenous vein. The left internal mammary artery (and occasionally the right internal mammary and gastroepiploic arteries) are completely mobilized. Cardiopulmonary bypass is established, and the saphenous vein is anastomosed from the ascending aorta to the coronary artery distal to the atherosclerotic obstruction. The left internal mammary artery is usually sewn only on the anterior surface of the heart—typically to the left anterior descending coronary artery. When all anastomoses are completed, the patient is weaned from cardiopulmonary bypass and the chest is closed.

14. What anatomic group of patients with coronary artery occlusive disease are at highest risk for postoperative problems?

Surprisingly, the number of diseased coronary arteries is not a factor in the risk of adverse outcome after CABG, provided that all vessels are revascularized at the time of surgery. Patients with diffuse disease, and poor run-off (diseased vascular beds that limit graft outflow) are at high risk for further problems. The dominant predictor of poor outcome remains depressed left ventricular function.

15. What technical problems are associated with CABG?

As is the case for most vascular procedures, the technical problems revolve around compromised proximal and distal anastomoses. If extensive atherosclerosis is present in either the aorta (proximal anastomosis) or coronary arteries (distal anastomosis), the anastomosis will be compromised and probably occlude. It is important to place the coronary anastomosis in a portion of the artery that is relatively free of atherosclerotic changes.

16. What are the risks of CABG?

Estimating operative risk is a critical component of developing operative therapy. Outcome has probably been analyzed more critically for CABG than for any other operation. The most comprehensive data for determining operative risk come from a large Veterans' Affairs database. Factors that increase the risk of CABG, in order of importance, are left ventricular ejection fraction, previous cardiac surgery, priority of operation (elective or emergent), New York Heart Association Function Class (NYHAFC), peripheral vascular disease, age, pulmonary rales, current diuretic use, and chronic obstructive pulmonary disease. Although the operative mortality rate of an elective CABG in patients with normal ventricular function was approximately 1% in the 1980s, the mortality rate of CABG has increased to roughly 3% in the 1990s. The explanation for this increase is not related to technical factors associated with CABG; rather, it reflects the older, sicker population that presently undergoes CABG. This observation makes a critical point about the shortcomings of raw mortality data. Surgeon A and surgeon B can perform identical operations but have very different raw mortality rates if surgeon A operates exclusively on triathletes and surgeon B exclusively on 2-pack-a-day cigarette-smoking couch potatoes.

17. What can be done if a patient cannot be weaned from cardiopulmonary bypass?

If a patient cannot maintain his or her own circulation without an external assist device (cardiopulmonary bypass), the surgeon in fact is treating shock. As with any kind of shock, management includes the following steps:

1. Replete volume until left- and right-sided filling pressures are adequate.

2. When intravascular volume is adequate, initiate pharmacologic support with inotropic agents. Commonly used agents include dobutamine, epinephrine, or amrinone.

3. When volume and drugs are insufficient, mechanical support devices, such as an intraaortic balloon or left and right ventricular assist devices, are used. Although once thought unimportant, the role of right ventricular failure in causing perioperative low cardiac output is now increasingly appreciated. Thus maintenance of arterial blood pH at ≥ 7.45 (alkalemia) and inhalation of nitric oxide hold promise as selective vasodilators (afterload reducers) in the pulmonary vascular circuit.

BIBLIOGRAPHY

1. Bolli R: Myocardial stunning in man. Circulation 86:1671, 1992.
2. Boylan MJ, Lytle BW, Loop FD, et al: Surgical treatment of isolated left anterior descending coronary stenosis. J Thorac Cardiovasc Surg 107:657–662, 1994.
3. Braunwald E, Rutherford JD; Reversible ischemic left ventricular dysfunction: Evidence for the hibernating myocardium. J Am Coll Cardiol 8:1467–1470, 1986.
4. CASS Principal Investigators, et al: Coronary artery surgery study (CASS): A randomized trial coronary artery bypass surgery: Quality of life data in patients randomly assigned to treatment groups. Circulation 68:951–960, 1983.
5. Doyle AR, Dhir AK, Moors AH, Latimer RD: Treatment of peri-operative low cardiac output syndrome. Ann Thorac Surg 59:S3–S11, 1995.
6. Grover FL, Hammermeister KE, Burchfiel C, Cardiac Surgeons of the Department of Veterans Affairs: Initial report of the Veterans Administration Preoperative Risk Assessment Study for Cardiac Surgery. Ann Thorac Surg 50:12–289, 1990.
7. Hamm CH, Reimers J, Ischinger T, and Investigators for the German Angioplasty Bypass Surgery Investigation: A randomized study of coronary angioplasty compared with bypass surgery in patients with symptomatic multivessel coronary disease. N Engl J Med 331:1037–1043, 1994.
8. Harken AH: The surgical treatment of cardiac arrhythmias. In Wilmore D, Harken AH, Holcraft J, Cheung L (eds): Scientific American Surgery. New York, Scientific American, 1993.
9. King SB, Lembo NJ, Weintraub WS, and Investigators for the Emory Angioplasty versus Surgery Trial (East): A randomized trial comparing coronary angioplasty with coronary bypass surgery. N Engl J Med 331:1044–1050, 1994.
10. Kirklin JW, Barratt-Boycs BG: Stenotic arteriosclerotic coronary artery disease. In Kirklin JW, Barratt-Boyes BG (eds): Cardiac Surgery, 2nd ed. New York, Churchill Livingstone, 1993, pp 285–383.
11. Lazar HL, Plehn JF, Schick EM, et al: Effects of coronary revascularization on regional wall motion. J Thorac Cardiovasc Surg 98:498–505, 1989.
12. Opie LH: Reperfusion injury and its pharmacologic modification. Circulation 80:12049–1062, 1989.
13. Rankin JS, Newman GE, Muhlbaier LH, et al: The effects of coronary revascularization on left ventricular function in ischemic heart disease. J Thorac Cardiovasc Surg 90:818–832, 1985.
14. RITA Trial Participants: Coronary angioplasty versus coronary artery bypass surgery: The randomised intervention treatment of angina (RITA) trial. Lancet 341:573–580, 1993.
15. Sonnenblick EH, Ross JR, Braunwald E: Oxygen consumption of the heart. Am J Cardiol 22:328–336, 1968.
16. Yusif S, Zucker D, Peduzzi P, et al: Effect of coronary artery bypass graft surgery on survival: Overview of 10-year results from randomised trials by the coronary artery bypass graft surgery trialists collaboration. Lancet 344:563–570, 1994.

72. MITRAL STENOSIS

Glenn J.R. Whitman, M.D., and David Fullerton, M.D.

1. What causes mitral stenosis?

By far the most common cause is rheumatic fever. Two-thirds of patients are female. Mitral stenosis usually does not develop for at least 10 years after acute rheumatic fever. Of all patients with rheumatic valvular disease, only one-third have pure mitral stenosis; the remainder have mitral regurgitation or combined mitral stenosis and mitral regurgitation. Rarely, mitral stenosis may result from collagen vascular diseases. Congenital stenosis is a rare lesion that is symptomatic in infancy; it is not an adult problem.

2. What is the pathophysiology of mitral stenosis?
For any given valve area, the Gorlin formula relates the transvalvular pressure gradient to the flow rate across the valve. The gradient across a stenotic valve increases with cardiac output. Because flow across the mitral valve occurs during diastole, a reduction in diastolic filling time (tachycardia) raises the transvalvular gradient for a given cardiac output. A higher transvalvular pressure gradient translates into a higher left atrial pressure, which in turn results in higher pulmonary venous and capillary pressures. With mitral stenosis, this process typically occurs with exertion (increased cardiac output and heart rate), with the resultant symptom of dyspnea.

3. What is the size of the typical mitral valve?
The circumference of the typical mitral valve is 10 cm. The valve area is normally 4–6 cm^2; with critical stenosis, < 1 cm^2. In critical stenosis flow may not increase, despite an increase in the pressure gradient across the valve.

4. What are the first symptoms of mitral stenosis?
The first symptom is usually dyspnea on exertion. For example, to maintain adequate left ventricular filling across a 1–2 cm^2 valve, a pressure gradient of 20 mmHg is required. A normal left ventricular end-diastolic pressure of 5 mmHg results in a left atrial pressure of 25 mmHg, which obviously is consistent with pulmonary venous congestion and shortness of breath. In addition, loss of a sinus mechanism with new-onset atrial fibrillation (as frequently occurs) leads to tachycardia, shorter diastolic intervals, and further elevation in left atrial pressure to maintain adequate transvalvular flow rates. Thus, atrial fibrillation may be associated with the acute onset of symptoms.

5. What precipitates symptoms in patients with mitral stenosis?
Any condition that increases cardiac output or decreases diastolic filling time (both of which increase flow across the stenotic valve).

6. Which patients with mitral stenosis should receive anticoagulation?
With time the increased left atrial pressure of mitral stenosis distends the left atrium, which leads to atrial fibrillation. Clot then may form in the fibrillating atrium, particularly in the left atrial appendage. Before anticoagulation and surgical therapy became routine, 25% of deaths in patients with mitral valve disease were caused by thromboemboli. Currently, 80% of patients with emboli are in atrial fibrillation. Any patient over 35 in atrial fibrillation, particularly with a low cardiac output and a large left atrial appendage, should be anticoagulated.

7. How does one make the diagnosis of mitral stenosis?
By auscultation one can hear an opening snap followed by a low-pitched diastolic rumble, which is best heard at the apex. The best noninvasive test is Doppler echocardiography, which can quantify the severity of the mitral stenosis.

8. What are the indications for surgery?
Symptomatic patients with a mitral valve area < 1 cm^2 should undergo surgery. Furthermore, surgery should be offered to patients with mitral stenosis and a prior history of emboli.

9. What types of procedures are available for the treatment of mitral stenosis?
Closed commissurotomy   Mitral valve replacement
Open commissurotomy   Balloon valvuloplasty

10. What are the benefits and drawbacks of each?

Closed commissurotomy (rarely performed in U.S.)

Benefits: (1) fast and inexpensive; (2) 1–2% mortality rate; and (3) one-third of patients derive long-term benefits.

Drawbacks: (1) poor results in valves with significant calcification, chordal fusion, or atrial thrombus; (2) severe mitral regurgitation may develop (1/200); and (3) 20–50% recurrence rate at 5 years.

Open commissurotomy

Benefits: (1) thrombi can be removed and the appendage oversewn; (2) extensive commissurotomy and chordal fenestration can be performed; and (3) mild-to-moderate mitral regurgitation can be treated with a valvuloplasty ring.

Drawbacks: none. If the valve is amenable to repair, this is far and away the best procedure. Recurrence rate: 1–2%/year.

Mitral valve replacement

Benefits: (1) totally corrects transvalvular gradient; (2) by preserving subvalvular apparatus, left ventricular function is preserved.

Drawbacks: (1) mortality, 8%; (2) 10-year survival, 65%; (3) 1–2% yearly: thromboembolic episodes, endocarditis, and mortality from anticoagulation; (4) removal of the entire mitral valve apparatus is detrimental to left ventricular function.

Balloon valvuloplasty

Benefits: comparable to a closed commissurotomy; possibly a better option in patients with high medical risk.

Drawbacks: (1) same as for a closed procedure; (2) 2–3% early mortality rate, 2–3% early stroke rate; (3) 30% residual atrial septal defect; (4) in poor-risk patients (thick immobile leaflet, calcification and fusion of leaflets and chordae) at 2 years the mortality rate is 30% and the incidence of valve replacement is 45%.

BIBLIOGRAPHY

1. Bowe JC, Bland F, Sprague HB, White PD: Course of mitral stenosis without surgery: 10 and 20 year perspectives. Ann Intern Med 52:741, 1960.
2. Olesen KH: The natural history of 271 patients with mitral stenosis under medical treatment. Br Heart J 24:349, 1962.
3. Hoit BD: Medical treatment of valvular heart disease. Curr Opin Cardiol 6:207, 1991.
4. Eguaras MG, Jimenez MAG, Calleja F, et al: Early open mitral commissurotomy: Long-term results. J Thorac Cardiovasc Surg 106:421–426, 1993.
5. Levine HJ: Which atrial fibrillation patients should be on chronic anticoagulation? J Cardiovasc Med 6:483, 1981.
6. Scott WC, Miller CD, Haverich A, et al: Operative risk of mitral valve replacement: Discriminant analysis of 1329 procedures. Circulation 72(Suppl II):108, 1985.
7. Rose EA, Oz MC: Preservation of anterior leaflet chordae tendineae during mitral valve replacement. Ann Thorac Surg 567:768–769, 1994.

73. MITRAL REGURGITATION

Glenn J.R. Whitman, M.D., and David Fullerton, M.D.

1. What causes mitral regurgitation?

As with mitral stenosis, the most common cause is rheumatic fever. Other causes include infective endocarditis with leaflet perforation or chordal rupture, senile annular calcification or annular dilatation with loss of leaflet coaptation, and collagen diseases that lead to severe annular dilatation and/or chordal rupture. Acute or chronic ischemia also may lead to mitral regurgitation due to papillary muscle dysfunction.

2. What is the pathophysiology of mitral regurgitation?

With mitral regurgitation, left ventricular ejection may occur via two routes, the aortic and the mitral valve. The greater the systemic afterload (i.e., blood pressure), the greater the regurgitant fraction. With chronic mitral regurgitation, the passive left atrium dilates slowly without significant increase in pressure, preventing early shortness of breath (as is so often seen in mitral stenosis). However, the chronic increase in left ventricular preload leads to left ventricular dilatation and contractile dysfunction. Thus, onset of symptoms is typically later than with mitral stenosis. Of course, acute mitral regurgitation is immediately symptomatic because left atrial pressure rises dramatically in the noncompliant left atrium.

3. What are the first symptoms of mitral regurgitation?

Acute mitral regurgitation leads to immediate elevations in left atrial pressures with shortness of breath. However, chronic mitral regurgitation frequently has only modest elevations in left atrial pressure. Fatigue and loss of exercise capacity are the main symptoms.

4. What is the role of anticoagulation in treatment of patients with mitral regurgitation?

As with stenosis, all patients with mitral regurgitation and atrial fibrillation should be anticoagulated. When patients are still in sinus rhythm, the need for anticoagulation is less clear. However, as the left atrium increases in size, flow becomes less laminar and formation of atrial thrombus is more likely.

5. How does one diagnose mitral regurgitation?

By auscultation a holosystolic murmur is best heard at the apex with radiation to the axilla. The best test is echocardiography, particularly transesophageal; only soft tissue lies between the probe and the valve, and the regurgitant jet may be easily seen head-on.

6. What are the indications for surgery?

The cornerstones of management of mitral regurgitation are afterload reduction (lowering of blood pressure) and decrease in preload (diuresis). Surgery is indicated when symptoms persist despite medical therapy or when left ventricular dysfunction occurs. In mitral regurgitation left ventricular contractility is increased because the two pathways by which blood can leave the ventricle result in decreased afterload and increased ejection fraction.

7. What procedures are available for treatment of mitral regurgitation?

In pure mitral regurgitation, mitral replacement should be required in only 30% of patients; mitral repair is successful in the remainder. A mechanical valve generally is used for replacement because tissue valve degeneration appears to be accelerated in the mitral as opposed to the aortic position. Mitral repair, in general, involves resection of the portion of the leaflet from which the chordae have ruptured, with plication and diminution of the annulus via placement of a prosthetic annular ring. Thus only leaflet tissue with chordal suspensions is left. As a result of leaflet resection, a decrease in annular circumference (via a ring or stent) is mandatory for good leaflet coaptation.

8. What are the benefits and drawbacks of replacement vs. repair?
Replacement

Benefits: (1) valve is guaranteed to be competent; (2) the procedure is easily taught and performed by a wide range of surgeons.

Drawbacks: (1) excision of subvalvular apparatus leads to systolic dysfunction; (2) anticoagulation is mandatory; (3) ever-present risk of prosthetic valve endocarditis and thromboemboli (although rate is < 3%/year); (4) mortality rate of 2–8%.

Repair

Benefits: (1) preservation of subvalvular apparatus maintains postoperative systolic function; (2) anticoagulation is optional; (3) endocarditis and thromboemboli are exceedingly rare; (4) mortality rate is low (2%).

Drawbacks: (1) takes longer intraoperatively; (2) difficult to teach, requiring an obligatory learning curve; (3) 1–3% yearly failure rate.

BIBLIOGRAPHY

1. Bowe JC, Bland F, Sprague HB, White PD: Course of mitral stenosis without surgery: 10 and 20 year perspectives. Ann Intern Med 52:741, 1960.
2. Hoit BD: Medical treatment of valvular heart disease. Curr Opin Cardiol 6:207, 1991.
3. Levine HJ: Which atrial fibrillation patients should be on chronic anticoagulation? J Cardiovasc Med 6:483, 1981.
4. Schneider RM, Helfant RH: Timing of surgery in chronic mitral and aortic regurgitation. In Frankl WS, Brest AN (eds): Valvular Heart Disease. Comprehensive Evaluation and Management. Philadelphia, F.A. Davis, 1986, pp 361–374.
5. Scott WC, Miller CD, Haverich A, et al: Operative risk of mitral valve replacement: Discriminant analysis of 1329 procedures. Circulation 72(Suppl II):108, 1985.
6. Galloway AC, Colvin SB, Baumann FG, et al: A comparison of mitral valve reconstruction with mitral valve replacement: Intermediate-term results. Ann Thorac Surg 47:655–662, 1989.
7. Rose EA, Oz MC: Preservation of anterior leaflet chordae tendineae during mitral valve replacement. Ann Thorac Surg 567:768–769, 1994.

74. AORTIC STENOSIS

David Campbell, M.D.

1. What are the two most common causes of aortic stenosis?
Congenital anomaly and rheumatic fever.

2. What is the most common anatomic anomaly in congenital aortic stenosis?
Bicuspid aortic valve.

3. What is the most common presentation in infancy?
Congestive heart failure.

4. What are the most common symptoms in adults with aortic stenosis?
Syncope, dyspnea on exertion, and angina.

5. What physical findings suggest aortic stenosis?
In infants, systolic crescendo-decresendo (diamond-shaped) murmur, poor peripheral pulses. **In adults**, systolic crescendo-decrescendo murmur, delayed pulse upstroke (pulsus parvus et tardus—this lingo will dazzle the medical chief resident on rounds).

6. What is the most feared complication of aortic stenosis?
Sudden death.

7. How is the diagnosis confirmed?
Aortic stenosis is confirmed by cardiac catheterization. **In critically ill infants**, the diagnosis may be made by Doppler echocardiography; then the child can be taken directly to the operating room for valvotomy. **In children**, associated lesions such as patent ductus arteriosus and coarctation of

thoracic aorta must be identified. **In adults,** the status of the coronary arteries is important to assess because atherosclerotic heart disease commonly coexists, especially in older patients with angina.

8. When is an operation indicated?
Development of symptoms, progression of left ventricular hypertrophy, or measured gradient of 50–60 mmHg.

9. Is aortic valvotomy for congenital aortic stenosis curative?
Usually not. Most children need aortic valve replacement later in life.

10. Can aortic valvotomy be used for calcific aortic stenosis?
No. Aortic valve replacement is the procedure of choice in adults (see question 17).

11. What are the technical details of aortic valve replacement?
Aortic valve replacement is done on cardiopulmonary bypass. Because the left ventricle is quite thickened, special care must be taken to avoid ischemic injury to the myocardium. The left ventricle should be vented to decrease wall tension, and the heart should be quieted with cold potassium cardioplegia. Care must be taken during debridement of the calcified valve and annulus to prevent dislodgement of calcium particles into the ventricle, which later may be ejected as calcium emboli. Finally, when suturing the valve, the surgeon must take care to avoid obstruction of the left coronary orifice.

12. If valve replacement is necessary in a child, what type of valve should be used?
A mechanical valve should be used in children under 15 years of age because of the high incidence of rapid calcification in porcine valves. Calcification of a porcine valve occurs rapidly in young adults between the ages of 15 and 30; therefore, use of a porcine valve in this group is controversial. Recently there has been a great deal of enthusiasm for the use of aortic allografts. Whether allograft valves will calcify early in children and young adults is not yet known.

13. What are the techniques to manage a small aortic annulus?
1. Konno aortoventriculoplasty. The ventricular septum is split along the aortic annulus. A patch is then sewn into the split to enlarge the aortic annulus, usually by two valve sizes or more.

2. Patch plasty through the aortic annulus toward the mitral valve. An incision is carried through the center of the noncoronary annulus toward annulus of the mitral valve but not onto the valve. A V-shaped patch is then sewn into position to enlarge the annulus about one valve size.

3. Manouguian patch plasty into the anterior leaflet of the mitral valve. The incision described above is extended onto the mitral valve. This allows the annulus to be enlarged about two valve sizes.

14. What is valve size?
Prosthetic valves are provided in numbers relating to the valve diameter. Thus, a no. 21 valve is 21 mm in diameter. Area increases exponentially with valve diameter; an increase of two valve sizes is a big deal.

15. What is the operative mortality rate?
In good-risk patients, less than 3%; in patients with poor ventricular function, 15–20%.

16. What are the complications of aortic valve replacement?
Low cardiac output (3–5%); higher for patients with preoperative congestive heart failure
Bleeding requiring reexploration (5%)
Heart block (1–2%)
Stroke (1%) due to air or calcium left in the heart after closure of aortotomy

17. What are the long-term results of aortic valve replacement?
Long-term results are excellent, unless the patient has had preoperative congestive heart failure or severe coronary artery disease. The 10-year survival rate ranges from 60–75%.

18. Can balloon valvotomy be used for adult calcific aortic stenosis?
No. Balloon valvotomy has been used for adult calcific aortic stenosis, but long-term results are very poor. Initially, it was hoped that balloon valvotomy could replace surgery and provide long-term palliation in older patients who are at higher surgical risk because of decreased ventricular function. However, it is exactly this group who do poorest after balloon valvotomy; fewer than 50% are alive at 1 year.

19. What are the indications for balloon valvotomy?
Because of the early hemodynamic deterioration, balloon valvotomy is used primarily as a bridge to aortic valve replacement or transplantation in critically ill patients. Temporary improvement in ventricular function suggests that the patient will benefit from aortic valve replacement. It also has been used to relieve symptoms of women in the second trimester of pregnancy who have severe aortic stenosis. The major use of balloon valvotomy remains in infants and young children who have congenital aortic stenosis, a pliable aortic fused valve, and a normal sized annulus. In such circumstances, the intermediate results are similar to surgical valvotomy.

CONTROVERSIES

20. Should valvotomy with inflow occlusion be used in infants under 3 months of age?
For:
1. Low mortality rate (20%).
2. Low incidence of low cardiac output.
Against:
1. Time-limited; procedure must be performed rapidly.
2. 20% incidence of significant aortic regurgitation.

21. Should knife valvotomy with cardiopulmonary bypass be used in infants under 3 months of age?
For: Allows plenty of time to perform operation.
Against: Higher postoperative incidence of low cardiac output.

22. Is balloon valvotomy in the catheterization lab appropriate for infants, children, and young adults?
For: Avoids an operation.
Against: Often not successful in infants with a small aortic annulus.

23. Should a tissue valve be used in young adults between ages 15 and 30?
For: Anticoagulation is not necessary; thus the risk of significant bleeding complications in active patients is avoided. For women in the childbearing years the advantages are obvious.
Against: There is a somewhat higher incidence of early valve dysfunction due to valve calcification; thus valve replacement may be necessary before 10 years.

BIBLIOGRAPHY

1. Aronow WS, Ahn C, Kronzon I, Nanna M: Prognosis of congestive heart failure in patients aged > or = 62 years with unoperated severe valvular aortic stenosis. Am J Cardiol 72:846, 1993.
2. Banning AP, Pearson JF, Hall RJ: Role of balloon dilatation of the aortic valve in pregnant patients with severe aortic stenosis. Br Heart J 70:544, 1993.
3. Burch M, Redington AN, Carvalho JS, et al: Open valvotomy for critical aortic stenosis in infancy. Br Heart J 63:37, 1990.

4. Crumbley AJ III, Crawford FA Jr: Long-term results of aortic valve replacement. Review article: 161 refs. Cardiol Clin 9:353, 1991.
5. Davidson CJ, Harrison JK, Leithe ME, et al: Failure of balloon aortic valvuloplasty to result in sustained clinical improvement in patients with depressed left ventricular function. Am J Cardiol 65:72, 1990.
6. Davidson CJ, Harrison JK, Pieper KS, et al: Determinants of one-year outcome from balloon aortic valvuloplasty. Am J Cardiol 68:75, 1991.
7. Elkins RC: Congenital aortic valve disease: Evolving management. Ann Thorac Surg 59:269, 1995.
8. Ettedgui JA, Tallman-Eddy T, Neches WH, et al: Long-term results of survivors of surgical valvotomy for severe aortic stenosis in early infancy. J Thorac Cardiovasc Surg 104:1714, 1992.
9. Isner JM: Acute catastrophic complications of balloon aortic valvuloplasty. The Mansfield Scientific Aortic Valvuloplasty Registry Investigators. J Am Coll Cardiol 17:1436, 1991.
10. Judge KW, Otto CM: Doppler echocardiographic evaluation of aortic stenosis. Review article: 46 refs. Cardiol Clin 8:203, 1990.
11. Keane JF, Driscoll EJ, Gersony WM, et al: Second natural history study of congenital heart defects. Results of treatment of patients with aortic valvar stenosis. Circulation 87:I16, 1993.
12. Konno S, Imai Y, Iida Y, et al: A new method for prosthetic valve replacement in congenital aortic stenosis associated with hypoplasia of the aortic valve ring. J Thorac Cardiovasc Surg 70:909, 1975.
13. Letac B, Cribier A, Eltchaninoff H, et al: Evaluation of restenosis after balloon dilatation in adult aortic stenosis by repeat catheterization. Am Heart J 122:55, 1991.
14. Logeais Y, Langanay T, Roussin R, et al: Surgery for aortic stenosis in elderly patients. A study of surgical risk and predictive factors. Circulation 90:2891, 1994.
15. Manouguian S, Abu-Aishah N, Neitzel J: Patch enlargement of the aortic and mitral valve rings with aortic and mitral double valve replacement. J Thorac Cardiovasc Surg 78:394, 1979.
16. Olsson M, Granstrom L, Lindblom D, et al: Aortic valve replacement in octogenarians with aortic stenosis: A case-control study. J Am Coll Cardiol 20:1512, 1992.
17. Pentely G, Morton M, Rahimtoola SH: Effects of successful, uncomplicated valve replacement on ventricular hypertrophy, volume, and performance in aortic stenosis and in aortic incompetence. J Thorac Cardiovasc Surg 75:383, 1978.
18. Pupello DF, Bessone LN, Hiro SP, et al: Aortic valve replacement: Procedure of choice in elderly patients with aortic stenosis. J Card Surg 9:148, 1994.
19. Rao PS: Balloon aortic valvuloplasty in children. Review article: 78 refs. Clin Cardiol 13:458, 1990.
20. Straumann E, Kiowski W, Langer I, et al: Aortic valve replacement in elderly patients with aortic stenosis. Br Heart J 71:449, 1994.

75. EMPYEMA AND TUBERCULOSIS

Marvin Pomerantz, M.D., and James M. Brown, M.D.

1. What is a pleural effusion?

Normal patients have approximately 1 ml/kg of lubricating fluid in the pleural spaces. There is a dynamic flux of this fluid through the pleural space; however, when production exceeds the clearance capacity of the pleural lymphatics, fluid accumulates. Sufficient fluid to be recognized by an astute clinician is termed an effusion. Pleural fluid is made at a rate of 5–10 L/24 hours.

2. What is an infected pleural effusion?

In 70% of instances when the pleural fluid becomes infected, the bacteria derive from adjacent infected lung (pneumonia).

3. Can an infected pleural effusion be sterile?

This finding is actually common. At presentation the patient may have already received a blast of antibiotics and the pleural fluid culture is negative. Look for bacterial fingerprints in the fluid—sugar (pleural fluid sugar should be less than $\frac{2}{3}$ the blood sugar) and pH (pleural fluid pH should be less than 7.2).

4. What is an empyema?

When an infected pleural effusion sits around, natural body defenses try to wall it off—just like any other abscess. A walled-off or loculated infected pleural effusion is an empyema. This diagnostic distinction is important because it is much tougher to drain adequately a loculated empyema than a free pleural effusion.

5. What are the basic principles in the treatment of empyema?

The principles of treating an empyema are the same as for any localized infection. First, the infection must be drained. Second, the space that the infection occupied must be obliterated. In the pleural space the lung usually fills the space, but if it is covered with filmous infection or inflammatory tissue or if it is abnormal to begin with, it may not fill the space.

6. What are the various techniques for drainage and treatment of an empyema?

Small uncomplicated empyema may be treated by thoracentesis. Larger effusions are best treated by insertion of a chest tube. If initial drainage is unsuccessful, streptokinase or urokinase may be of therapeutic value. If, however, after trying these procedures the lung remains trapped with significant restrictive disease or sepsis persists, decortication should be performed either by video-assisted thoracic surgery or open thoracotomy.

7. What is decortication?

The cortex is the outside wall or peel of an orange. Thus, decortication is the surgical release and removal of the abscess cavity walls. After successful decortication, healthy lung should expand and fill the entire pleural space.

8. Postresectional empyema presents a difficult problem. What are the options for management after lobectomy and pneumonectomy with and without bronchopleural fistula?

All postresectional empyemas should be drained by a large-bore chest tube immediately after the diagnosis is made. After lobectomy without bronchopleural fistula, prompt drainage and appropriate antibiotics are often sufficient. This approach also may lead to closure of small bronchopleural fistulas; if not, closure may require muscle flaps, omental flaps, or thoracoplasty. Further resection also may be required. Following pneumonectomy without bronchopleural fistula after drainage, an Eloesser flap should be performed, followed by irrigation of the pleural cavity with eventual closure of the chest wall and instillation of antibiotic solution. With postpneumonectomy empyema and bronchopleural fistula, treatment is more difficult. Irrigation cannot be carried out because the patient will aspirate the irrigation fluid through the fistula. Closure of the fistula has to be done by muscle or omental flaps, thoracoplasty, and, if feasible, transmediastinal approach.

9. Under what two conditions should an empyema not be surgically drained?

Pure tuberculous empyema and poststaphylococcal pneumonia empyema in children.

10. What percent of the world's population is infected with tuberculosis?

Approximately 33%, or 3.0 billion people.

11. How many people die yearly from tuberculosis?

2.8 million.

12. What is a Ghon complex?

A Ghon complex consists of the peripheral tubercular lung lesion accompanied by hilar adenopathy.

13. What is the standard medical treatment of drug-sensitive tuberculosis?

Treatment of drug-sensitive tuberculosis consists of 6 months of therapy with isoniazid (INH) and rifampin with 2 months of pyrazinamide (PZA).

14. Does surgery play a role in the treatment of tuberculosis?

Surgery is reserved for the complications of tuberculosis, including bronchopleural fistula, massive hemoptysis, and bronchostenosis. The most common indication in the U.S. is multidrug-resistant tuberculosis with localized disease. In addition, a solitary pulmonary nodule in a patient who is PPD-positive can still be lung cancer.

15. How are organisms that cause tuberculosis classified?

The most significant clinical distinction is between typical and atypical tuberculosis. Typical strains include *Mycobacterium tuberculosis, M. bovis,* and *M. africanum.* Atypical organisms include *M. fortritum, M. chelonei, M. scrofulaton,* and many others, especially *M. avium intracellulare* or MAI. This distinction is important because atypical infections like MAI can be inherently resistant to medical therapy. In the microbiology lab tuberculous organisms can be classified according to growth characteristics such as growth rate and need for light. This approach led to the original Runyon classification (I-IV), which is probably not clinically helpful.

16. What is the significance of drug-resistant tuberculosis?

M. tuberculosis that is resistant to two or more of the first-line drugs is called multidrug resistant (MDRTB) and implies high rates of failure when treated solely with medications.

BIBLIOGRAPHY

1. Blum BR, Murray CJL: Tuberculosis: Commentary on a re-emergent killer. Science 257:1055–1062, 1992.
2. Clagett OT, Gelaci JE: A procedure for the management of post-pneumonectomy empyema. J Thorac Cardiovasc Surg 45:141, 1963.
3. DeMeester TR: The pleura. In Sabiston DC, Spencer RC (eds): Gibbon's Surgery of the Chest, 4th ed. Philadelphia, W.B. Saunders, 1983.
4. Elliot AM: The medical management of disease caused by drug susceptible *Mycobacterium tuberculosis.* In Chest Surg Clin North Am 3:707–713, 1993.
5. Girod CE, Neff TA: Daily monitoring of drainage is key to success: How to manage parapneumonic effusion/empyema. J Respir Dis 15:35–44, 1994.
6. Pomerantz M, Madsen L, Goble M, Iseman M: Surgical management of resistant mycobacterial tuberculosis and other mycobacterial pulmonary infections. Ann Thorac Surg 52:1108–1112, 1991.
7. Pothula V, Krellenstein DJ: Early aggressive surgical management of parapneumonic empyemas. Chest 105:832–836, 1994.
8. Robinson LA, Moulton AL, Fleming WH, et al: Intrapleural fibrinolytic treatment of multiloculated thoracic empyemas. Ann Thorac Surg 57:830–814, 1994.
9. Samson PC: Empyema thoracis. Ann Thorac Surg 112:210, 1971.

76. LUNG CANCER

James M. Brown, M.D., and Marvin Pomerantz, M.D.

1. How common is lung cancer?

In 1992 lung cancer caused 168,000 deaths in the United States alone, with a steadily increasing incidence of approximately 190,000 new cases annually. Although the male-to-female ratio was 8:1 in 1980, the incidence in women has increased to such a degree that the ratio is now less than 2:1. Indeed, the only group of people within U.S. society in whom the incidence of smoking is increasing is teenaged girls. Although the incidence of lung cancer is increasing, the mortality rate has not declined; less than 10% of patients live for 5 years. Furthermore, lung cancer has increased in nonsmokers.

2. What risk factors are thought to be important in the development of lung cancer?
The most prominent risk factors are smoking and age; 90% of patients have a smoking history. Previously smoking was thought to be associated only with squamous cell carcinoma of the lung; recently, however, there has been an alarming increase in the incidence of adenocarcinoma, especially in nonsmokers. Other potential inciting agents include chemicals (aromatic hydrocarbons, vinyl chloride), radiation (radon gas and uranium), asbestos and metals (chromium, nickel, lead, and arsenic), and environmental factors (air pollution, coal tar, petroleum products).

3. Do familial or acquired genetic alterations contribute to lung cancer?
The expression of the *ras* oncogene has been related to poor prognosis in lung cancer. In addition, tumor suppressor genes such as the p53 gene are frequently lost in lung cancer.

4. What are the major histologic types of lung cancer and their relative frequency?
Non–small-cell carcinomas   80%
1. Adenocarcinoma   45%
   This ominous type of lung cancer is increasing dramatically in nonsmokers.
2. Squamous cell carcinoma   40%
   This type of lung cancer, also referred to as epidermoid, is associated histologically with keratin pearls and is promoted by smoking and other inhaled irritants.
3. Large-cell carcinoma   15%
   Bronchoalveolar carcinoma is the lung cancer associated with frothy bronchorrhea on "multiple-guess" examinations. It is a subtype of adenocarcinoma. Intuitively malignant overgrowth of surfactant-secreting cells produces frothy sputum. Although this symptom is rarely encountered clinically, it is common on examinations.

Small-cell carcinoma   20%
The most important distinction is between small-cell and non–small-cell carcinoma because of fundamental differences in tumor biology and clinical behavior. Patients with small-cell lung cancer are classified as having either limited or extensive disease. **Limited** means that all known disease is confined to one hemithorax and regional lymph nodes, including mediastinal, contralateral hilar, and ipsilateral supraclavicular nodes. **Extensive** describes disease beyond these limits, including brain, bone marrow, and intraabdominal metastases.

5. Does lung cancer screening make sense?
Unfortunately, no. Even chest radiographs performed in 40–60-year-old male smokers have not increased the curability rate of patients presenting with lung cancer.

6. How do patients with lung cancer present?
Increasingly, primary lung cancer is discovered on routine chest radiograph. Occasionally patients have a cough, streaky hemoptysis, or recurrent pneumonia. As many as 10% of patients complain of a paraneoplastic syndrome.

7. What is a paraneoplastic syndrome?
Paraneoplastic syndromes of lung cancer may be **metabolic** (hypercalcemia, Cushing's syndrome), **neurologic** (peripheral neuropathy, polymyositis, or Lambert-Eaton syndrome, which is like myasthenia gravis), **skeletal** (clubbing, hypertrophic osteoarthropathy), **hematologic** (anemia, thrombocytosis, disseminated intravascular coagulation), or **cutaneous** (hyperkeratosis, acanthosis nigricans, dermatomyositis). Of interest, the presence of a paraneoplastic syndrome does not influence the ultimate curability of the lung cancer.

8. Does the staging system for lung cancer have prognostic and therapeutic importance?
Yes. The classification system is based on clinical and pathologic data for non–small-cell lung cancer. Patients often are staged clinically in conjunction with CT scans.

Stage I: Intraparenchymal disease with or without extension to the visceral pleura, at least 2 cm from the carina and no lymph node or metastatic spread.

Stage II: Primary tumor is similar to that of stage I but with extension to inter-bronchial lymph nodes (N1).

Stage IIIa: Extension of tumor into the parietal pleura, chest wall, or mediastinal pleura, and/or extension into hilar or mediastinal (N2) lymph nodes.

Stage IIIb: All elements of IIIa plus extension to mediastinal structures (heart or great vessels) and/or contralateral hilar, paratracheal, or supraclavicular lymph nodes (N3).

Stage IV: Malignant pleural effusion or metastatic disease (M1).

9. Describe the work-up of a patient with a mass on chest radiographs.

Surgical resection remains the most effective way to cure lung cancer. Therefore, early evaluation stresses the patient's candidacy for a thoracotomy and subsequently focuses on the diagnosis and staging of the pulmonary neoplasm. The diagnosis can be made only 60% of the time by sputum cytology; less than 85% of the time by bronchoscopy with biopsy; and only 80–90% of the time with CT scan-guided needle biopsy. Thus, the mainstay of diagnosis is wedge resection of the pulmonary lung mass. CT scanning of the chest (looking for mediastinal lymph nodes) and abdomen (looking for adrenal metastases) is standard. Other procedures, such as bone or brain scanning, are omitted unless the patient complains of specific symptoms. The patient's ability to withstand a thoracotomy requires cardiac evaluation (history of myocardial infarction, congestive failure, and angina) and pulmonary reserve (bedside spirometry determines FEV_1).

10. What are the lower limits of pulmonary functional reserve that allow resection of lung cancer?

1. The forced expiratory volume in one second (FEV_1) should be more than 1 liter/second; the room air arterial blood gas indicates that the partial pressure of oxygen (PO_2) and partial pressure of carbon dioxide (PCO_2) are on the proper side of 50 (PO_2 above 50 and PCO_2 below 50).

2. The patient should be able to walk up one flight of stairs.

3. In borderline cases, ventilation perfusion scanning can be used to predict how much functioning lung will remain after operation.

11. How is lung cancer treated?

The most effective treatment for lung cancer is surgical resection. Unfortunately, 50% of patients initially present with clearly advanced disease, and only 25% of all patients are candidates for resection. Fortunately, preoperative chemotherapy with a cisplatinum-containing regimen has increased the number of stage III patients who are candidates for resection. This recently innovative therapy may translate into improved survival rates.

12. Does radiation therapy have a place in the therapy of lung cancer?

Radiation therapy is effective palliative but not curative therapy for lung cancer. Specifically, patients who present with a superior vena cava syndrome or a blocked bronchus with distal pneumonia frequently can be "opened up" with radiation therapy. Radiation is also excellent for the palliation of pathologic bone pain.

13. What is the survival rate of patients treated for lung cancer?

For stage I, non–small-cell carcinoma, the 5-year survival rate is 60–80% after complete resection. The 5-year survival rates for stage II, stage IIIa, and IIIb are 50%, 15%, and 5%, respectively. The 5-year survival for small-cell carcinoma remains dismal; 7% of patients with limited disease and only 1% of patients with extensive disease survive 5 years.

14. What is a mediastinoscopy?

Mediastinoscopy is a staging procedure in which the paratracheal, subcarinal, and proximal peribronchial lymph nodes are sampled from a small incision made in the suprasternal notch.

15. What are the indications for mediastinoscopy?

Mediastinal staging is indicated in patients with either apparent or documented lung cancer who have:

1. Known lung cancer with mediastinal lymph nodes accessible by cervical mediastinal exploration and > 1 cm, as assessed by CT scan.

2. Adenocarcinoma of the lung and multiple mediastinal lymph nodes < 1 cm.

3. Central or large (> 5 cm) lung cancers with mediastinal lymph nodes < 1 cm.

4. Lung cancer in patients who are high risks for thoracotomy and lung resection.

If the mediastinoscopy is negative, the surgeon should proceed with thoracotomy, biopsy, and curative lung resection. A mediastinoscopy benefits only a patient who is proved to have unresectable lung cancer. A positive mediastinoscopy spares the patient a thoracotomy.

16. Is malignant pleural effusion and/or recurrent nerve involvement with tumor an absolute contraindication to surgical resection for lung cancer?

A malignant pleural effusion is an absolute contraindication to surgical resective therapy. Conversely, both King George V and Arthur Godfrey had successful surgical resections in the face of recurrent nerve involvement with tumor.

BIBLIOGRAPHY

 1. American Joint Committee on Cancer (AJCC): Lung. In Beahrs OH, et al (eds): Manual for Staging Cancer, 4th ed. Philadelphia, J.B. Lippincott, 1992, pp 115–121.
 2. American Thoracic Society: Clinical staging of primary lung cancer. Am Rev Respir Dis 127:1–6, 1983.
 3. Boring CC, et al: Cancer statistician. Cancer 42:19, 1992.
 4. Deslauriers J, et al: Current operative morbidity associated with elective surgical resection for lung cancer. Can J Surg 31:335, 1989.
 5. Dristin L: The Price of Prevention. Sci Am:124–127, 1995.
 6. Johnston MR: Selecting patients with lung cancer for surgical resection. Semin Oncol 15:246–254, 1988.
 7. Martini N, Flelinger BJ: The role of surgery in N2 lung cancer. Surg Clin North Am 67:1037, 1987.
 8. McGee JM: Screening for lung cancer. Semin Surg Oncol 5:179, 1989.
 9. Minna JD, Pass H, Glatstein E, Ihde DC: Cancer of the lung. In Devita VT, Hellman S, Rosenberg SA (eds): Cancer: Principles and Practice of Oncology, 2nd ed. Philadelphia, J.B. Lippincott, 1989.
10. Moossa AR, Schimpff SC, Robson MD (eds): Comprehensive Textbook of Oncology. Baltimore, William & Wilkins, 1991, pp 732-785.
11. Pass HI: Adjunctive and alternate treatment of bronchogenic lung cancer. Chest Surg Clin North Am 1:1, 1991.
12. Shields TW: General Thoracic Surgery, 4th ed. Baltimore, Williams & Wilkins, 1994, pp 1095–1277.

77. SOLITARY PULMONARY NODULE

James M. Brown, M.D., and Marvin Pomerantz, M.D.

1. What is a solitary pulmonary nodule?

A solitary pulmonary nodule or "coin lesion" is ≤ 3 cm and discrete on chest radiograph. It is usually surrounded by lung parenchyma.

2. What causes a solitary pulmonary nodule?

The most common causes of a pulmonary nodule are either neoplastic (carcinoma) or infectious (granuloma). Pulmonary nodules also may represent lung abscess, pulmonary infarction, arteriovenous malformation, resolving pneumonia, pulmonary sequestration, hamartoma, and others. As a general rule of thumb, likelihood of malignancy is comparable to the patient's age. Thus, lung cancer is rare (although it does occur) in 30-year-olds, whereas in 50–60-year-old smokers the chances of malignancy may be as high as 50–60%.

3. How does a solitary pulmonary nodule present?
Typically, a solitary pulmonary nodule is picked up incidentally on a routine chest radiograph. In several large series, more than 75% of lesions were surprise findings on routine chest radiographs. Less than 25% of patients had symptoms referable to the lung.

4. How frequently does a solitary pulmonary nodule represent metastatic disease?
Less than 10% of solitary nodules represent metastatic disease. Accordingly, an extensive work-up for a primary site of cancer other than the lung is not indicated.

5. Can a tissue sample be obtained by fluoroscopic or CT-guided needle biopsy?
Yes, but the results do not change the treatment. If the needle biopsy tissue indicates cancer, the nodule must be removed. If the needle biopsy is negative, the nodule still must be removed.

6. Are radiographic findings important?
Only relatively. The resolution of modern CT scanners allows the best identification of characteristics that suggest cancer:
1. Indistinct or irregular spiculated borders of the nodule.
2. The larger the nodule, the more likely it is to be malignant.
3. Calcification in the nodule is generally associated with benign disease. Specifically central, diffuse, or laminated calcifications are typical of a granuloma, whereas calcifications with more dense and irregular popcorn patterns are associated with hamartomas. Unfortunately, eccentric foci of calcium or small flecks of calcium may be found in malignant lesions.

7. What social or clinical findings suggest that a nodule is malignant rather than benign?
Unfortunately, none of the findings are sufficiently sensitive or specific to influence the work-up. Both increasing age and a long smoking history predispose to lung cancer. Winston Churchill should have had lung cancer—but he did not. Thus, the fact that the patient is the president of the spelunking club (histoplasmosis), has a sister who raises pigeons (cryptococcosis), grew up in the Ohio River Valley (histoplasmosis), works as sexton for a dog cemetery (blastomycosis), or just took a hiking trip through the San Joaquin Valley (coccidioidomycosis) is interesting associated history but does not affect the work-up of a solitary pulmonary nodule.

8. What is the most valuable bit of historic data?
An old chest radiograph. If the nodule is new, it is more likely to be malignant, whereas if the nodule has not changed in the past 2 years, it is less likely to be neoplastic. Unfortunately, even this observation is not absolute.

9. If a patient presents with a treated prior malignancy and a new solitary pulmonary nodule, is it safe to assume that the new nodule represents metastatic disease?
No. Even in patients with known prior malignancies, less than 50% of new pulmonary nodules are metastatic. Thus, the work-up should proceed exactly as for any other patient with a new solitary pulmonary nodule.

10. How should a solitary pulmonary nodule be evaluated?
A complete travel and occupational history is interesting but does not affect the evaluation. Because of the peripheral location of most nodules, bronchoscopy has a diagnostic yield of less than 50%. Even in the best hands, sputum cytology has a low yield. CT scanning is recommended because it can identify other potentially metastatic nodules and delineate the status of mediastinal lymph nodes. As indicated above, percutaneous needle biopsy has a diagnostic yield of approximately 80% but rarely alters the subsequent management.

The critical step in the evaluation is to determine whether the patient is capable of withstanding curative surgical therapy. Cardiac, lung, hepatic, renal, and neurologic function must be deemed stable. If the patient is not likely to survive for several years, there is simply no point in surgical excision of an asymptomatic pulmonary nodule.

The mainstay of management in patients who can tolerate surgery is resection of the nodule for diagnosis by either a minimally invasive thoracoscopic approach or a limited thoracotomy.

11. If the lesion proves to be cancer, what is the appropriate surgical therapy?
Although several series have suggested that wedge excision of the nodule is sufficient, an anatomic lobectomy remains the procedure of choice. Local recurrence of cancer is higher and 5-year survival rates are lower after wedge excision than after lobectomy.

BIBLIOGRAPHY

1. Cummings SR, Lillington GA, Richard RJ: Managing solitary pulmonary nodules: The choice of strategy is a "close call." Am Rev Respir Dis 134:453–460, 1986.
2. Higgins GA, Shields TW, Keehn RJ: The solitary pulmonary nodule: Ten-year follow-up of Veterans Administration-Armed Forces Cooperative Study. Arch Surg 110:570–575, 1975.
3. Khouri NF, Meziane MA, Zerhouni EA, et al: The solitary pulmonary nodule: Assessment, diagnosis and management. Chest 91:128–133, 1987.
4. McKenna RJ, Libshitz HI, Mountain CE, McMurtrey MJ: Roentgenographic evaluation of mediastinal nodes for preoperative assessment in lung cancer. Chest 88:206–210, 1985.
5. Mountain CF: Value of the new TNM staging system for lung cancer. Chest 96:47s–49s, 1989.
6. Neff TA: When the x-ray shows a "spot" on the lung. Med Times 106:65–69, 1978.
7. Neff TA: The science and humanity of the solitary pulmonary nodule. Am Rev Respir Dis 134:433–434, 1986.
8. Ray JF, Lawton BR, Magnin GE, et al: The coin lesion story: Update 1976. Chest 70:332–336, 1976.

78. DISSECTING AORTIC ANEURYSM

David Neil Campbell, M.D.

1. Why is the term "dissecting aortic aneurysm" really incorrect in patients with acute dissection?
The correct term should be "dissecting aortic hematoma" because the lesion is not an aneurysm. Blood dissects the middle and outer layers of the media of the aorta.

2. How is the diagnosis made?
An index of suspicion is the most important factor because no one feature is common to patients presenting with aortic dissections. In any patient who presents with severe "knifelike, ripping" chest and back pain, the diagnosis of aortic dissection should be considered.

3. Once the diagnosis is entertained, how should the patient be managed?
The other diagnosis to be strongly considered is acute myocardial infarction. Therefore, the patient should be placed in an intensive care unit, monitored closely, and stabilized. Two-thirds of patients may be hypertensive, and blood pressure must be controlled. An electrocardiogram often rules out an infarction, but some aortic dissections tear off a coronary artery and thus involve both acute infarction and aortic dissection.

4. What is the most significant diagnostic clue?
The most significant clue is a new aortic valvular diastolic murmur, indicating aortic valvular regurgitation. Neurologic findings, including paraplegia and hemiplegia, also may be present. Hypertension is common, as are differential blood pressures in the four extremities. Blood flow

from the dissecting hematoma encircles the lumen of the blood vessel and constricts it or actually cleaves the takeoff of the subclavian or femoral vessels.

5. What chest radiograph findings are helpful in diagnosis?
Widened mediastinum and loss of aortic knob silhouette.

6. How is the diagnosis confirmed? What is the role of transesophageal echocardiography?
Many articles in the literature now (see Bibliography) report the high accuracy of transesophageal echocardiography (TEE) in the diagnosis of aortic dissections. In some institutions patients undergo operation with this diagnostic tool only. However, the aortogram is still the gold standard. If there is time and the patient is stable, an aortogram should be obtained to confirm the diagnosis, type of dissection (ascending vs. descending), status of the aortic valve, status of the coronary arteries, and extent of involvement of the major branches of the aorta. In fact, both modalities may be complementary: the TEE confirms the diagnosis while the aortogram defines location, aortic valve, and coronary arteries.

7. What are the types of dissection?
  Type A involves only the ascending or both the ascending and descending aorta.
  Type B involves only the descending aorta.

8. Why is the type of dissection important?
  Type A dissections involve the ascending aorta, although the tear may be anywhere in the aorta. Usually they should undergo early surgical correction.
  Type B or descending dissections do not involve the ascending aorta and may be managed medically or surgically (see Controversies).

9. What is the key to medical management?
Blood pressure should be lowered to 100–110 mmHg (systolic) with a combination of sodium nitroprusside and propranolol. Propranolol is particularly important because it decreases the contractility of the myocardium (DP/DT), thereby decreasing the shearing force and preventing propagation of the dissection down the aorta.

10. Can trimethaphan camsylate (Arfonad) be used instead of propranolol or nitroprusside?
No.

11. What are the principles and advantages of surgical management?
  Type A
  1. To close off the hematoma by obliterating the most proximal intimal tear.
  2. To restore competency of the aortic valve.
  3. To restore flow to any branches of the aorta that have been sheared off and receive blood flow from a false lumen.
  4. To protect the heart during these maneuvers and possibly to restore coronary blood flow if coronary has been sheared off.
  5. To look for tears in the transverse aortic arch.
  Technique: Use of deep hypothermia circulatory arrest with or without retrograde cerebral perfusion is in vogue at present. This technique allows the arch to be inspected and the distal anastomosis of the dacron graft to be sewn accurately to the distal ascending aorta in open fashion. Whether to replace or repair the aortic valve is controversial.
  Type B
  1. To close off the hematoma by obliterating the most proximal intimal tear.
  2. To restore blood flow to branches of the aorta fed by the false channel.
  Technique: Surgery can be done using partial cardiopulmonary bypass, Gott shunt, or the Crawford technique, in which the aorta is cross-clamped and the graft is sewn in as fast as possible (see Controversies).

12. Describe the Gott shunt.

A Gott shunt is a hollow plastic tube that is tapered at both ends; it has an internal coating of TDMA-C bound with heparin, which allows blood to flow through the shunt without clotting. One end is placed in the aorta proximal to the aneurysm, and the other is placed distal to the aneurysm. The Gott shunt allows removal or repair of the aneurysm without interrupting the flow of blood beyond the aneurysm.

13. What are the operative complications?

    1. Hemorrhage (10–20%). Very common because of the use of heparin and the poor quality of the aortas, which do not hold sutures well.

    2. Renal failure (21%).

    3. Pulmonary insufficiency (30% higher in type B repair).

    4. Paraplegia. Often presents before operation. As a surgical complication, it usually occurs only with type B.

    5. Acute myocardial infarction or low cardiac output (5–40%), chronic dissection repairs (6–20%).

    6. Bowel infarction (5%).

    7. Death (8–25%). Higher for acute than chronic dissections and for type A than type B.

14. What are the long-term results?

Of patients who survive operation, two-thirds die within 7 years because of comorbid cardiac and cerebral disease.

CONTROVERSIES

15. Surgical or medical management of type B dissections?

Initial surgical management

    1. Approximately 25% of patients initially treated medically eventually need an operation.

    2. Operative mortality is much less today (20%) than in the past.

    3. Medical management has the same in-hospital mortality (20%).

Initial medical management

    1. Avoids unnecessary operation and its attendant cost and complication rate.

16. Management of aortic insufficiency in type A dissections.

Replacement of aortic valve

    1. Easy (valved conduits now available).

    2. Eliminates aortic insufficiency completely.

    3. Should always be done in patients with Marfan's syndrome.

Repair of aortic valve

    1. With native valve reconstruction, when done correctly, the need to replace the valve at a later time is 5–10% in some series.

    2. Avoids need for anticoagulation, which is necessary when a mechanical valve is used to replace the aortic valve.

17. Repair of type B dissections.

Partial femorofemoral or aortofemoral bypass

For:

    1. Allows unloading of the heart.

    2. Allows distal perfusion to avoid ischemia.

    3. Allows as much time as needed to complete anastomosis.

Against: Requires heparinization.

Gott shunt
For:
1. Allows unloading of the heart.
2. Allows distal perfusion to avoid ischemia.
3. Does not require heparinization.
4. Allows as much time as needed to accomplish the anastomosis.

Against: May injure the aorta in placement.

Simple aortic cross-clamping
For: Fast.

Against: Placement of the graft has to be done in less than 30 minutes or the complication rate, particularly paraplegia, increases significantly.

BIBLIOGRAPHY

1. Adachi H, Omoto R, Kyo S, et al: Emergency surgical intervention of acute aortic dissection with the rapid diagnosis by transesophageal echocardiography. Circulation 84:III14, 1991.
2. Asfoura JY, Vidt DG: Acute aortic dissection. Chest 99:724, 1991 [published erratum appears in Chest 100:L1480, 1991].
3. Bachet JE, Termignon JL, Dreyfus G, et al: Aortic dissection. Prevalence, cause, and results of late reoperations. J Thorac Cardiovasc Surg 108:199, 1994.
4. Banning AP, Masani ND, Ikram S, et al: Transesophageal echocardiography as the sole diagnostic investigation in patients with suspected thoracic aortic dissection. Br Heart J 72:461, 1994.
5. Blanchard DG, Kimura BJ, Dittrich HC, DeMaria AN: Transesophageal echocardiography of the aorta. JAMA 272:546, 1994.
6. Chirillo F, Cavallini C, Longhini C, et al: Comparative diagnostic value of transesophageal echocardiography and retrograde aortography in the evaluation of thoracic aortic dissection. Am J Cardiol 74:590, 1994.
7. Cigarroa JE, Isselbacher EM, DeSanctis RW, Eagle KA: Diagnostic imaging in the evaluation of suspected aortic dissection. Old standards and new directions. N Engl J Med 328:35, 1993.
8. Coselli JS, Buket S, Djukanovic B: Aortic arch operation: Current treatment and results. Ann Thorac Surg 59:19, 1995.
9. Crawford ES: The diagnosis and management of aortic dissection. JAMA 264:2537, 1990.
10. Deeb GM, Jenkins E, Bolling SF, et al: Retrograde cerebral perfusion during hypothermic circulatory arrest reduces neurologic morbidity. J Thorac Cardiovasc Surg 109:259, 1995.
11. Ergin MA, Phillips RA, Galla JD, et al: Significance of distal false lumen after type A dissection repair. Ann Thorac Surg 57:820, 1994.
12. Glower DD, Fann JI, Speier RH, et al: Comparison of medical and surgical therapy for uncomplicated descending aortic dissection. Circulation 82:IV39, 1990.
13. Lourie JK, Appelbe A, Martin RP: Detection of complex intimal flaps in aortic dissection by transesophageal echocardiography. Am J Cardiol 69:1361, 1992.
14. Masuda Y, Yamada Z, Morooka N, et al: Prognosis of patients with medically treated aortic dissections. Circulation 84:III7, 1991.
15. Nienaber CA, von Kodolitsch Y, Nicolas V, et al: The diagnosis of thoracic aortic dissection by noninvasive imaging procedures. N Engl J Med 328:1, 1993.
16. Ueda Y, Miki S, Okita Y, et al: Protective effect of continuous retrograde cerebral perfusion on the brain during deep hypothermic systemic circulatory arrest. J Cardiovasc Surg 9:584, 1994.
17. Weiss P, Weiss I, Zuber M, Ritz R: How many patients with acute dissection of the thoracic aorta would erroneously receive thrombolytic therapy based on the electrocardiographic findings on admission? Am J Cardiol 72:1329, 1993.
18. Wheat MW Jr, Shumacker HB Jr: Dissecting aneurysm: Problems of management. Chest 70:6450, 1976.
19. Wheat MW Jr, Palmer RF, Bartley TB, Seelman RC: Treatment of dissecting aneurysms of the aorta without surgery. J Thorac Cardiovasc Surg 50:364, 1965.

IX. Pediatric Surgery

---

79. HYPERTROPHIC PYLORIC STENOSIS

Frederick M. Karrer, M.D., and Denis D. Bensard, M.D.

---

1. What is the incidence of pyloric stenosis?
Hypertrophic pyloric stenosis (HPS) occurs in 1:300 to 1:900 births. The male-to-female ratio is 4:1. It has been suggested that first-born siblings are more commonly affected, but the data are inconclusive. In contrast, a familial pattern is well documented.

2. Describe the typical presentation of HPS.
A healthy infant who initially fed normally presents at 2–6 weeks of age with a history of progressive vomiting. Vomiting may be intermittent at first but soon progresses to projectile vomiting after each feeding. The emesis is nonbilious, although blood or "coffee grounds" may be observed because of associated esophagitis. After vomiting the infant appears hungry and will refeed immediately. With time dehydration and malnutrition worsen, leading the parents to seek medical evaluation. The parents also may report multiple formula changes with no apparent improvement in symptoms.

3. What are the physical findings?
Affected infants are dehydrated to variable degrees. The abdomen is nondistended, and occasionally gastric peristalsis is observed through the abdominal wall. A palpable pyloric tumor, known as the "olive," confirms the diagnosis. The pyloric tumor is palpable in 75–90% of patients, depending on the experience and persistence of the examiner. Associated findings include inguinal hernia (10%) and mild scleral icterus due to reduced glucuronyl transferase activity (2–8%).

4. How is the diagnosis made?
A palpable "olive" in patients with a suggestive history is sufficient to make the diagnosis of HPS. If doubt exists, ultrasonography confirms the presence of a pyloric tumor. Ultrasonographic criteria include pyloric diameter > 1.4 cm, wall width > 4 mm, and pyloric canal length > 1.6 cm. Alternatively, a barium upper gastrointestinal (UGI) examination may be used to confirm the diagnosis. Diagnostic criteria include gastric outlet obstruction, a "string" sign demonstrating pyloric channel narrowing, "shoulder" sign, or "pyloric tit' in high-grade obstruction. If a UGI study is used, a nasogastric tube should be placed and the stomach irrigated with saline to remove the barium before surgery.

5. Describe the likely electrolyte abnormalities?
Hypokalemic, hypochloremic metabolic alkalosis is the classic electrolyte abnormality associated with HPS. The repeated vomiting of gastric acid, generally replaced with inadequate electrolyte solutions results in significant loss of chloride and hydrogen ion. The kidneys attempt to compensate by preserving hydrogen ions at the expense of potassium. If the condition remains uncorrected, the ability of the kidneys to compensate is lost. Alkalosis and hypokalemia worsen, and paradoxical aciduria demonstrates the kidney's inability to conserve hydrogen ions. Adequate fluid resuscitation begins with intravenous administration of 0.45% saline solution. Once urinary flow has been established, 20–20 mEq/L of potassium chloride is added to the intravenous solution to correct the potassium deficit. Severely dehydrated patients may require fluid resuscitation for 24–48 hours before proceeding to the operating room.

6. What procedure is recommended for the correction of HPS?

The Fredet-Ramstedt pylorotomy is generally accepted as the procedure of choice. Medical management, although reportedly effective in some patients, is associated with a higher failure rate and longer hospitalization compared with surgical management. Recently endoscopic balloon dilation and laparoscopic pyloromyotomy have been reported to be efficacious, but they need to achieve the 99% success rate of operative pyloromyotomy before either can be advocated. The standard pyloromyotomy is performed through a supraumbilical transverse incision over the right rectus muscle. The pylorus is delivered through the muscle-splitting incision and a superficial incision made longitudinally over the pyloric muscle in an avascular area. The incision encompasses all of the pylorus and extends to the antrum for a short distance. The muscle fibers are then carefully spread, resulting in complete separation with exposure of the underlying mucosa. At the conclusion of the pyloromyotomy, the gastric mucosa should bulge upward into the cleft, and the pyloric muscle walls should move independently of one another. The duodenum should be milked in a retrograde direction, and the pyloromyotomy should be inspected for leak, which suggests inadvertent mucosal entry.

7. What should be done if a leak is identified?

If the duodenum has been inadvertently entered, the mucosa should be closed with several fine sutures and covered with an omental patch. If the myotomy is compromised or the mucosal injury too extensive, the myotomy should be closed with sutures, and a second, parallel myotomy should be made at 45–180° from the original myotomy.

8. When can postoperative feeding begin? What are the limitations?

Gastric ileus persists for 8–12 hours after the procedure, and a variable degree of gastric atony is found in all patients. Therefore, dextrose and water or electrolyte solutions may be started 6–8 hours postoperatively. It is necessary to begin with frequent, small-volume feedings (15–30 ml every 2–3 hours). The volume and formula strength are gradually advanced over the ensuing 24 hours. Small amounts of vomiting are not unusual (20%) and should not cause alarm unless persistent. Incomplete pyloromyotomy is generally not considered unless symptoms of gastric outlet obstruction continue for 10–14 days postoperatively.

9. Describe several hypotheses about the pathogenesis of HPS.

Although the cause of HPS remains unknown, several hypotheses have been proposed. In 1960 Lynn suggested that milk curds passing through the narrowed pyloric channel result in edema and swelling, which progress to complete occlusion. If this hypothesis is correct, why are not all infants affected? Thus a familial or genetic predisposition must also exist. Postnatal work hypertrophy in response to congenital delay in the opening of the pyloric sphincter also has been suggested as a possible mechanism. More recently, investigators have implicated a defect in the production of nitric oxide in the pathogenesis of HPS. Nitric oxide, a smooth muscle relaxant, appears to be important in the relaxation of the mammalian digestive tract. In a study of pyloric tissue obtained from 9 infants with HPS, Vanderwinden et al. found a reduction in nitric oxide synthase activity. The investigators proposed that a reduction in nitric oxide production may account for the pylorospasm observed in HPS.

BIBLIOGRAPHY

1. Breaux CW, Hood JS, Georgeson KE: The significance of alkalosis and hyperkalemia in hypertrophic pyloric stenosis. J Pediatr Surg 24:1250–1252, 1989.
2. Forman HP, Leonides JC, Kronfeld GD: A rational approach to the diagnosis of hypertrophic pyloric stenosis: Do the results match the claims? J Pediatr Surg 25:262–266, 1990.
3. Georgeson KE, Corbin TJ, Griffen JW, et al: An analysis of feeding regimens after pyloromyotomy for hypertrophic pyloric stenosis. J Pediatr Surg 28:1478–1480, 1993.
4. Hernanz-Schulman M, Sells LL, Ambrosin MM, et al: Hypertrophic pyloric stenosis in the infant without . a palpable olive: Accuracy of sonographic diagnosis. Radiology 193:771–776, 1994.
5. Pollock WF, Norris WJ: Dr. Conrad Ramstedt and pyloromyotomy. Surgery 42:966, 1057.
6. Spicer RD: Infantile hypertrophic pyloric stenosis: A review. Br J Surg 69:128, 1982.

7. Vanderwinden JM, Mailleux P, Schiffman SN, et al: Nitric oxide synthetase activity in infantile hyper-trophic pyloric stenosis. N Engl J Med 327:511–515m 1992.
8. Wooley MM, Felsher BF, Asch MJ, et al: Jaundice, hypertrophic pyloric stenosis, and glucuronyl trans-ferase. J Pediatr Surg 9:359, 1974.

80. NEONATAL INTESTINAL OBSTRUCTION

Luis A. Martinez-Frontanilla, M.D.

1. Which are the common types of neonatal bowel obstruction?

1. Atresia at any level from duodenum to rectum. Rare at the large-bowel level.

2. Obstructions of the duodenum related to intestinal malrotation and/or abnormal fixation (midgut volvulus or Ladd's bands).

3. Ileal obstruction due to meconium ileus.

4. Obstruction at the level of the colon due to Hirschsprung's disease, small left colon syn-drome, or meconium plug syndrome.

5. Obstruction at the anorectal level due to congenital atresia (imperforate anus).

2. What is the clinical presentation of neonatal intestinal obstruction?

Vomiting, usually bilious, commonly in the first week of life. Depending on the level of obstruc-tion: abdominal distention, obstipation, or failure to pass meconium.

3. How is an infant with neonatal intestinal obstruction properly studied and diagnosed?

Careful physical examination including aspiration of the stomach with a nasogastric tube. Rectal examination. A two-way plain x-ray film of the abdomen. If the obstruction appears located at the duodenal or high jejunal level, a limited contrast study of the upper gastrointestinal tract should follow. If the obstruction appears to lie beyond the jejunum, a barium enema is indicated. Gastrografin may be the appropriate contrast medium if meconium ileus is suspected (see Con-troversies). Presently, a large number of obstructions are diagnosed with antenatal ultrasound.

4. Do all atresias of the alimentary canal share a common etiology?

No. Probably there are different entities. Anorectal and esophageal atresia may have a a similar background. They may be part of a broad constellation of abnormalities (VACTER syndrome, see chapter 81). Duodenal atresias may be related to Down's syndrome. Some jejunoileal atresias result from an acquired form of in utero mesenteric artery occlusion or other vascular accidents. These are rarely associated with other syndromes or anomalies; exceptions to these are the asso-ciation with cystic fibrosis in 10% of cases of jejunoileal atresia, and the familial occurrence of "apple peel" jejunal atresia. Hirschsprung's disease has been reported in families.

5. How are jejunoileal atresias classified?

1. **Membrane or diaphragm type:** There is interruption of the intestinal lumen, which can also be partial. There is external continuity of the intestine.

2. **Cord type:** A string of solid tissue is interposed between the atretic ends of the intestine.

3. **Gap type:** Loss of tissue between the atretic ends. Multiplicity and combinations of these three types can occur in the same patient.

4. **"Apple peel" type:** Described in question 6.

6. What is "apple peel" jejunal atresia?

A severe form of atresia with loss of significant length of intestine. Only a short segment of je-junum remains proximal to the atresia. The distal intestine, totally separated, is represented by the entire colon and a coiled segment of the terminal ileum, the vascular supply of which is a marginal artery derived from the middle colic artery. These infants have a worse prognosis than infants with the other varieties of jejunal atresia. Familial incidence and association with other malformations have been reported.

7. How is intestinal malrotation diagnosed?
By the demonstration on a contrast x-ray film of the GI tract of an abnormal position and configuration of the duodenum or the cecum (barium enema or upper GI x-rays; see Controversies).

8. What is meconium ileus and how is it diagnosed?
It is a neonatal gastrointestinal manifestation of cystic fibrosis. The meconium is extremely thick and plugs the ileum, producing an intraluminal obstruction. The diagnosis is made with a contrast study of the lower gastrointestinal tract or intraoperatively.

9. Is the sweat test useful in the diagnosis of meconium ileus?
Only retrospectively; the test is inaccurate in the neonatal period when this disease manifests.

10. What is the treatment for neonatal intestinal obstructions?
For the majority, the treatment is surgical (either bypass or removal of the obstruction). Some cases of meconium ileus resolve with the administration of Gastrografin enema, and most cases of small left colon syndrome and meconium plug syndrome resolve spontaneously. See chapter 82, Hirschsprung's disease.

11. What are the surgical options?
1. Duodenojejunal anastomosis bypassing or resecting a duodenal atresia.
2. For jejunoileal atresia: "End-to-back" anastomosis. Frequently requires resection of a proximal segment (see Controversies).
3. For meconium ileus: Evacuation of the inspissated meconium through an opening in the ileum. Further treatment of the intestine is described under Controversies.
4. For malrotation-related obstructions: Detorsion of the midgut volvulus, if present, followed by division of all adhesions and bands between the cecum and over the duodenum (Ladd's bands).
5. For Hirschsprung's disease and imperforate anus: See chapters 82 and 85, respectively.

12. What are possible complications of operations to correct intestinal obstruction in the neonate?
The stretched-out and dilated intestine proximal to an atresia may fail to provide peristaltic function after the anastomosis, frequently requiring reoperation with either resection or enteroplasty to reduce the diameter of the intestine. Short-gut syndrome and anastomotic leak are also possible complications.

CONTROVERSIES

13. Are contrast studies of the gastrointestinal tract necessary, or are plain films sufficient to make the diagnosis?
On many occasions plain x-ray films of the abdomen may give a high suspicion of a diagnosis, particularly in duodenal atresia. This, added to the small risk that a contrast study may represent for the infant, weighs in favor of avoiding contrast studies. However, a barium enema or upper gastrointestinal radiographic study done by a radiologist familiar with neonates may provide useful information such as malrotation, Hirschsprung's disease (and level of transition), meconium ileus, or transient colonic obstructions. Some of these may respond to medical treatment or dictate different surgical approaches or priorities.

14. Upper versus lower gastrointestinal x-ray films for the diagnosis of malrotation.
Traditionally a barium enema had been the x-ray of choice to show the malposition of the cecum. However, this can be challenged, because occasionally malrotation of the midgut with volvulus

can occur with a normally rotated cecum. An upper gastrointestinal study may have also the advantage of showing other possible causes of upper intestinal obstruction.

15. Primary versus deferred anastomosis for jejunoileal atresia.
Frequently the dilated proximal loop of jejunum leading to the atresia has a very impaired peristaltic action. This has been the reason why diverting the intestinal flow as cutaneous enterostomies has been used as a temporizing method of treatment. However, employing the techniques of resection of the dilated intestine or plication to reduce its diameter with primary anastomosis has been shown to overcome this problem.

16. Primary anastomosis versus cutaneous enterostomy for meconium ileus.
Although primary anastomosis after evacuation of the thick obstructing meconium has been used by some, most pediatric surgeons favor some type of enterostomy. These vary from a Bishop-Coop (end-to-side) "chimney," to the Santulli (side-to-end) "chimney," to a Mickulicz enterostomy. There are minor variations in the end result, and the controversy is merely a matter of personal preference.

BIBLIOGRAPHY

1. Benson CD, Loyd JR, Smith JD: Resection and primary anastomosis in the management of stenosis and atresia of the jejunum and ileum. Pediatrics 26:265, 1960.
2. deLorimier AA, Fonkalsrud EW, Hays DM: Congenital atresia and stenosis of the jejunum and ileum. Surgery 65:819, 1969.
3. Grosfeld JL: The small intestine. In Ravitch MM, Welch KJ, Benson CB, et al (eds): Pediatric Surgery, Vol. 2. Chicago, Year Book, 1979, p 933.
4. Louw JH, Barnard CN: Congenital intestinal atresia: Observations on its origin. Lancet 2:1065, 1955.
5. Nixon HH: Intestinal obstruction in the newborn. Arch Dis Child 30:13, 1955.
6. Puri P, Fujimoto T: New observations on the pathogenesis of multiple intestinal atresia. J Pediatr Surg 23:221, 1988.
7. Robertson FM, Crombleholme TM, Paidas M, et al: Prenatal diagnosis and management of gastrointestinal anomalies. Semin Perinatol 18:182, 1994.
8. Santulli TV, Blanc WA: Congenital atresia of the intestine: Pathogenesis and treatment. Ann Surg 154:939, 1961.
9. Simpson AJ, Leonidas JC, Krasna HH, t al: Roentgen diagnosis of midgut malrotation: Value of upper gastrointestinal radiographic study. J Pediatr Surg 7:243, 1972.
10. Weiss RG, Ryan DP, Ilstad ST, et al: A complex case of jejunocolic atresia. J Pediatr Surg 25:560, 1990.

81. TRACHEOESOPHAGEAL MALFORMATIONS

Luis A. Martinez-Frontanilla, M.D.

1. Which are the common types of congenital tracheoesophageal malformations?
Single or combined forms of esophageal atresia and tracheoesophageal fistula. The fistula may connect the trachea with one or both atretic ends of the esophagus.

2. What are the possible combinations?
1. Esophageal atresia with fistula to the distal pouch.
2. Esophageal atresia with tracheoesophageal fistula to the proximal pouch.
3. Esophageal atresia with two fistulas, one to each esophageal pouch.
4. Esophageal atresia without fistula.
5. Tracheoesophageal fistula without atresia, the so-called H type.

(See figure, following page.)

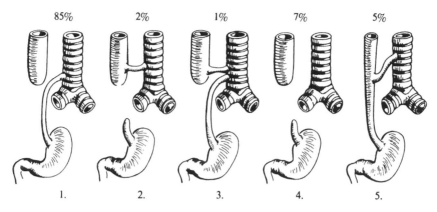

Relative incidence of various types of esophageal atresia/tracheoesophageal fistula. (Modified from Myers MA, Aberdeen E: The esophagus. In Ravitch MM, Welch KJ, Benson CD, et al (eds): Pediatric Surgery, Vol. 1. Chicago, Year Book, 1979, p 450.)

3. What is the relative incidence of each variety?

Very unequal. The most frequent one is the combination of esophageal atresia with tracheo-esophageal fistula to the distal atretic pouch of the esophagus (85%) (no. 1 in above figure).

4. Are there other anomalies associated with tracheoesophageal fistulas?

In over 30% of cases there are associated anomalies of other organs and systems. The most frequent ones are cardiovascular malformations, followed by gastrointestinal ones consisting of imperforate anus and duodenal atresia.

5. What is the VACTER syndrome?

A "package" of multisystem malformations, of which the esophageal ones are most important. VACTER is an acronym descriptive of the malformations: **V**ertebral, **A**norectal, **C**ardiac, **T**racheo**E**sophageal, **R**enal, and limb (usually on the radial side of the upper extremity). Two or more of these varieties should be present to constitute the syndrome. The importance of this syndrome is that the presence of one malformation can lead to the suspicion and investigation of others that are possibly fatal if unrecognized.

6. What is the clinical presentation?

Usually related to inability to swallow (in cases of atresia). Excess salivation: "mucousy baby." Episodes of coughing and cyanosis in the first 2–3 days of life. In cases of pure fistula the symptoms present later in infancy and resemble those of aspiration pneumonia.

7. How is the diagnosis made?

Clinically. Most times the diagnosis is confirmed by the inability to pass a nasogastric tube beyond a distance of about 12 cm from the nose. This should be accompanied by a plain x-ray film of the entire baby ("Babygram").

8. What information is obtained from a Babygram?

- The position of the nasogastric tube is observed.
- Vertebral and other skeletal anomalies are noted.
- Status of the lungs: pneumonia, lobar collapse, etc.
- Intestinal gas pattern: increased in cases of fistula and absent in atresia without a fistula to the distal pouch; typical "double-bubble" if associated with duodenal atresia; abnormal in more distally located intestinal atresia that may be associated.

9. Is the use of x-rays with contrast material in the upper esophageal pouch indicated?
The use of air as contrast is safe and can be helpful. The use of liquid contrast (barium or Gastrografin) carries a high risk of aspiration and pneumonia. It should be reserved for cases of unclear diagnosis and it should be done under fluoroscopy using a very small amount of contrast material (less than 1 ml) (see Controversies).

10. What is the treatment for these malformations?
The ultimate goal is to interrupt the fistula and to restore esophageal continuity. It varies for the different combinations.

11. How is the most common variety (esophageal atresia with distal tracheoesophageal fistula) treated?
The definitive treatment consists of surgical division of the tracheoesophageal fistula and anastomosis of the atretic esophagus. This can be achieved in a primary or a staged fashion. The creation of a tube gastrostomy can be part of the treatment (see Controversies). Indications for staging are severe prematurity and/or pneumonia, deterioration during the initial stages of surgical treatment, and technical difficulties in approximating the ends of the esophagus. The stages consist of gastrostomy, ligature of the fistula via thoracotomy, and esophageal anastomosis or replacement.

12. Discuss the treatment of other varieties of esophageal atresia with tracheoesophageal fistula.
Atresia without fistula to the distal pouch or without fistula at all usually presents the difficulty of a long gap between the atretic ends of the esophagus. For these varieties the approach of delayed esophageal repair is used. A gastrostomy is created early in all of these infants. This is used for feedings. A period of observation and/or instrumental stretching of the atretic pouches of about 8 weeks follows. The esophageal gap is reevaluated radiographically. A thoracotomy can then be performed and anastomosis attempted. If still unsuccessful, further treatment is delayed until the infant is approximately 1 year old, at which time the esophageal gap is bridged with a piece of colon or stomach (see Controversies).

13. Which are the complications of these operations?
Immediate: Anastomotic leak, empyema, and pneumothorax. **Delayed:** Esophageal stricture usually requiring dilatations and occasionally reoperation; food impaction can occur repeatedly at the level of the anastomosis; fistula recurrence; gastroesophageal reflux, which may require surgical treatment; cases in which interposition of other organs to replace the esophagus is required are more complicated.

14. What are the results of the treatment of congenital esophageal atresia with tracheoesophageal fistula?
The mortality can be heavily increased by two factors: prematurity and presence of major associated anomalies. In the absence of these factors, survival currently approaches 100%. In the long term, many patients require esophageal dilatations, and some require reoperation.

CONTROVERSIES

15. Use of contrast x-rays in the diagnosis of esophageal atresia
This procedure provides the most reliable confirmation of diagnosis, may demonstrate a proximal fistula, and may differentiate a traumatic pseudodiverticulum of the esophagus. Most pediatric surgeons, however, avoid contrast procedures because of the danger of aspiration.

16. Primary versus staged repair in premature babies with or without pneumonia or other malformations
Creation of a gastrostomy tube followed by a period of observation has the advantage of providing an opportunity to treat or evaluate associated conditions or of allowing time for some aggravating

conditions to improve. However, it carries a risk of continuous soiling of the lungs with gastric acid through the fistula. Currently, there is a tendency toward earlier definitive treatment in smaller and smaller babies as pediatric anesthesia, neonatal intensive care, and nutritional support have improved in recent years.

17. Gastrostomy
Some surgeons prefer to use gastrostomy selectively as part of the treatment of these fistulas, avoiding its use particularly in term babies with no associated conditions. Advantages of gastrostomy are access to gastric decompression, access to feeding, and access to retrograde dilatation in case of stricture.

18. Colon versus gastric or jejunal interposition for long-gap atresia of the esophagus
The ideal organ to replace the esophagus is still to be found. Both colon and reverse or direct gastric tube are plagued with complications. Most pediatric surgeons seem to favor the former. For these reasons, all attempts should be made to reapproximate and repair the patient's esophagus, leaving interpositions as the very last resort.

19. Transpleural versus extrapleural thoracotomy
Transpleural approach is easier technically. However, anastomotic leaks are better tolerated after extrapleural operations.

BIBLIOGRAPHY

1. Ein SM, Shandling B, Wesson D, et al: Esophageal atresia with distal tracheoesophageal fistula: Associated anomalies and prognosis in the 1980s. J Pediatr Surg 24:1055, 1989.
2. Holder TM, Cloud DP, Lewis GE Jr, et al: Esophageal atresia and tracheoesophageal fistula. A survey of its members by the Surgical Section of the American Academy of Pediatrics. Pediatrics 34:542, 1964.
3. Martinez-Frontanilla LA, Janik J, Meagher DP Jr: Colon esophagoplasty in the orthotopic position. J Pediatr Surg 23:1215, 1988.
4. Myers MA, Aberdeen E: The esophagus. In Welch KJ, Ravitch MM, Aberdeen E (eds): Pediatric Surgery, 4th ed. Chicago, Year Book, 1979.
5. Spitz L, Kiely EM, Morecroft JA, et al: J Pediatr Surg 29:723, 1994.

82. HIRSCHSPRUNG'S DISEASE

Luis A. Martinez-Frontanilla, M.D.

1. What is Hirschsprung's disease?
A form of distal intestinal obstruction of functional type caused by lack of peristaltic activity of the area of the affected intestine.

2. Which histologic changes can be demonstrated in the affected intestine?
Absence of ganglion cells in the submucosal and myenteric plexus. Also increased nerve fibers in the same area.

3. What are the location and extent of the disease?
It always affects at least the lower rectum. From there it may extend to a variable distance in a continuous involvement (see Controversies). In more than 75% of cases, the extent is confined to the left colon. In less than 10% of patients, it involves the entire colon. Very rarely it involves the entire gastrointestinal tract.

4. How is the diagnosis made?
Clinical suspicion. Usually a lifelong history of constipation that goes back to the nursery (90% of normal newborn infants have their first bowel movement within 48 hours of birth). Poor growth and development. Distended, prominent abdomen. Rectal ampulla usually empty, as opposed to patients with psychogenic constipation.

5. How is the diagnosis confirmed?
The most reliable modality is a rectal biopsy usually done transanally. Anorectal manometry has been used by some authors as an acceptable alternative (see Controversies).

6. What is the role of a barium enema in the diagnosis?
To reinforce the clinical suspicion and to help determine the area of transition between normal and aganglionic intestine. It should not be used as a definitive diagnostic modality.

7. Discuss the differential diagnosis.
In the neonate: meconium plug syndrome (not meconium ileus) and small left colon syndrome. Both are self-limited forms of transient obstruction identified with barium enema examination. **In the older child:** psychogenic constipation, which is characterized by soiling and a fecal mass in the rectal ampulla. Manometrics and rectal biopsy are both diagnostic.

8. Which are the complications of untreated Hirschsprung's disease?
Chronic constipation, failure to thrive, acute enterocolitis, intestinal perforation, and death.

9. Describe the treatment of Hirschsprung's disease.
Surgical. Usually staged starting with a diverting colostomy at a site uninvolved with the disease (verified by biopsy). This is followed several months later by a definitive operation that either removes or bypasses the affected area of the intestine. Occasionally in very short segment Hirschsprung's disease, an anorectal myectomy (removal of a posterior strip of muscularis) can be curative (see also Controversies).

10. Which are the accepted surgical techniques for definitive treatment?
  Swenson: removal of the entire affected area and anastomosis of the normal intestine near the anal level.
  Soave: endorectal pull-through, preserving the external layer of the affected rectum into which the normal intestine is telescoped.
  Duhamel: "back-to-back" anastomosis of uninvolved end of the intestine to the rectum down to the anal level.

11. What are possible complications of these operations?
Rectal stenosis with constipation, which may result from ischemia or local infection; recurrent obstruction and enterocolitis; soiling or diarrhea; and genitourinary neurologic dysfunction.

12. What are the results of these operations?
Good results, with normal intestinal function in 75–90%.

CONTROVERSIES

13. "Skip area" of aganglionosis
There have been occasional reports of patients with more than one area without ganglion cells separated by a normal segment of intestine, or an area of aganglionosis proximal to the rectum with normal ganglion cells distally. The difficulties in diagnosis and treatment in these instances are obvious. The existence of this variant is, however, strongly disputed by most pediatric surgeons.

14. Rectal biopsy versus manometry to confirm the diagnosis
Both modalities seem to give equally good results, and preference and accuracy seem to vary according to the experience of the authors. Rectal biopsy is more widely accepted.

15. Primary versus staged surgical treatment
Diverting colostomy as a first stage is the treatment of choice for newborn infants and patients with severe enterocolitis as the presenting event. A small number of older patients with only mild or chronic symptoms who can be adequately decompressed can be treated primarily with one of the accepted definitive procedures.

BIBLIOGRAPHY

1. Aaronson I, Nixon HH: A clinical evaluation of ano-rectal pressure studies in the diagnosis of Hirschsprung's disease. Gut 13:138, 1972.
2. Harrison MW, Deitz DM, Campbell JR, et al: Diagnosis and management of Hirschsprung's disease. A 25-year perspective. Am J Surg 152:49, 1986.
3. Klein MD, Philipart AI: Hirschsprung's disease: Three decades experience at a single institution. J Pediatr Surg 28:1291, 1993.
4. MacIver AG, Whiteside R: Zonal colonic aganglionosis, a variant of Hirschsprung's disease. Arch Dis Child 47:233, 1972.
5. Sieber WK: Hirschsprung's disease. In Welch JJ, Ravitch MM, Aberdeen E, et al (eds): Pediatric Surgery, 4th ed. Chicago, Year Book, 1986, pp 995–1013.
6. Swenson O, Sherman JO, Fisher JH: Diagnosis of congenital megacolon: An analysis of 501 patients. J Pediatr Surg 8:587, 1973.
7. Tiffin ME, Chandler FR, Faber HK: Localized absence of the ganglion cells in the myenteric plexus in congenital megacolon. Am J Dis Child 59:1071, 1940.
8. Tobon F, Schuster M: Megacolon: Special diagnostic and therapeutic features. Johns Hopkins Med J 135:91, 1974.

83. INTUSSUSCEPTION

Denis D. Bensard, M.D., and Frederick M. Karrer, M.D.

1. At what ages is idiopathic intussusception most likely to occur? Is there a seasonal variation in the incidence?
Idiopathic intussusception is a disease of infancy. Nearly two-thirds (63%) of the cases occur within the first 2 years of life. Intussusception in neonates and older children is uncommon. The number of reported cases peaks in the summer months. However, this seasonal fluctuation does not coincide with the peak incidence of respiratory or gastrointestinal viral illnesses, which more commonly peak in the midwinter months.

2. What is the cause of intussusception?
The cause remains unknown, but investigators have hypothesized that viral infection leads to lymphoid hyperplasia. The hypertrophied Peyer's patches, primarily in the terminal ileum, then serve as a lead point, resulting in intussusception of the ileum into the colon. This form of intussusception, known as idiopathic intussusception, accounts for approximately 90% of reported cases. The remaining 10% of cases consist of intussusception due to an identifiable lead point.

3. When should a lead point be suspected?
A pathologic lead point should be suspected in children over the age of 2 years. Bruce et al. reported that a pathologic lead point was identified in only 10% of patients under 2 years of age; in contrast, 75% of children over the age of 5 demonstrated a pathologic lead point.

4. Name several pathologic lead points that may result in intussusception.
Meckel's diverticulum is the most commonly reported lead point (>75%), followed by **intestinal polyps** (juvenile polyp, Peutz-Jeghers syndrome), **hematoma** (abdominal trauma, hemophilia, blood dyscrasia, Henoch-Schönlein purpura), and **malignancy** (lymphoma, lymphosarcoma). Rare lead points include enteric duplications, ectopic gastric mucosa, foreign body, intramural fecalith, and suture line.

5. Intussusception occurs most frequently in which area of the intestine?
Because idiopathic intussusception is the most frequent type and involves primarily the terminal ileum, the most frequent location of intussusception is ileocolic. Colocolic and ileoileal intussusceptions typically occur when a lead point is present and thus are less common.

6. Which is the intussusceptum and which is the intussuscipiens?
The advancing telescoping inner segment of intestine is defined as the intussusceptum and associated with a lead point, if present. The outer segment of the intestine, in which the inner telescoping segment of intestine advances, is defined as the intussuscipiens.

7. What is the typical presentation of a child with intussusception?
A previously healthy, well-nourished infant presents with the sudden onset of abdominal pain. The crampy abdominal pain characteristically produces paroxysms of crying, sweating, and drawing up of the lower extremities. When the pain subsides, the infant initially appears well, but if the attacks persist, exhaustion follows and the infant becomes somnolent. As the bowel obstruction progresses, vomiting and fever ensue. The passage of a stool with blood and mucus, often described as currant jelly, is considered pathognomonic for the diagnosis of intussusception. Unfortunately, the classic triad of intermittent bloody stool, vomiting, and crampy pain is present in fewer than 25% of patients. The physical examination depends on the duration of the intussusception; various degrees of dehydration and abdominal distention are present. A palpable sausage-shaped mass in the right upper quadrant or mid-upper abdomen is present in about one-half of patients. Rectal examination reveals grossly bloody stool or guaiac-positive stool; in rare patients, the intussusception may even be palpable. A plain radiograph of the abdomen may demonstrate the absence of viscera in the right lower quadrant of the abdomen, known as **Dance's sign**. The presence of free air in the abdomen suggests hollow visceral perforation; no further tests are necessary, and the patient is prepared for exploratory laparotomy.

8. How is the diagnosis confirmed? What should be done before the study? What are the contraindications?
Barium enema is considered the diagnostic test of choice. However, the infant has a potential surgical problem and must be prepared accordingly. Intravenous fluids, antibiotics, and appropriate sedation are given. The operating room and the surgeon in attendance for the barium enema should be notified. A positive study demonstrates distal obstruction with the absence of reflux into the terminal ileum. Barium enema should not be performed in patients in septic shock or with evidence of peritonitis on physical examination or pneumoperitoneum on plain radiograph of the abdomen.

9. What are the therapeutic options?
Once the diagnosis is established, hydrostatic reduction with barium enema is the preferred initial treatment—if there are no compelling reasons to proceed directly to surgery. In experienced centers, hydrostatic reduction is successful in 70–85% of patients. To reiterate, absolute contraindications to attempted hydrostatic reduction include clinical shock, peritonitis, or pneumoperitoneum. Relative contraindications include duration of symptoms for longer than 24 hours and age greater than 6 years.

10. What are the principles of successful hydrostatic reduction?
The principles of successful nonoperative management emerged from the seminal work of Mark Ravitch and are typically referred to as Ravitch's rules:

1. The patient is prepared for the operation (intravenous line, hydration, blood type and cross-match, antibiotics, and nasogastric tube if obstruction is present).

2. The surgeon in attendance constantly reevaluates the patient and the progress of the attempted hydrostatic reduction.

3. The barium reservoir should not exceed a height of 1 meter above the patient.

4. Visible reflux of barium into the terminal ileum ensures successful reduction.

11. What are the operative principles?

Operative reduction is indicated in patients for whom barium enema is contraindicated or fails to reduce the intussusception. Once the need for operative reduction has been established, it should be done as expeditiously as possible to avoid ischemic necrosis of the bowel. A right-sided transverse supraumbilical incision is preferred and provides adequate access to the intussuscepted bowel; if necessary, the incision may be easily extended across the midline to provide greater exposure. Once the intussusception is mobilized, gentle milking of distal bowel against the leading edge permits reduction. To prevent perforation, traction must not be applied to the proximal bowel. If the intussuscepted bowel is nonviable or perforated, no attempts at reduction are made and the bowel is resected. If operative reduction is unsuccessful, bowel resection and primary anastomosis are indicated. If reduction is successful, the bowel must be assessed for viability and irreversible ischemic injury must be excluded before closure of the incision.

12. Once nonoperative or operative reduction is successful, what is the risk of recurrent intussusception?

The risk of recurrent intussusception is 5–10%, regardless of the method of reduction. Thus patients must be observed for recurrence 24–48 hours after successful reduction.

CONTROVERSIES

13. Is ultrasound a useful diagnostic modality or just another test?

Investigators have demonstrated the efficacy of ultrasonography in the diagnosis of intussusception. Ultrasound may demonstrate a target lesion (transverse section) or a pseudokidney (longitudinal section) suggestive of intussusception. In a study of patients with presumptive intussusception, Pracros reported 100% sensitivity and specificity for diagnostic ultrasound. Unlike barium enema, however, ultrasound cannot be used therapeutically, depends on the experience and skill of the sonographer, and may lead to therapeutic delay in the presence of threatened bowel. Given these limitations and the climate of medical cost-consciousness, ultrasound cannot be recommended.

14. Is air enema an advance in nonoperative treatment or just more hot air?

Air enema appears to be highly successful in the nonoperative management of intussusception. Developed in mainland China, air enema has been used to achieve successful reduction in 80–90% of patients. Air is insufflated at an initial pressure 60 mmHg and incrementally increased to a pressure of 120 mmHg. Successful reduction is characterized by radiographic demonstration of the intussusception, flow of air into the small bowel, and clinical improvement. The risk of perforation (0.5–1.5%) does not appear to be significantly different from that of hydrostatic reduction (0.5–2%); if perforation occurs, it is not complicated by barium contamination of the peritoneal cavity. Reported advantages of air enema over hydrostatic enema include shorter fluoroscopic times with concomitant decrease in radiation exposure, greater facility in reduction of the intussusception due to the characteristics of air, and reduced rate of recurrent intussusception. Therefore, air enema appears to be an emerging alternative to hydrostatic enema for the nonoperative management of intussusception.

BIBLIOGRAPHY

1. Bruce J, Huh YS, Cooney DR, et al: Intussusception: Evolution of current management. J Pediatr Gastroenterol Nutr 6:663–764, 1987.

2. Ein SH, Palder SB, Alton DJ, et al: Intussusception: Toward less surgery? J Pediatr Surg 29:433–435, 1994.
3. Ong NT, Beasley SW: The leadpoint in intussusception. J Pediatr Surg 25:640–643, 1990.
4. Palder SB, Ein SH, Stringer DA, et al: Intussusception: Barium or air? J Pediatr Surg 26:271–275, 1991.
5. Pracros JP, Tran-Minh VA, Morin De Finfe CH, et al: Acute intestinal intussusception in children: Contribution of ultrasonography. Ann Radiol 30:525–530, 1987.
6. Ravitch MM: Intussusception in Infants and Children. Springfield, IL, Charles C Thomas, 1959.
7. Zheng JY, Frush DP, Guo JZ: Review of pneumatic reduction of intussusception: Evolution not revolution. J Pediatr Surg 29:93–97, 1994.

84. CONGENITAL DIAPHRAGMATIC HERNIA

Denis D. Bensard, M.D., and Frederick M. Karrer, M.D.

1. What is the most common type of congenital diaphragmatic hernia?

Congenital abnormalities of the diaphragm include a posterolateral defect (Bochdalek hernia), an anteromedial defect (Morgagni hernia), and eventration (central weakening) of the diaphragm. The most common congenital diaphragmatic hernia (CDH) is the posterolateral defect, which occurs in 1 in 3600 live births; 80% occur on the left side, 19% on the right side, and 1% are bilateral. The Bochdalek hernia is thought to arise from failure of the septum transversum and pleuroperitoneal folds to fuse at 8 weeks of gestation. This failure allows herniation of the bowel into the thorax, compression of the developing lung, and resultant lung hypoplasia. The anteromedial defect arises through an area of the diaphragm normally traversed by the internal mammary and epigastric vessels. The Morgagni hernia, which is 20 times less common than the Bochdalek hernia, is rarely symptomatic in neonates. If the defect enlarges, children present with episodic coughing, choking, vomiting, and/or epigastric complaints. Eventration of the diaphragm may be congenital or acquired. If the hemidiaphragm consists only of the pleuroperitoneal membrane, the distinction from CDH becomes arbitrary. In contrast, acquired eventration generally occurs secondary to a CNS disorder (Werdnig-Hoffman or Erb-Duchnenne syndrome) or after injury to the phrenic nerve. Like Bochdalek hernia, eventration is typically recognized when the neonate develops respiratory distress; a chest roentgenogram reveals abnormal elevation of the diaphragm with paradoxical motion.

2. What signs and symptoms suggest congenital diaphragmatic hernia?

Neonatal respiratory distress is the most common manifestation of CDH. At birth or shortly thereafter, the infant develops severe dyspnea, retractions, and cyanosis. On physical examination, breath sounds are diminished on the ipsilateral side, heart sounds can be heard more easily in the contralateral chest, and the abdomen is scaphoid because of the herniation of abdominal viscera into the chest. As the infant struggles to breathe, air enters the bowel, which becomes distended and results in further compromise of ventilation. If the herniation is allowed to progress, the mediastinum shifts, impairing venous return and cardiac output. Typically, the infant is mottled and hypotensive.

3. How is the diagnosis confirmed?

If CDH is suspected, a plain chest roentgenogram is obtained. The radiograph may demonstrate multiple loops of air-filled intestine in the ipsilateral thorax. If, however, films are obtained before entry of significant amounts of air into the bowel, a confusing pattern of mediastinal shift, cardiac displacement, and opacification of the hemithorax may be observed. Insertion of a nasogastric tube, injection of air or contrast, and repeat chest roentgenogram should confirm the diagnosis.

4. Are other anomalies associated with CDH?

Major congenital malformations are typically associated with other anomalies. The reported incidence of associated anomalies in CDH varies from 40–60%. Fewer than 10% of patients with multiple major anomalies survive. Postmortem studies of stillbirths with CDH demonstrate the presence of associated anomalies in 95% of cases. Wilson suggests that the disparate variability of reported anomalies results from the **inclusion** or **exclusion** of certain anomalies (patent ductus arteriosus, intestinal malrotation, pulmonary hypoplasia), of stillborns or deaths before arrival at a referral center, and of autopsy results. He also suggests that the timing of diagnosis of CDH affects the detection of associated anomalies. Although Wilson reported the overall incidence of associated anomalies to be 39%, the incidence was higher in patients in whom an antenatal diagnosis of CDH was made, and if CDH was diagnosed before 25 weeks, the anomalies were often more severe and life-threatening. Consequently, the true incidence is likely underestimated; the more critically affected subset of patients is not recognized because of fetal demise or early postnatal death. Excluding intestinal malrotation and pulmonary hypoplasia, cardiac anomalies (63%) are the most frequent, followed by genitourinary (23%), gastrointestinal (17%), central nervous system (14%), and pulmonary (5%) anomalies.

5. What therapeutic measures should be initiated before transport or operation?
Perhaps the easiest and most effective palliative intervention is the placement of a nasogastric tube with continuous suction. This maneuver permits decompression of the stomach, prevents further distention of the bowel, and thus improves ventilation. Endotracheal intubation follows with a twofold purpose: (1) adequate ventilation and oxygenation and (2) prevention of bowel distention due to crying or mask ventilation. Because the lungs are hypoplastic and at risk for further injury from barotrauma, ventilatory pressures are kept low (< 30 mmHg) and the infant is ventilated with a rapid ventilatory rate (40–60 breaths/minute). Venous access is rapidly obtained, fluids administered, and acidosis corrected. Once such measures are completed, the infant is prepared for emergent transport to a neonatal center.

6. What is the "honeymoon period"?
A spectrum of presentations is seen in patients with CDH. Up to 65% of neonates with CDH are stillborn or die shortly after birth, whereas 5–25% of patients with CDH are discovered after the neonatal period. If the patient develops symptoms after the first 24 hours of life, the survival rate is nearly 100%. On the other hand, if respiratory symptoms develop within the first 24 hours of life, the survival rate decreases to 50–60%. The degree and rapidity of respiratory symptoms appear to be related to the degree of lung hypoplasia. Minimally symptomatic or asymptomatic neonates have demonstrated sufficient lung volume compatible with survival. Conversely, profound respiratory distress implies insufficient lung volume to ensure survival without maximal medical therapy; a subset of patients succumbs from pulmonary insufficiency despite all interventions. The honeymoon period describes the interval of time in which a neonate demonstrates adequate oxygenation and ventilation in the absence of maximal medical therapy. Regardless of subsequent deterioration, a honeymoon period suggests that pulmonary function is compatible with survival.

7. Describe the operative approach.
The infant must be stabilized before surgical repair is attempted, but the optimal timing of surgery remains unclear. In a prospective study of 32 patients with CDH randomized to early (< 6 hours) or delayed repair (> 96 hours), Nio et al. found that survival rates and use of extracorporeal membrane oxygenation (ECMO) were the same, whether repair was early or delayed. This study and others confirm that repair of CDH is not a surgical emergency. A transthoracic or transabdominal approach may be used for surgical repair of CDH. The transabdominal approach is the favored initial approach for the following reasons: (1) reduction of the herniated abdominal viscera is simplified; (2) the diaphragmatic defect may be repaired with unobstructed vision and without tension; (3) malrotation with or without obstruction is easily identified and corrected; and (4) if the abdominal cavity does not initially accommodate the reduced viscera, it may be stretched or a ventral hernia may be created with either a prosthetic patch or silo. The transthoracic approach is generally reserved for repair of recurrent diaphragmatic hernia or for older children (age > 1 year). Adhesions are easily taken down and diaphragmatic closure is better achieved because of the excellent exposure provided by the larger hemithorax.

8. What is the most feared complication of diaphragmatic hernia? Is it correctable? If so, how?

In congenital diaphragmatic hernia, one or both lungs are hypoplastic, the pulmonary vascular bed is reduced, and the pulmonary arteries demonstrate thickened muscular walls that are hyper-reactive to mediators of pulmonary vasoconstriction (hypoxia, hypercarbia, acidemia). Thus, patients with CDH are particularly prone to the development of pulmonary hypertension. If CDH is uncorrected, the infant rapidly develops persistent fetal circulation (PFC), the most feared complication. PFC arises from a sustained increase in pulmonary artery pressure. Blood is shunted away from the lungs, and the unoxygenated blood is diverted to the systemic circulation through the patent ductus arteriosus and patent foramen ovale. PFC results in profound acidosis, shock, and, if irreversible, death. PFC is triggered by acidosis, hypercarbia, and hypoxia, all potent vaso-constrictors of the pulmonary circulation. Various strategies are used to prevent the onset of PFC:

1. Oxygen monitoring or arterial sampling (preductal in the right upper extremity, postductal in the lower extremity) detects the shunting of unoxygenated blood to the systemic circulation.

2. Optimal ventilation to prevent hypercarbia is enhanced by rapid, low-pressure mechanical ventilation, adequate sedation, and, if necessary, pharmacologic paralysis.

3. Similarly hypoxemia is avoided by adequate ventilation and high concentrations of inspired oxygen (generally $FiO_2 = 100\%$).

4. Metabolic acidosis is managed by restoring adequate perfusion with intravenous fluids or blood, inotropes, and appropriate administration of sodium bicarbonate.

If these maneuvers fail, alternate therapies include administration of pulmonary vasodilators via the ventilatory circuit (nitric oxide) or systemic circulation (priscoline, prostaglandin E_2), high-frequency ventilation, and finally ECMO. Additional early complications include lung injury and pneumothorax due to barotrauma and bleeding, particularly if repaired on ECMO. In follow-up studies of patients with CDH who require ECMO, the most common late complications appear to be failure to thrive, gastroesophageal reflux, chronic lung disease, abnormal neurocognitive development, and recurrent diaphragmatic hernia.

9. What is the survival rate among patients with CDH?

Accurate survival data in CDH are confounded by a number of variables. Although the overall survival rate appears to be 50–60%, a wider range may be reported in centers with the ability to care for more critically affected neonates. The major determinants of survival are the degree of pulmonary hypoplasia and associated major congenital anomalies. Among infants surviving the early newborn period without significant lung dysfunction, the survival rate is 70–100%. In contrast, severely affected infants with severe lung dysfunction often die shortly after birth. As Harrison suggests, such patients represent the hidden mortality of CDH. Moreover, in centers at which salvage therapies, such as ECMO or nitric oxide are used, survival rates have not improved; in fact, they have decreased because of inclusion of more severely affected patients who previously died shortly after birth. At the University of Michigan, examination of survival data before and after the introduction of ECMO demonstrates a fall in the overall rate from 75% to 59%. Furthermore, expansion of inclusion criteria for ECMO resulted in only a 27% increase in survival for patients who were previously considered unsalvageable. Clearly, patients with severe lung hypoplasia due to CDH will die regardless of application of current therapies, and overall survival rates will not change unless experimental therapies, such as lung transplantation or fetal surgery, prove to be efficacious.

10. Does in-utero intervention have a role in treatment of CDH?

To date, fetal surgery for CDH remains experimental. Harrison, a pioneer in fetal surgery, has accrued the most extensive experience in in-utero repair of CDH. In 1993 he reported the results of in-utero repair of 14 patients. Five fetuses died intraoperatively; of 9 patients successfully repaired, 4 (29%) survived. During the same period, 47 additional patients underwent evaluation for in-utero repair but were not considered candidates; of these, 40% survived. Such data suggest that, as in ECMO, accurate identification of patients most likely to benefit from aggressive intervention remains undefined. Given the difficulties of in-utero repair of CDH, Harrison reported an alternative approach in animals, using in-utero tracheal occlusion. In an animal model of CDH, tracheal occlusion resulted in lung growth and reduction of the herniated viscera, permitting uncomplicated postnatal repair of the CDH. No results have yet been reported in humans.

BIBLIOGRAPHY

1. Bealer JF, Skarsgard ED, Hedrick MH, et al: The "PLUG" odyssey: Adventures in experimental fetal tracheal occlusion. J Pediatr Surg 30:361–365, 1995.
2. Breaux CW, Rouse TM, Cain WS, et al: Improvement in survival of patients with congenital diaphragmatic hernia utilizing a strategy of delayed repair after medical and/or ECMO stabilization. J Pediatr Surg 26:333–338, 1991.
3. D'Agostino JA, Bernbaum JC, Gerdes M, et al: Outcome for infants with congenital diaphragmatic hernia requiring extracorporeal membrane oxygenation: The first year. J Pediatr Surg 30:10–15, 1995.
4. Fauza DO, Wilson JM: Congenital diaphragmatic hernia and associated anomalies: Their incidence, identification, and impact on prognosis. J Pediatr Surg 29:1113–1117, 1994.
5. Gleeson F, Spitz L: Pitfalls in the diagnosis of congenital diaphragmatic hernia. Arch Dis Child 66:670–671, 1991.
6. Gross RE: Congenital hernias of the diaphragm. In Surgery of Infancy and Childhood. Philadelphia, W.B. Saunders, 1953.
7. Harrison MR, Adzick NS, Flake AW, et al: Correction of congenital diaphragmatic hernia in-utero. VI: Hard-learned lessons. J Pediatr Surg 28:1411–1418, 1993.
8. Nio M, Haase G, Kennaugh J, et al: A prospective randomized trial of delayed versus immediate repair of congenital diaphragmatic hernia. J Pediatr Surg 29:618–621, 1994.
9. Steimle CN, Meric F, Hirschl RB, et al: Effect of extracorporeal life support on survival when applied to all patients with congenital diaphragmatic hernia. J Pediatr Surg 29:997–1001, 1994.
10. Weinstein S, Stolar CJ: Newborn surgical emergencies: Congenital diaphragmatic hernia and extracorporeal membrane oxygenation. Pediatr Clin North Am 40:1315–1333, 1993.

85. IMPERFORATE ANUS

Kennith H. Sartorelli, M.D., and Frederick M. Karrer, M.D.

1. How common is imperforate anus? Is it associated with other anomalies?

Anorectal malformations occur in 1/5000 live births and are part of the **VACTERL** (vertebral, anorectal, cardiac, tracheoesophageal, renal, and limb) complex of defects. Ten percent of patients have tracheoesophageal fistula, 15% have cardiac defects, 10–50% have renal anomalies, 40% have vertebral anomalies, and up to 14% have spinal dysraphism. Infants with imperforate anus must be carefully screened for these other defects.

2. What are the types of imperforate anus? How are they differentiated?

Anorectal malformations can be classified into high and low lesions. High lesions are much more common in boys (75% of cases), whereas low lesions predominate in girls. Low lesions are characterized by perineal or Fourchette fistulas in girls. Meconium in the urine, pneumaturia, bifid scrotum, and a "flat bottom" are indicative of high lesions. When the level of the lesion is not clear, a prone or inverted abdominal radiograph may reveal a column of rectal gas and aid in determining the height of the defect.

3. Does treatment differ for high and low lesions?

Low anorectal malformations may be treated by immediate anoplasty (with the exception of Fourchette fistulas). High lesions require a colostomy and later pull-through procedure. High lesions are also more likely than low lesions to have associated anomalies. Of boys with high anorectal malformations, 60–80% have a rectourinary fistula that must be fixed at the time of pull-through.

4. What is a cloaca?
This complex defect accounts for 10% of anorectal malformations in girls and is characterized by a common external opening for the rectum, urethra, and vagina. Up to 90% of patients have other urinary tract anomalies.

5. Do children with anorectal malformations achieve normal continence?
Children with low imperforate anus should have normal continence, although they are prone to constipation. Voluntary bowel function with high malformations is proportional to the level of the lesion. Of children with moderately high defects, 60–70% have voluntary bowel movements, whereas only 10–20% with rectums ending at the level of the bladder have voluntary bowel movements. Bowel management with dietary modifications and enemas allows most children with poor continence to minimize soiling.

CONTROVERSY

6. What type of colostomy should be performed in infants with high imperforate anus?
Traditionally loop colostomies have been performed, although divided colostomies have been advocated. A divided colostomy prevents the formation of a blind-ending megarectum from stool spillover, separates the urinary tract from the fecal stream when a rectourinary fistula is present, and allows access to the distal rectum for radiographic imaging.

BIBLIOGRAPHY

1. Pena A: Atlas of Surgical Management of Anorectal Malformations. New York, Springer Verlag, 1992.
2. Pena A: Anorectal malformations. Semin Pediatr 4:35–47, 1995.

86. ABDOMINAL MASSES AND TUMORS

Kennith H. Sartorelli, M.D., and Frederick M. Karrer, M.D.

1. What is the most common abdominal mass in a newborn infant?
An obstructed kidney (usually from uteropelvic junction obstruction) is the most frequent cause of an abdominal mass in a newborn infant. Other causes include congenital mesoblastic nephromas, mesenteric cysts, ovarian masses, benign and malignant hepatic tumors, neuroblastomas, and Wilms' tumors (rare).

2. What are the most common malignant solid abdominal tumors in children? Where do they originate?
Neuroblastomas, Wilms' tumors, hepatoblastomas, and hepatocellular carcinomas are the most common solid abdominal malignancies in children. Neuroblastomas are derived from neural crest tissue; in the abdomen they originate from the adrenal glands and paraspinal sympathetic ganglia. Wilms' tumors originate from the kidney. Hepatoblastomas and hepatocellular carcinoma originate in the liver.

3. How are Wilms' tumors differentiated from neuroblastomas?
Both tumors often present as an asymptomatic mass. Wilms' tumors rarely cross the midline, whereas midline extension is common with neuroblastomas. Neuroblastomas are more common in 1–2-year-old children, whereas Wilms' tumors are most common in 3–4-year-old children. Wilms' tumors often present with painless hematuria. Neuroblastomas may have diverse associated

symptoms, including flushing and hypertension from catecholamine release, watery diarrhea, periorbital ecchymoses, and abnormal ocular movements. On radiographs neuroblastomas often show calcification.

4. What is the treatment of Wilms' tumor and neuroblastomas?
Surgical resection is the primary treatment for both types of tumor. Adjunctive chemotherapy has been instrumental in dramatically increasing the cure rate for Wilms' tumor but has had little effect on survival in patients with neuroblastoma.

5. What are the major prognostic factors in neuroblastomas?
Age at presentation is an important prognostic factor in neuroblastomas. Children younger than 1 year have an overall survival rate greater than 70%, whereas the survival rate in children older than 1 year is under 35%. Shimada proposed a prognostic classification based on evaluation of histologic parameters (tumor differentiation, mitosis-karyorrhexis index) as well as age. Aneuploid tumors and tumors with fewer than 10 copies of the n-*myc* gene also have been associated with better outcomes.

6. What are the differences between hepatoblastomas and hepatocellular carcinomas? How are these tumors treated?
Hepatoblastomas usually occur in infants and young children, whereas hepatocellular carcinoma usually occurs in children over 10 years of age. Hepatocellular carcinoma is associated with cirrhosis and hepatitis B and is histologically identical to the adult form. Surgical resection is the primary therapy for both types of tumor. Hepatoblastomas often have a good response to adjunctive chemotherapy, whereas hepatocellular carcinoma rarely responds to chemotherapy.

CONTROVERSY

7. Should patients with hepatoblastoma receive preoperative chemotherapy to shrink the tumor?
Preoperative chemotherapy has been reported to shrink tumors, resulting in easier hepatic resection and lower surgical morbidity. This benefit must be weighed against the morbidity related to the toxicity of chemotherapeutic agents.

BIBLIOGRAPHY

1. D'Angio GJ, Breslow N, Beckwith JB, et al: Treatment of Wilms' tumor—results of the third National Wilms' Tumor Study. Cancer 64:349–360, 1989.
2. Grosfeld JL, Rescorla FJ, West KW, et al: Neuroblastoma in the first year of life: Clinical and biological factors influencing outcome. Semin Pediatr Surg 2:37–46, 1993.
3. Pierro A, Langevin AM, Filler RM, et al: Preoperative chemotherapy for "unresectable" hepatoblastoma. J Pediatr Surg 24:24–29, 1989.

87. CONGENITAL CYSTS AND SINUSES

Kennith H. Sartorelli, M.D., and Frederick M. Karrer, M.D.

1. What are the most common masses in the necks of children?
Lymphadenitis is very common in children and must be differentiated from thyroglossal duct cysts, branchial cleft cysts, and cystic hygromas, which are common congenital neck cysts.

2. What is a thyroglossal duct cyst? Why should it be removed?

Thyroglossal duct cysts represent failure of the thyroid migration tract to close. The thyroid normally descends from the foramen cecum to its anatomic position in the lower neck. Thyroglossal duct cysts should be removed to prevent infection. Successful removal depends on resection of the central portion of the hyoid bone (Sistrunk procedure), through which the thyroglossal duct cyst passes.

3. Do thyroglossal duct cysts contain thyroid tissue?

Thyroid tissue is frequently found in thyroglossal duct cysts. If the thyroid gland is not palpable, an ultrasound or nuclear thyroid scan should be obtained. If the cyst represents the entire thyroid, treatment options include splitting the gland surgically, cyst removal with thyroid hormone supplementation, autotransplantation, or no operative treatment.

4. What is a branchial cleft cyst?

Branchial cleft cysts are malformations due to incomplete obliteration of the first, second, or third branchial cleft.

5. How do branchial cleft malformations present clinically?

Branchial cleft malformations may be a cyst, sinus, or complete fistulous tract. Cysts often present with a mass, sinuses and fistulas sometimes have clear or mucoid drainage, and all types may become infected. First branchial cleft anomalies present in front of the ear along the lower edge of the mandible and originate in the external auditory canal. Second branchial cleft cysts, which are the most common branchial cleft malformation, present along the anterior border of the sternocleidomastoid muscle. Second branchial cleft cysts originate in the tonsillar fossa and usually pass between the carotid bifurcation. Third branchial cleft cysts are rare; they present in the same areas but lower than second branchial cleft cysts. Third branchial cleft cysts originate from the pyriform sinus.

6. What are the major operative hazards of branchial cleft excisions?

The facial nerve is at risk during excision of first branchial cysts, whereas carotid artery and hypoglossal nerve injuries may occur during repair of second branchial cleft cysts.

7. What are cystic hygromas?

Cystic hygromas are malformations of the lymph system that result in lymph-filled cysts. Cystic hygromas are often intimately involved with neurovascular structures. Because they are benign, important neurovascular structures should not be sacrificed in an attempt at excision.

CONTROVERSY

8. How should lingual thyroids be treated?

Lingual thyroids (thyroid present in the tongue) may be treated by resection, resection with autotransplantation, or thyroid extract, which causes and maintains shrinkage of the lingual thyroid gland.

BIBLIOGRAPHY

1. Knight PJ, Hamoudi AB, Vassay LE: The diagnosis and treatment of midline neck masses in children. Surgery 93:603–611, 1983.
2. Tapper D: Head and neck masses. In Holder TM, Ashcraft KW (eds): Pediatric Surgery. Philadelphia, W.B. Saunders, 1993, pp 923–933.

X. Transplantation

88. LIVER TRANSPLANTATION

Mark D. Stegall, M.D., Frederick M. Karrer, M.D., and Igal Kam, M.D.

1. When and by whom was the first successful human liver transplant performed?
On March 1, 1963, Thomas Starzl performed the first human liver transplant at the University of Colorado in Denver.

2. How many liver transplants are performed each year in the U.S.?
Currently more than 2500 liver transplants are performed annually. However, this number is less than half of the estimated 5000 people for whom liver transplantation is the optimal treatment.

3. What are the most common indications for liver transplantation?
Postnecrotic cirrhosis, primary biliary cirrhosis, and sclerosing cholangitis account for more than 75% of the adult diagnoses. Biliary atresia accounts for over one-half of liver transplants in children.

4. What is the cost of a liver transplant?
The average initial cost is about $125,000, with follow-up costs of $10,000 /year.

5. What is the survival rate of patients who undergo liver transplantation?
The 1-year survival rate is 77%, whereas the 5-year survival rate is 65%. High-risk patients (preoperative encephalopathy, intensive care, renal failure) have a high early mortality rate with a 6-month survival rate of only 22% compared with 96% for low-risk patients.

6. Name the most common "weirdo" infections that occur in transplant recipients.
Cytomegalovirus (CMV), herpes simplex virus (HSV), and Epstein-Barr virus (EBV) are common in transplant recipients. Fungal infections such as aspergillosis pneumonia and candidal esophagitis are more common in immunosuppressed patients.

7. Are transplant recipients more likely to develop cancer?
Yes—especially skin and cervical cancers. EBV infection is closely linked to a B-cell lymphoma that usually responds to antiviral therapy and a reduction in immunosuppression.

CONTROVERSIES

8. Should patients with alcoholic liver disease receive a liver transplant?
The recidivism rate of alcoholics who receive transplants is only 11%, and the cost of repeated hospitalizations for end-stage alcoholic liver disease may easily exceed the cost of a liver transplant. Most centers offer transplants to alcoholics who have abstained from drinking for at least 6 months and have good family support.

9. Should infants with biliary atresia initially undergo a Kasai portoenterostomy or a liver transplant?

Infants with adequate bile ducts for a successful Kasai operation have a 70% chance of survival into childhood (5–10 years) and a 25% chance of indefinite survival with adequate liver function. The mortality rate for liver transplantation is high in children under the age of 1 year (60–80%). Consequently, the current recommendation is to attempt the Kasai portoenterostomy and to resort to liver transplantation only if it fails.

10. Did someone transplant a baboon liver into a human?

Yes. In June 1992 and again in January 1993, baboon-to-human liver transplants were performed at the University of Pittsburgh. Both grafts functioned initially and then were lost. In the future, xenografts (transplants between species) may be used to solve the organ shortage if the problems of xenograft rejection can be overcome.

11. What are the indications for liver transplant from a living relative?

Most recipients of liver transplants from living relatives are children for whom a donor cannot be found. A parent is usually the donor, and only a small portion of the donor's liver is removed (usually the left lateral segment). Despite an apparent increase in complications, especially bile leaks and strictures of the bile duct, the 1-year survival rate for both patient and graft is greater than 90%.

BIBLIOGRAPHY

1. Belle SH, Beringer KC, Detre DM: Trends in liver transplantation in the United States. In Terasaki PI, Cecka JM (eds): Clinical Transplantation 1993. Los Angeles, UCLA Tissue Typing Laboratory, 1994, pp 19–36.
2. Broelsch C, Emond J, Thistlewaite J, et al: Liver transplantation, including the concept of reduced-size liver transplants in children. Ann Surg 208:410, 1988.
3. Gish RG, Lee AH, Keeffe EB, et al: Liver transplantation with alcoholism and end-stage liver disease. Am J Gastroenterol 88:1337, 1993.
4. Penn I: The problem of cancer in organ transplant recipients: An overview. Transplant Sci 4:23, 1994.
5. Starzl TE, Fung J, Tzakis A, et al: Baboon to human liver transplantation. Lancet 341:65, 1993.
6. Starzl TE, Gordon RD, Tzakis AG, et al: Liver transplantation. In Sabiston DC (ed): Textbook of Surgery. Philadelphia, W.B. Saunders, 1991, pp 423–433.
7. Staschak S, Wagner S, Block D, et al: A cost comparison of liver transplantation with FK506 and CyA as the primary immunosuppressive agent. Transplant Proc 22(Suppl 1):47, 1990.

89. KIDNEY TRANSPLANTATION

Mark D. Stegall, M.D.

1. List the most common causes of renal failure leading to kidney transplantation.

Diabetes, glomerulonephritis, and hypertension are the leading causes. In many cases, the cause is not determined.

2. How many hours can a kidney be preserved outside the donor before transplantation?

Using the University of Wisconsin solution, a kidney can be stored for up to 72 hours and still function. In practice, however, most kidneys function best if transplanted within 24 hours of procurement.

3. List the common immunosuppressive agents and their mechanism of action.

Cyclosporine: a cyclic polypeptide that acts by inhibiting the synthesis of interleukin-2 (IL-2), a cytokine necessary for T-helper cell activation.

Azathioprine: a purine analog that prevents lymphocyte proliferation.

Corticosteroids: inhibit cytokines, especially IL-1.

Tacrolimus (FK506): like cyclosporine, inhibits IL-2 production and may be especially beneficial in liver transplantation.

Mycophrenic mofetil: inhibits the purine salvage pathway that is important to dividing lymphocytes; may replace azathioprine.

4. What is OKT3?

OKT3 is a mouse monoclonal antibody directed against the CD3 molecule present on all T-cells. OKT3 may be given as induction immunosuppression (i.e., initially from the time of transplant), but its main use is in the treatment of rejection episodes that do not respond to corticosteroid treatment. OKT3 is the most powerful antirejection treatment available, but its efficacy is limited if the recipient develops antimouse antibodies.

5. Do transplant recipients have to take immunosuppressive medicines indefinitely?

A very small number of patients have been able to stop taking immunosuppressive medicines without rejecting the transplanted kidney, but most patients reject the kidney if they stop their medicine. Presently, there is no way to predict who needs to be immunosuppressed, and late graft loss due to chronic rejection is common even in immunosuppressed patients.

6. How many kidney transplants are performed each year?

In 1992, 6244 transplants from cadaver donors and 1616 from living donors were performed in the United States.

7. What is the graft survival rate of kidney transplants?

The 1-year graft survival rate is approximately 84% for cadaver donors. The 3-year graft survival rate is approximately 70%. In hundreds of patients kidney grafts have functioned more than 20 years, and one patient transplanted in 1964 still has a functioning cadaver graft.

CONTROVERSIES

8. Who can get a kidney-pancreas transplant?

Any diabetic with renal failure is a possible candidate for both kidney and pancreas transplants. Most centers perform kidney-pancreas transplants only in type I diabetic patients with few secondary complications. A successful pancreas transplant leads to normal serum glucose levels without insulin treatment and greatly improves the recipient's quality of life.

9. Who can be a living donor for a kidney transplant?

Most living donors of transplanted kidneys are siblings or parents of the recipient. However, grafts from living unrelated donors (spouses, distant relatives, or significant others) have excellent survival rates: 92% at 1 year and 85% at 3 years. There seems to be no long-term health risks to living donors.

10. Does HLA matching improve renal graft survival?

There is a small but significant improvement in graft survival with better HLA matching. The 3-year graft survival is 84% with no mismatches and 75%, 71%, and 67%, respectively, with 1 or 2, 3 or 4, and 5 or 6 mismatches.

BIBLIOGRAPHY

1. Barker CF, Naji A, Dafoe DC, et al: Renal transplantation. In Sabiston DC (ed): Textbook of Surgery. Philadelphia, W.B. Saunders, 1991, pp 374–393.
2. Cecka JM, Terasaki PI: The UNOS scientific renal transplant registry. In Terasaki PI (ed): Clinical Transplants 1994. Los Angeles, UCLA Tissue Typing Laboratory, 1995, pp 1–18.

3. Marshall SE, Waldmann H: Monoclonal antibody therapy in clinical transplantation. In Kupiec-Weglinski JW (ed): New Immunosuppressive Modalities and Anti-rejection Approaches in Organ Transplantation. Austin, TX, R.G. Landes, 1994, pp 107–124.
4. Matas AJ, Sutherland DER, Najarian JS: The impact of HLA matching on graft survival. Transplantation 54:568, 1992.
5. Ploeg RJ, Goossens D, McAnulty JF, et al: Successful 72-hour cold storage of dog kidneys with UW solution. Transplantation 46:191, 1988.
6. Ploeg RJ, Pirsch JD, Stegall MD, et al: Living unrelated kidney donation: An underutilized resource? Transplant Proc 25:1532, 1993.
7. Sollinger HW, Stegall MD: Pancreas transplantation. In Sabiston DC (ed): Textbook of Surgery. Philadelphia, W.B. Saunders, 1991, p 433.
8. Takemoto S, Terasaki PI, Cecka JM, et al: Survival of nationally shared HLA-matched kidney transplants from cadaveric donors. N Engl J Med 327:834, 1992.
9. Young CJ, Sollinger HW: Mycophenolate mofetil (RS-61443). In Kupiec-Weglinski JW (ed): New Immunosuppressive Modalities and Anti-rejection Approaches in Organ Transplantation. Austin, TX, R.G. Landes, 1994, pp 1–18.

90. HEART AND LUNG TRANSPLANTATION

Daniel R. Meldrum, M.D., and Frederick L. Grover, M.D.

HEART TRANSPLANTATION

1. Who performed the first human heart transplant and when?
C.N. Bernard performed the first human heart transplant in December, 1967, although Norman Shumway set the stage by developing the technique in animals. Shumway and the Stanford group also accomplished the first successful clinical series.

2. Approximately how many heart transplants are performed annually? Is the number increasing or decreasing?
In 1983 approximately 500 heart transplants were performed. By 1988 the number had rapidly increased to approximately 3000 and remains relatively stable at about 3000.

3. Who is a candidate for a heart transplant?
Although candidate selection is evolving as a result of improved techniques and outcomes, the following criteria are standard: age between newborn and 65 years; irremediable New York Heart Association Functional Class IV cardiac disease; normal renal, hepatic, pulmonary, and CNS function; pulmonary vascular resistance less than 6–8 Wood units; and absence of malignancy, infection, recent pulmonary infarction, and severe peripheral vascular or cerebrovascular disease. Diabetes is a relative contraindication; the steroids frequently used in posttransplant immunosuppression make diabetes difficult to manage.

4. What are the most common indications for heart transplant?
In adults, coronary artery disease (ischemic cardiomyopathy) and idiopathic cardiomyopathy are the most common indications for heart transplantation, each accounting for approximately 45% of transplants.

In children, congenital heart disease and cardiomyopathy are the most common indications for heart transplantation; hypoplastic left heart is the most common congenital malformation requiring heart transplantation.

5. What percent of potential recipients die while waiting for a heart transplant?
20%.

6. Does HLA mismatch influence the incidence of rejection after heart transplantation? Is HLA typing routinely done before heart transplantation?

Yes and no. In a multiinstitutional, multivariate analysis of 1719 cardiac transplant recipients by Jarcho et al., HLA mismatch increased the incidence of rejection, but HLA typing is not routinely performed before heart transplantation because it takes too long. In addition, with 3 of 6 mismatches there was still only a trend toward increased rejection-related deaths (p = 0.14). If longer organ preservation times can be achieved, donor/recipient HLA matching will become feasible and should improve survival rates.

7. How is cardiac allograft rejection prevented?

Pharmacologically induced immunosuppression is performed by using one of two protocols. The first is triple therapy, which combines cyclosporine, azathioprine, and prednisone. The second major protocol incorporates the monoclonal antibody OKT3 into the triple therapy protocol. OKT3 is substituted for cyclosporine for the first 2 weeks after transplant.

8. What is OKT3?

OKT3 is a mouse monoclonal antibody that binds to and blocks the T-cell CD3 receptor. A monoclonal antibody is an antibody generated from the clones of a single cell. For instance, a single B-cell, which recognizes the CD3 receptor as an antigen (foreign), is immortalized in cell culture and able to secrete the monoclonal antibody OKT3 in limitless supply. The CD3 receptor, which is common to all T-cells, is important for antigen recognition and T-cell activation; therefore, OKT3 is highly immunosuppressive. OKT3 may have severe side effects, including pulmonary edema and high fevers, that are thought to result from transient cytokine release, which may occur when OKT3 binds to the T-cell activation site. Because OKT3 is an antigen, patients develop anti-OKT3 antibodies fairly quickly; the result is desensitization. Therefore, OKT3 is used judiciously.

9. What is cardiac preconditioning?

Cardiac preconditioning, first termed ischemic preconditioning, is a phenomenon by which a brief antecedent ischemic or hypoxic episode renders the heart more tolerant of a subsequent ischemic event. Pharmacologic preconditioning is based on using drugs to access the same endogenous protective mechanisms that occur during ischemic and hypoxic preconditioning. Alpha-1 adrenergic (norepinephrine and phenylephrine) and purinergic (adenosine A_1) agonists have shown promise experimentally. Pharmacologic induction of protective cardiac preconditioning may have profound implications for preservation of cardiac allografts.

10. At what point does donor heart ischemic time influence mortality?

Donor ischemic time greater than 6 hours definitely increases mortality. Ischemic times between 4 and 6 hours stun the donor heart. Most transplant teams try to keep ischemic times (from donor harvest to perfusion in the recipient) to less than 4 hours.

11. What are the major complications of heart transplantation?

Allograft rejection (days to weeks)
Infection (months)
Transplant coronary artery disease (years)

12. How is cardiac allograft rejection diagnosed?

Clinical suspicion is raised by new-onset cardiac arrhythmia, fever, or hypotension. Diagnosis depends on endomyocardial biopsy, which is performed at regular intervals to detect histologic evidence of rejection before signs or symptoms occur. Radionuclide ventriculography and echocardiography are useful adjuncts in following the hemodynamic manifestations of rejection. ECG is **not** useful in the diagnosis of rejection.

13. Can one heart be successfully transplanted twice?
Yes. Meiser et al. transplanted the same heart twice on March 19, 1991, 42 hours after the initial transplantation. Double transplant has since been reported by others.

14. What is "domino heart transplant"?
The good heart from a heart-lung recipient is transplanted into a patient requiring a heart transplant. Some patients with primary lung dysfunction have secondary irreversible cardiac dysfunction (i.e., Eisenmenger's syndrome); others, however, such as patients with cystic fibrosis, have good cardiac function. Patients with good cardiac function may serve as donors and increase the donor pool.

15. What is the overall 30-day mortality rate after heart transplant? What is the breakdown in mortality between adult and pediatric patients?
The registry of the International Society for Heart and Lung Transplantation, which has data about approximately 18,000 heart transplants, has recorded a 30-day mortality rate of 10%. The 30-day mortality rate for adult recipients is 8.5%; for pediatric recipients it is slightly higher (14%).

16. What are the 5- and 10-year actuarial survival rates for heart transplant recipients?
75% and 50%, respectively.

LUNG TRANSPLANTATION

17. What are the general types of lung transplants?
Single, double (bilateral), and heart-lung.

18. Which human organ transplant was performed first, the heart or the lung?
Although heart transplantation progressed more rapidly at first and therefore seems to outdate lung transplantation, the first lung transplant actually preceded the first heart transplant.

19. Who performed the first lung transplant and when?
James Hardy performed the first human lung transplant in 1963; however, more then 20 years passed before lung transplantation was performed routinely in clinical practice. This delay was due to problems with initial graft failure secondary to inadequate organ preservation, long ischemic times, lack of good immunosuppressants, and technical difficulties.

20. Who is a candidate for a lung transplant?
Patients with no other medical or surgical alternative who are likely to die of pulmonary disease within 12–18 months, are younger than 65 years, are not ventilator-dependent, and do not have a history of previous malignancy.

21. What are the most common indications for single lung transplant?
Emphysema (40%)
Idiopathic pulmonary fibrosis (17%)
Alpha-1 antitrypsin deficiency (17%)
Primary pulmonary hypertension and pulmonary hypertension secondary to correctable congenital heart disease (10–20%)

22. What are the most common indications for a double-lung transplant?
Cystic fibrosis (40%)
Emphysema (15%)
Alpha-1 antitrypsin deficiency (15%)
Primary pulmonary hypertension and pulmonary hypertension secondary to correctable congenital heart disease (15%)

23. What are the most common indications for heart-lung transplant?
Primary pulmonary hypertension (30%) and cystic fibrosis (16%) are instances in which bad lungs have ruined a good heart. Conversely, with congenital heart disease (27%), a bad heart has destroyed good lungs.

24. Which diagnoses carry the best results for single lung transplants?
Patients with emphysema and alpha-1 antitrypsin deficiency do significantly better, with 1-year survival rates of 80%.

25. How many single lung transplants are performed annually? Is the number increasing or decreasing?
Nearly 600 were performed in 1993; the number has rapidly increased from approximately 50 single lung transplants in 1988.

26. Why is the number of heart-lung transplants performed annually decreasing?
Approximately 225 heart-lung transplants were performed in 1989; the number decreased to approximately 150 in 1993. As the results of single and double lung transplant improved, the need to perform heart-lung transplants in patients with isolated pulmonary disease has been obviated.

27. What are the most common complications after lung transplant?
   Airway surgical healing defects (early)
   Rejection (early)
   Bacterial and cytomegalovirus infection (weeks to months)
   Bronchiolitis obliterans (months to years)

28. What is bronchiolitis obliterans?
Bronchiolitis obliterans, a major cause of long-term morbidity after lung transplantation, is a process in which membranous and respiratory bronchioles demonstrate histologic evidence of subepithelial scarring that eventually progresses to occlusion of the bronchiolar lumen. The pathogenesis is thought to be chronic rejection. It is clinically characterized by dyspnea and airflow obstruction.

29. How is rejection of the transplanted lung diagnosed?
Unlike hearts, the diagnosis of rejection in the transplanted lung is imprecise and based on a collection of symptoms and signs. Decreased oxygen saturation, fever, decreased exercise tolerance, and radiologic infiltrate suggest rejection. Sequential quantitative lung perfusion scans that demonstrate a decrease in perfusion are helpful in the diagnosis of rejection after single lung transplants. Transbronchial lung biopsy is useful after single and double lung transplants.

30. What percent of pulmonary blood flow goes to the transplanted lung after single lung transplant?
50–95% (predictably almost all), depending on the pulmonary vascular resistance of the contralateral native lung.

31. Is living-related lung transplant possible?
Yes. Living-related lobe transplants are an innovative approach to increasing the donor pool.

32. Is the 3-year actuarial survival rate different for single and double lung transplants?
No. The 3-year actuarial survival rate is about 50% for each.

33. What are the major types of preservation solutions for heart and lung grafts?
Euro-Collins (EC) solution and University of Wisconsin (UW) solution for lung, and crystalloid cardioplegia and UW solutions for hearts.

34. What are the main differences in composition between Euro-Collins solution and University of Wisconsin solution?

Euro-Collins solution is a glucose-based solution with an ionic composition that approximates that of the intracellular environment.

University of Wisconsin solution does not contain glucose but includes the following components not found in EC solution: hydroxy-ethyl starch (prevents expansion of interstitial space), lactobionate and raffinose (suppress hypothermia-induced cell swelling), glutathione and allopurinol (reduce cytotoxic injury from oxygen free radicals), and adenosine (substrate for adenosine triphosphate and a vasodilator).

BIBLIOGRAPHY

1. Arcidi JM, Patterson GA: Technique of bilateral lung transplantation. In Patterson CA, Couraud L (eds): Current Topics in General Thoracic Surgery, vol. 3. New York, Elsevier Science, 1995.
2. Calhoon JH, Grover FL, Gibbons WJ, et al: Single lung transplantation: Alternative indications for the technique. J Thorac Cardiovasc Surg 101:816–825, 1991.
3. Cohen RG, Barr ML, Schenkel FA, et al: Living-related donor lobectomy for bilateral lobar transplantation in patients with cystic fibrosis, Ann Thorac Surg 57:1423–1427, 1994.
4. Costanzo-Nordin MR, Swinnen LJ, Fisher SG, et al: Cytomegalovirus infections in heart transplant recipients: Relationship to immunosuppression. J Heart Lung Transplant 13:561–570, 1994.
5. Fremes SE, Furukawa RD, Zhang J, et al: Cardiac storage with University of Wisconsin solution and a nucleoside-transport blocker. Ann Thorac Surg 59:1127–1133, 1995.
6. Fullerton DA, Campbell DN, Jones SD, et al: Heart transplantation in children and young adults: Early and intermediate term results. Ann Thorac Surg 59:804–812, 1995.
7. Hopkinson DN, Odom NJ, Bridgewater BJM, Hooper TL: University of Wisconsin solution: Which components are important? J Heart Lung Transplant 13:990–997, 1994.
8. Hosenpud JD, Novick RJ, Breen TJ, Daily OP: The Registry of the International Society for Heart and Lung Transplantation: Eleventh official report—1994. J Heart Lung Transplant 13:561–570, 1994.
9. Jarcho J, Naftel DC, Shroyer TW, et al: Influence of HLA mismatch on rejection after heart transplantation: A multiinstitutional study. J Heart Lung Transplant 13:583–596, 1994.
10. Jeevanadam V, Barr ML, Auteri JS, et al: University of Wisconsin solution versus crystalloid cardioplegia for human donor preservation. A randomized blinded perspective trial. J Thorac Cardiovasc Surg 103:194–199, 1991.
11. Mitchell MB, Meng X, Ao L, et al: Preconditioning of isolated rat heart is mediated by protein kinase C. Circ Res 76:73–81, 1995.
12. O'Connell JB, Bourge RC, Costanzo-Nordin MR, et al: Cardiac transplantation: Recipient selection, donor procurement, and medical follow-up. Circulation 86:1061–1079, 1992.
13. Ortho Multicenter Transplant Study Group: A randomized clinical trial of OKT3 monoclonal antibody in cardiac transplant recipients. N Engl J Med 313:337–342, 1985.
14. Patterson GA: Double lung transplantation. Clin Chest Med 11:227–233, 1990.
15. Starnes VA, Lewiston NJ, Luikart H, et al: Current trends in lung transplantation: Lobar transplantation and expanded use of single lungs. J Thorac Cardiovasc Surg 104:1060–1066, 1992.
16. Starnes VA, Stinson EB, Oyer PE, et al: Single lung transplantation: A new therapeutic option for patients with pulmonary hypertension. Transplant Proc 23:1209–1210, 1991.

XI. Health Care

91. HEALTH REFORM

John Ogunkeye, MSC, Jeanne Nozawa, and Alden H. Harken, M.D.

1. What is fee for service?

The doctor establishes the price, and the patient agrees to pay it. This traditional system of exchange has great merit if both parties understand the value of the service provided. If either (usually the patient) cannot estimate the service value, it is possible (even likely) that the doctor will honestly escalate the service value in a fashion unchecked by the patient's perceptions. Thus, medical prices tend to rise.

2. What is discounted fee for service?

The patient gets together with a group of friends, and they come to the doctor with the following proposition: "Hey, doc, you can dazzle us with your fancy medical talk, but we still think that your prices are too high. How about me and my pals will pay you 80% of what you charge us?"

3. Is there a difference between hospital costs and hospital charges?

Absolutely. Hospital cost is the sum of the expenses (sutures, nurse's salaries, electricity, instrument sterilization, and band-aids) that are expended in suturing a laceration. The hospital typically charges about twice the cost (100% mark-up) for repairing a cut finger. This mark-up is highly industry-specific. Thus, intensely competitive food chains may make a profit of only 1 penny on a loaf of bread, whereas hospitals and liquor stores usually charge twice the cost.

4. What is cost shifting?

Up to one-third of patients (in some university hospitals) or as few as 1% of patients (in some private hospitals) do not pay. Moreover, some services, like the morgue and the dean's office, make no money. Thus, dollars from profitable hospital sites are shifted to subsidize poor sites in true Robin Hood fashion.

5. What are fixed costs?

After accounting for light, heat, and staff (nurses, housekeepers, administrators) at a hospital but **before** seeing a single patient, the doctor has already spent a huge amount of money. Doctors must pay fixed costs whether or not they provide medical services.

6. What are actual costs?

The incremental costs of actually providing a service in a hospital (in addition to the fixed costs of light and heat). Thus, the patient shows up in the emergency department at midnight complaining of a lump on the tip of his nose. The doctor, with characteristic erudition, says, "Yep, you have a wart on your nose," and sends the patient home with a bill for $500. The actual cost of this encounter is obviously negligible. The patient is really paying for the fixed costs of nurses and emergency resuscitative equipment should he have a cardiac arrest (when he sees the bill).

7. Is hospital accounting a precisely scientific and objective analysis of financial data?

No. Accounting is an art form that requires abundant imagination.

8. What is health insurance?
Traditionally, individuals can purchase insurance that may pay either all or a portion of their hospital and physician charges if they become ill. Insurance companies make a profit, therefore, only if the patient stays healthy. Insurance companies have elaborate tables to predict who will get sick and they prefer to sell policies exclusively to young decathlon champions. (This practice is termed "skimming"). In this model the insurance company takes all the risk—and they like to keep it low. Conversely, hospitals must cover fixed costs—and the more expensive the health care that physicians provide, the better for them.

9. So along came the HMOs. What are they?
Health maintenance organizations (HMOs) are complex systems composed, in their most comprehensive form, of a hospital(s), doctors plus offices, and an insurance company. HMOs contract with large groups of people (potential patients) to maintain their health. The enrollee pays a monthly fee (just like health insurance) so that all hospital and physician charges are covered if the enrollee becomes ill. Unlike health insurance, however, in the HMO model hospitals and physicians get paid whether or not the enrollee gets sick. So it is better for everyone if enrollees stay healthy—and out of the hospital.

10. Initially, a lot of physicians did not like HMOs. Why not?
Because physicians are fiercely independent. They did not want a bunch of business managers telling them how to manage patients.

11. Why are physicians fiercely independent?
Probably they were born that way.

12. Is that good?
Probably not. Eventually everyone will need to work together and not hit each other when they are mad.

13. Do HMO administrators really dictate how physicians manage their patients?
Yes and no. Physicians have developed medically effective and optimally efficient strategies—termed clinical pathways—for caring for many common illnesses. Although physicians must treat each patient individually, when they adhere to predetermined treatment guidelines (as encouraged by the HMO administrators), patients usually get better faster and cheaper.

14. Do physicians follow these clinical pathways?
Traditionally they have not.

15. So where do the HMO managers come in?
They evaluate each physician's utilization of expensive resources (within the predetermined clinical pathways) relative to the health of the physician's patients.

16. Do physicians welcome this kind of scrutiny?
No.

17. What is a PPO?
A preferred provider organization (PPO) is a group of doctors who have elected to remain legally independent of a hospital and insurance company (if they joined together, they would be an HMO)—and, most of all, patients. But PPOs maintain their independence as physicians, even though most PPOs require administrators to coordinate programs, keep the books, and keep the doctors from hitting each other. PPOs have the perception of independence, however.

18. Is health care expensive?

Unfortunately, yes. Physicians argue that patients pay a lot but also get a lot. In the United States, patients expect unlimited access to liver transplantation and an MRI for every headache. Americans believe that fancy, expensive health care is not just a privilege—it is a right.

19. So what is the problem?

The CEOs of big American corporations argue that the mandatory expense of health care is driving up the cost of U.S. products and making American companies less competitive in the global market—"there is more health care than steel in a new Chevrolet."

20. Does big business have a solution?

They think so. The CEOs still want unlimited access to the most modern health care for themselves and their families. Indeed, they typically want to keep their granny on dialysis (even though she spends her days tied in a nursing home wheelchair). Without sounding cynical, the CEOs want to save health care dollars spent on their employees and "other people's families." They want to limit access to health care (even for their own granny), but they do not want to wield the ax personally. So they have developed the idea of capitation.

21. What is capitation?

The CEOs of large businesses come to hospitals, HMOs, or PPOs and say: "Why don't you provide *all* the health care for *all* my employees at a fixed price (say, $180 per month per head)?" Hence capitation. In this model physicians make the decisions about who gets how much medical care (satisfying their urge for independence), but they also promise to provide *all* the necessary medical care for a prearranged price. Thus they take *all* the risk. The CEOs like this because they can still offer health care as an employee benefit and budget the cost in advance.

22. Why do physicians not like capitation?

All of a sudden physicians may have acquired a little more independence than they bargained for. Now they are paid in advance so that all costs of patients' health care are subtracted from the bag of money that they negotiated up front. Now they must advise against an MRI for every headache and break the news to Granny that she will not think better if they dialyze her BUN down to 50. This is the reverse of the good old days when physicians were rewarded if their patients got sick and stayed sick. Physicians could ply them with a smorgasbord of miracle drugs and technologies. Now physicians are trying to control health care costs.

23. Is all this change good?

Absolutely. Medicine has always changed—and the faster the better. Physicians were initially attracted to medicine as an intellectually stimulating discipline because medicine and surgery evolve rapidly.

24. Can physicians keep up with all this change?

Absolutely.

25. Despite all of the medical Chicken Littles who sonorously declare that the sky is falling, is medicine (and even more clearly, surgery) still the most gratifying, stimulating, and rewarding profession?

Absolutely.

INDEX

Page numbers in **boldface type** indicate complete chapters.

Bite wounds, 26
  to face, 78, 79
  to hand, 81
Bladder, injury and rupture of, 87–88
Blastomycosis, 262
Blood
  deoxygenated, equilibration with alveolar gas, 11
  oxygen-binding capacity of, 13
  pulmonary, without oxygen or carbon dioxide
      exchange, 12
Blood circulation, in cardiopulmonary resuscitation, 2–4
Blood dyscrasia, 277
Blood flow, venous, stasis of, 238
Blood oxygen content (cO_2), 39
Blood oxygen saturation, apnea-related decrease of, 1
Blood pressure, emergency room assessment of, 229
Blood transfusions
  hematocrit as indication for, 14
  use in shock management, 3–4, 8
"Blue toe syndrome", 217
Blunt injury
  arterial, 228, 229, 230
  duodenal, 73
  hepatic, 68, 69
  pancreatic, 73
  renal, 86
  thoracoabdominal, **57–59**
Body fluids, electrolyte content of, 15
Body secretions, daily volume and electrolyte content
    of, 15
Bogros' space, 167
Bone injury, repair of, 230
Bone resection, in parotid tumor treatment, 202
Bowel sounds, in acute abdomen, 45
Bowel viability, in intestinal ischemia, 143
Brain
  gunshot wounds to, 97
  impaired posterior circulation in, 223
  traumatic injury to, **94–98**
Brainstem, ischemia of, 223
Branchial cleft, cysts of, 212, 214, 284, 285
Breast
  cystic disease of, 187, 188
  normal anatomy of, 185, 186, 188
Breast cancer
  diagnostic techniques for, 185–190
  inoperable, 193
  in males, 189
  metastases of, 190–191, 192
  as mortality cause, 154
  neoadjuvant therapy for, 193
  noninvasive (in situ) compared with invasive, 190
  primary therapy for, 189–194
  risk factors for, 187
  staging of, 190
Breast-conservation therapy, 192
Breast examination, 185–186
Breast masses, **185–189**
Breast reconstruction, following mastectomy, 192
Breathing, energy expenditure during, 9
Bretylium, as ventricular arrhythmia therapy, 6
Bretylium tosylate, use in cardiopulmonary
    resuscitation, 5
Bronchoscopy, for evaluation of neck injuries and
    masses, 76, 213

Brooke ileostomy, 149
Brown-Sequard syndrome, 100
Bruit, carotid, 222
Bullets. See also Gunshot wounds
  entry and exit wounds caused by, 64
  kinetic energy of, 228
Burns, **90–94**

Cachexia strumipriva, 177
Calcium channel antagonists, as angina therapy, 245
Calcium chloride, use in cardiopulmonary
    resuscitation, 5
Calf cramps, sporadic, differentiated from claudication,
    217
Calorimetry, indirect, 19
Calot, triangle of, 108
Cancer patients. See also specific types of cancer
  parenteral nutrition in, 24
Candida infections, in liver transplantation recipients,
    287
Cannulation, arterial, 32–34
Capillaries, pulmonary
  fluid influx across, 10
  leakage of, 10–11
Capitation, 297
Carbon monoxide poisoning, 91–92
Carcinoid tumors
  appendiceal, 105
  gastric, 136
  rectal, 156
Carcinoma
  as large bowel obstruction cause, 145, 146
  undifferentiated, of neck, 214
Carcinoma in situ, colorectal polyp-associated, 159
Cardiac arrest
  end-tidal CO_2 monitoring in, 4–5
  in thoracic trauma patients, 61
Cardiac compression, open versus closed, 4
Cardiac output
  relationship to shock, 7
  Swan-Ganz catheter measurement of, 37–38
Cardiac preconditioning, 291
Cardiac tamponade, 60, 61
Cardiomyopathy, as heart transplantation indication, 290
Cardiopulmonary bypass
  with knife valvotomy, 255
  weaning from, 248–249
Cardiopulmonary resuscitation (CPR), **1–6**
Carotid artery
  bifurcation of, 224
  occlusion/stenosis of, 223, 224, 242
Carotid body
  function of, 224
  tumors of, 212
Carotid disease, **222–226**
Carotid endarterectomy, 225, 244
Carotid sinus, function of, 224
Carpal tunnel syndrome, 81
Catheters
  for central venous pressure monitoring, 34–36
  Fogarty, 227, 236
  Foley, 37, 44, 96
  pulmonary arterial, for oxygen delivery and
      consumption determination, 30
  radial arterial, 33